Yearbook of

CRITICAL CARE 2024

HICS Initiative

Yearbook of
CRITICAL CARE 2024
HICS Initiative

Editors

Srinivas Samavedam
MD DNB FRCP FNB EDIC FICCM
Chief Intensivist
Ramdev Rao Hospital
Hyderabad, Telangana, India

Ganshyam Jagathkar
MD FNB FICCM
Director
Department of Critical Care
Medicover Hospitals
Hyderabad, Telangana, India

JAYPEE

JAYPEE BROTHERS MEDICAL PUBLISHERS
The Health Sciences Publisher
New Delhi | London

JAYPEE **Jaypee Brothers Medical Publishers (P) Ltd**

Headquarters
Jaypee Brothers Medical Publishers (P) Ltd
EMCA House, 23/23-B
Ansari Road, Daryaganj
New Delhi 110 002, India
Landline: +91-11-23272143, +91-11-23272703
+91-11-23282021, +91-11-23245672
Email: jaypee@jaypeebrothers.com

Corporate Office
Jaypee Brothers Medical Publishers (P) Ltd
4838/24, Ansari Road, Daryaganj
New Delhi 110 002, India
Phone: +91-11-43574357
Fax: +91-11-43574314
Email: jaypee@jaypeebrothers.com

Overseas Office
JP Medical Ltd.
83, Victoria Street, London
SW1H 0HW (UK)
Phone: +44 20 3170 8910
Fax: +44 (0)20 3008 6180
Email: info@jpmedpub.com

Website: www.jaypeebrothers.com
Website: www.jaypeedigital.com

Inquiries for bulk sales may be solicited at: jaypee@jaypeebrothers.com

Yearbook of Critical Care 2024

First Edition: **2025**

ISBN: 978-93-6616-228-7

Printed in India

Dedicated to

This edition of the book on critical care is the result of the hard work and commitment of a lot of people and teams.
The editors wish to dedicate this edition to (Late) Professor Luciano Gattinoni.
Professor Gattinoni changed the practices of mechanical ventilation for acute respiratory distress syndrome (ARDS) with his persistent and dedicated work. A lot of refinements and newer concepts have found their roots in the pioneering work of Professor Gattinoni.
The spirit of Professor Gattinoni serves as a driving force for all of us and shows us how basic research can be translated to highly effective and practice-changing clinical practices.

Contributors

SECTION EDITORS

Deven Juneja DNB FNB EDIC FCCP
Director
Institute of Critical Care Medicine
Max Super Specialty Hospital
New Delhi, India
(Section 12: Guidelines)

Gunjan Chanchalani
MD IFCCM FNB EDIC FICCM
Chief Intensivist
Department of Critical Care
KJ Somaiya Hospital and Research Center
Mumbai, Maharashtra, India
(Section 8: Hematology)

Jaicob Varghese
MD (General Medicine) DM (Critical Care) EDIC
Senior Consultant and Head
Department of Critical Care
Rajagiri Hospital
Kochi, Kerala, India
(Section 2: Respiratory/Ventilation/ARDS)

Kanwalpreet Sodhi
DA DNB IDCCM EDIC FICCM
Director and Head
Department of Critical Care
Deep Hospital
Ludhiana, Punjab, India
(Section 5: Nephrology Section)

Ketan Kargirwar MD FNB EDIC IDCCM
Senior Consultant
Department of Critical Care Medicine
Sir HN Reliance Foundation Hospital and Research Centre
Mumbai, Maharashtra, India
(Section 11: Nutrition/Metabolic)

Lalita Gouri Mitra DA MD DNB FICCM
Professor and Officer In-charge
Department of Anesthesia, Critical Care, and Pain
Homi Bhabha Cancer Hospital
and Research Centre
Medicity Mullanpur (New Chandigarh)
Punjab, India
(A Unit of Tata Memorial Centre, Mumbai and Department of Atomic Energy, Government of India)
(Section 4: Gastroenterology/Hepatobiliary)

Manoj Y Singh
MD (Medicine) FNB (Critical Care) EDIC PG Dip (Perioperative) AFRACMA FCICM
Clinical Director and Senior
Intensive Care Physician
The Canberra Hospital
Garran, Australian Capital Territory, Australia
(Section 7: Sepsis)

Prashant Nasa
MD FNB (Critical Care Medicine)
EDIC SCE (Acute Medicine)
Senior Clinical Fellow
Department of Anesthesia and Critical Care Medicine
New Cross Hospital
The Royal Wolverhampton Trust
Wolverhampton, UK
(Section 9: Ethics, Organization, and Outcomes in Intensive Care Unit)

Shrikanth Srinivasan MD DNB FNB EDIC FICCM
Chairman
Manipal Institute of Critical Care Medicine
Manipal Hospitals
New Delhi, India
(Section 10: Sonography/Imaging)

Sivakumar MN DA DNB IDCCM EDIC FICCM
Head
Institute of Critical Care Medicine
Royalcare Superspeciality Hospitals
Coimbatore, Tamil Nadu, India
(Section 3: Neurocritical Care)

Sumesh Arora FCICM EDIC MD
Senior Staff Specialist
Department of Intensive Care
Prince of Wales Hospital
Randwick, New South Wales, Australia
Director, gotheextramile.com, and
'Critical Care MCQ' the App
(Section 6: Antimicrobials)

Supradip Ghosh
DNB (General Medicine) MRCP (UK) EDIC FICCM
Director
Department of Critical Care
Max Super Speciality Hospital
Lucknow, Uttar Pradesh, India
(Section 1: Cardiac/Hemodynamics/Fluids)

ASSOCIATE EDITORS

Amandeep Singh MD (General Medicine) IDCCM
Director
Department of Critical Care
Max Super Speciality Hospital
Lucknow, Uttar Pradesh, India

Atul Phillips MD FNB (Critical Care Medicine)
Assistant Professor
Department of Critical Care Medicine
Christian Medical College
Ludhiana, Punjab, India

Biji Thomas Philip MD PDCC EDIC
Senior Consultant
Department of Critical Care
Rajagiri Hospital
Kochi, Kerala, India

Garima Arora DNB (Anesthesiology) FNB (Critical Care)
Registrar
Department of Intensive Care Medicine
Werribee Mercy Hospital
Victoria, Australia

Harsimran Singh Walia MD IDCCM FNB (CCM)
Associate Professor
Department of Anesthesia
Critical Care, and Pain
Homi Bhabha Cancer Hospital
and Research Centre
Medicity Mullanpur (New Chandigarh)
Punjab, India

Jagdeep Sharma MD DNB DESAIC
Associate Professor
Department of Anesthesia
Critical Care and Pain
Homi Bhabha Cancer Hospital and
Research Centre
Medicity Mullanpur (New Chandigarh)
Punjab, India

Lakshmikanth Charan S
MD IDCCM EDIC EDAIC FNCC
Consultant Intensivist
Institute of Critical Care Medicine
Royalcare Superspeciality Hospitals
Coimbatore, Tamil Nadu, India

Magesh Parthiban MD DM
Consultant Intensivist
KMCH Hospital
Coimbatore, Tamil Nadu, India

Manu Gupta MD (Medicine) IDCCM
Consultant
Department of Critical Care
St Stephen's Hospital
New Delhi, India

Melwin George MD IDCCM EDIC DrNB
Consultant
Department of Critical Care
Rajagiri Hospital
Kochi, Kerala, India

Nilanjan Umesh
DNB (Respiratory Medicine) FNB (Critical Care) IFCCM
Consultant
Department of Critical Care
Rajagiri Hospital
Kochi, Kerala, India

Ripenmeet Salhotra
MD (Anesthesiology) IDCCM IFCCM EDIC
Senior Consultant
Department of Critical Care
Amrita Hospital
Faridabad, Haryana, India

Sahil Kataria MD DrNB
Associate Consultant
Department of Critical Care Medicine
Holy Family Hospital
New Delhi, India

Sanket Hansora MBBS CTCCM IDCCM
Associate Consultant
Sir HN Reliance Foundation Hospital and Research Centre
Mumbai, Maharashtra, India

Saurabh Kumar Rai DNB (Emergency Medicine)
Final Year DrNB (Critical Care Medicine) Fellow
Fortis-Escorts Hospital
Faridabad, Haryana, India

Shrirang Nagorao Bamne
MD DM (CCM) FNB (CCM) EDIC
Head
Department of Critical Care Medicine
NMC Speciality Hospital
Abu Dhabi, UAE

Sonali Ghosh DCH MRCPCH IDPCCM
Principal Consultant
Department of Pediatric Intensive Care Unit
Max Super Speciality Hospital
Lucknow, Uttar Pradesh, India

Velmurugan Selvam MD DM
Associate Professor
Sri Ramachandra Institute of Higher Education and Research
Chennai, Tamil Nadu, India

Vishal Khandelwal
MD (Anesthesiology) FNB (Critical Care)
PGDMLE (NLU, Bengaluru)
Consultant
Department of Critical Care
Sarvodaya Hospital
Faridabad, Haryana, India

Preface

We are happy to introduce this edition of the book. The last edition was well received and got good reviews from senior teachers.

The team has taken motivation from the feedback and has embarked upon the task of compiling the literature related to Critical Care for the year 2024. The authors of the previous edition did a wonderful job and the same team has worked on the book this year as well.

We have fallen behind the timelines due to reasons beyond our control. But it's always better late than never. The compilations this year have been analyzed meticulously and the opinions expressed by the authors would go a long way in guiding the readers in understanding the publications while suggesting whether the conclusions should change current practices.

The editorial team wishes to thank all the authors who took time out to go through the voluminous published data and select the best of the lot for analysis. The team of M/s Jaypee Brothers Medical Publishers (P) Ltd, New Delhi, India, deserves utmost commendation for the diligence and commitment with which they have executed this publication. The biggest thanks are reserved for all of you as readers and patrons of this book which motivates the editorial team to continue this year after year.

Srinivas Samavedam
Ganshyam Jagathkar

Contents

SECTION

1

Cardiac/Hemodynamics/Fluids

Section Editor: *Supradip Ghosh*

Associate Editors: *Vishal Khandelwal, Amandeep Singh, Atul Phillips, Saurabh Kumar Rai, Ripenmeet Salhotra, Sonali Ghosh, Garima Arora*

Fluid Balance Control in Critically Ill Patients: Results from POINCARE-2 Stepped Wedge Cluster-Randomized Trial[1]

Bollaert PE, Monnier A, Schneider F, Argaud L, Badie J, Charpentier C, et al. Fluid balance control in critically ill patients: results from POINCARE-2 stepped wedge cluster-randomized trial.

Crit Care. 2023;27(1):66.

CLINICAL QUESTION

As compared to the present standard of care, does an effective fluid balance control strategy help in reducing all-cause mortality at 60 days?

WHAT IS ALREADY KNOWN?

- Most of the critically ill patients are in positive fluid balance owing to the resuscitation, optimization, and stabilization phases of fluid therapy. The evacuation phase is often neglected.
- Studies have shown that patients are in a positive cumulative balance of about 4–10 L at the end of the first week of hospital stay, which is detrimental in cases of acute respiratory distress syndrome (ARDS), sepsis, and renal failure.
- Large fluid volumes eventually translate into tissue edema which leads to impaired diffusion of gases and metabolites and hampers the microcirculation.

STUDY DESIGN

- This study was a stepped-wedge cluster open-label randomized trial conducted at 12 intensive care units (ICUs) (clusters) of nine French hospitals.
- The trial period was from June 2016 to May 2019.

POPULATION STUDIED

- *Inclusion criteria:*
    - Aged 18 years or older
    - On invasive mechanical ventilation support
    - Admitted in one of the 12 recruiting ICUs for >48 hours and <72 hours with expected length of stay for >24 hours postinclusion
- *Exclusion criteria:*
    - Clinical conditions impeding weighing
    - Nonavailability of bedside weighing scale
    - Multiple trauma

- Pregnant patients
- Expected withdrawal of life-sustaining therapy within 7 days
- Admitted in another ICU >24 hours immediately before the index admission
- Patients' refusal for personal data collection/use
- *Past history of ICU:* Stay in one of the 12 recruiting ICUs during the recruitment period.
- Patients under guardianship

INTERVENTION

(POINCARE-2 strategy group)

- Daily weighing of patients from day 2 of admission to day 14 by trained nurses using: beds with integrated weighing scales if available, ceiling hoist scales, or bed scales
- Weight gain was considered as a marker of fluid retention.
- Based on the daily weight gain, the decision was taken about salt and water restriction, receipt of diuretics (furosemide 1 mg/kg) or administration of albumin (20% 100 mL/8 hours for maximum 24 hours).
- Decision was taken by a senior intensivist or a resident doctor supervised by an intensivist.
- Strategy was stopped until recovery, systolic BP <90 mm Hg and/or vasopressor use, at the discretion of intensivist, serum sodium >155 mmol/L, serum potassium <2.8 mmol/L, worsening renal function with acute kidney injury (AKI) as defined by RIFLE criteria or any adverse event.

COMPARATOR

- Patients received usual standard care as per the routine care given by each ICU.
- Weighing on day 0, day 7, and day 14 (more frequently if it was part of routine care)

OUTCOME

Following are the outcomes:

- Cluster-randomized analysis (CRA) and randomized before-and-after analysis (RBAA) were done; both intentions are to treat.
- Out of 10,272 patients 1,361 were included in RBAA (643 in strategy group and 718 in control group) and 905 were included in CRA (433 in strategy and 472 in control group).
- Mean daily weight was lower in the strategy group. However, the difference was statistically not significant.
- Cumulative fluid balance from day 0 to day 14 was lower in the strategy group but statistically nonsignificant.
- The median total dose of furosemide in the strategy group was 220 mg [interquartile range (IQR) 80–520 mg] versus 305 mg (IQR 80–727) in the control group. (In RBAA, it was 233 mg in the strategy group vs. 220 mg in the control group).
- The median total dose of albumin infused was 550 mL (IQR 300–1,000) in the strategy group versus 400 mL (IQR 300–1,000) in the control group.

Types of Outcomes

- *Primary outcome:* No statistically significant difference in the 60-day mortality rates (30.5% in the strategy group vs. 33.9% in the control group).
- *Secondary outcomes:* The study could not prove statistically significant between the group difference in mechanical ventilator-free days, vasopressor-free days, renal replacement therapy (RRT)-free days, 28-day mortality, and in-hospital mortality.
- *Safety outcomes:* No significant difference among the groups in terms of occurrence of hypotension, hypokalemia,

renal worsening, and myocardial and mesenteric infarction.

- Hypernatremia (Na >155) which was more frequent in the strategy group.

AUTHORS' VIEWPOINT

- Authors feel that their study could not find statistical significance in primary or any of the secondary outcomes because either the strategy could be ineffective or they failed to prove the actual effectiveness of the strategy using intention-to-treat analysis.
- Authors feel that, since standard care too has components of the POINCARE-2 strategy (infrequent weighing, diuretics, and albumin)—this may have contaminated the control group.
- Contamination during the control period and suboptimal application of the POINCARE-2 strategy may have underestimated the effect of the strategy group.
- Finally, the authors concluded that based on intention-to-treat analysis, the POINCARE-2 strategy did not reduce mortality in critically ill patients, but an as-treated analysis might help address the contamination effect and shed light on the actual effectiveness of the strategy.

STRENGTHS OF THE STUDY

- Multicenter, randomized study design
- Intention-to-treat analysis
- Pragmatic approach
- *Wedge-stepped design:* It tries to avoid contamination of control with intervention
- Timely enrollment of patients which is critical in wedge step design trial.
- Thorough data monitoring
- Preplanned additional process evaluation, as-treated analysis in the protocol
- Training period to ensure maximal adherence to the intervention under scrutiny

DRAWBACKS OF THE STUDY

- The trial was powered to detect a 15% absolute difference in mortality which was quite high.
- Intraperiod correlation coefficient lower than intracluster coefficient
- *Similar interventions used in both control and strategy groups:* Possible contamination of the control group which was unavoidable.
- The accuracy of the patient's weight being used as a marker of fluid accumulation is questionable.

REVIEWERS' VIEWPOINT

- The findings of the trial suggest no statistical difference in mortality and any of the secondary outcomes, but the following facts should be considered before concluding:
  - There was neither a major difference in the median total dose of diuretics used nor a major difference in the use of albumin between the two groups.
  - There was a trend toward lower mean daily weight in the strategy group but statistically insignificant.
  - Observed cumulative fluid balance was lower in the strategy group but again insignificant.
- These findings indicate that the standard of care used nowadays is already toward maintaining a restricted cumulative balance due to which there has been a significant contamination of the control group leading to undermining the effects of the POINCARE-2 strategy.

Fluid Balance Control in Critically Ill Patients: Results from As-Treated Analyses of POINCARE-2 Randomized Trial[2]

Mansouri A, Buzzi M, Gibot S, Charpentier C, Schneider F, Louis G, et al. Fluid balance control in critically ill patients: results from as-treated analyses of POINCARE-2 randomized trial.

Crit Care*. *2023;27:(1)426.

CLINICAL QUESTION

Does actual exposure to the POINCARE-2 strategy reduce all-cause mortality at day 60?

WHAT IS ALREADY KNOWN?

- POINCARE-2 stepped-wedge randomized controlled trial (RCT) aimed to assess the effectiveness of fluid balance control (conservative strategy) in critically ill patients, results of which were inconclusive.[1]
- Intention-to-treat analysis of the trial showed no difference in mortality at day 60 and no difference in secondary outcomes
- Strategy under scrutiny consisted of daily weighing of the patients from day 2 to day 14, subsequently daily decision for salt and water restriction, administration of diuretics, albumin and or RRT was taken in case of weight gain (weight gain was equated with fluid accumulation).[1]
- The control group too received diuretics, albumin, and RRT as part of standard care, which led to unavoidable contamination of the control group.
- Relying only on the intention-to-treat analysis might discredit a strategy that could be beneficial; hence, the need for an as-to-treat analysis.

STUDY DESIGN

- This study was a stepped-wedge cluster open-label randomized trial.
- The trial period was from June 2016 to May 2019 and was done at 12 ICUs (clusters) of nine French hospitals.
- The main analysis conducted was the intention to treat. To study the magnitude of the concerned intervention, the as-to-treat analysis was planned before the protocol administration.

POPULATION STUDIED

Same as Article 1.

INTERVENTION

Same as Article 1.

COMPARATOR

Same as Article 1.

ASSESSMENT OF EXPOSURE TO THE STRATEGY

- Authors developed a crude score of deviation (based on actual deviation from the strategy algorithm)
- Score was from 0 to 100 (0 meaning POINCARE-2 strategy not administered at all; 100 meaning strategy optimally administered).
- After discussion with experts, they considered that patients were actually exposed to strategy if their score was ≥75 and as unexposed otherwise.
- Score was calculated for every patient irrespective of their group (whether control or strategy) to see for the patients who were actually exposed to the POINCARE-2 strategy.

OUTCOME

- Overall, 69.4% patients in strategy group versus 24.8% patients in control group had score of exposure to strategy ≥75 and were considered exposed to strategy.
- Average daily fluid intake did not vary with exposure to strategy ($p = 0.031$).
- Highest dose of diuretics was received in patients who were in the class of exposure to strategy (75–100 score).
- Patients exposed to the POINCARE-2 strategy were more likely to be:
  - Older patients ($p < 0.001$)
  - Had a higher McCabe score at admission ($p = 0.016$)
  - Cancer patients ($p = 0.031$)
  - Chronic kidney disease patients under RRT (0.008)
- Patients exposed to the strategy (score >75) had higher mortality at day 60. However, the difference was not statistically significant when adjusted for confounders.
- Subgroup analysis showed that exposure to the strategy was associated with increased 60-day mortality in case of ARDS and septic shock. However, these results were not significant when adjusted for confounders.
- No significant association of the exposure to POINCARE-2 strategy with mechanical ventilator-free days, vasopressor-free days, any unexpected harmful events, and worsening of renal failure.

AUTHORS' VIEWPOINT

- Authors conclude that as-treated analysis showed no statistically significant association between exposure to the POINCARE-2 strategy and 60-day all-cause mortality and the results are in line with their previous findings.[1]
- Authors stressed on the fact that in studies related to fluid balance control, it is highly unlikely that the control group does not receive any component of the strategy and vice versa that the strategy group receives optimal exposure due to factors such as dehydration and anuria. Hence, it is very difficult to prove the actual effectiveness of fluid balance control.
- Authors feel that further research such as target trial emulation might help.

STRENGTHS OF THE STUDY

- Thorough data monitoring
- Additional process evaluation
- As-to-treat analysis
- Instrumental variable analysis is to take into account measured and unmeasured confounders.

DRAWBACKS OF THE STUDY

- Consensus was reached on the point regarding a score >75 as exposed to the strategy but the expert's agreement with lower scores indicated low. Exposure to strategy was less consensual. The possibility that results are biased toward null.
- Different ICUs had different weighing scales—the possibility of measurement bias.
- Process evaluation conducted after the trial. Ideally should be conducted along with the trial so that the shortcomings are addressed simultaneously.

REVIEWERS' VIEWPOINT

- Results from the as-treated analysis are on similar lines with the previous results.
- This study did not find any statistical significance between fluid balance control and 60-day mortality, but the study has highlighted that even after a rigorous

attempt and troublesome statistical analysis, it is very difficult to prove the beneficial effect of fluid balance control.

- The interventions done in the standard care are more or less the same as compared to the strategy group, which is evident by almost the same dosages of diuretics and albumin administered in both groups. There was no statistical difference in the cumulative fluid balance as well.
- *This study further strengthens our belief that we have already moved toward a more conservative approach in fluid management.*

Association of Sublingual Microcirculation Parameters and Capillary Refill Time in the Early Phase of ICU Admission[3]

Huang W, Xiang H, Hu C, Wu T, Zhang D, Ma S, et al. Association of Sublingual Microcirculation Parameters and Capillary Refill Time in the Early Phase of ICU Admission.

Crit Care Med. 2023;51(7):913-23.

CLINICAL QUESTION

What is the relationship between capillary refill time (CRT) and microcirculatory abnormalities in critically ill patients during the early phase of ICU admission?

WHAT IS ALREADY KNOWN?

- CRT is an indirect tool used to monitor peripheral perfusion in critically ill patients.
- Altered sublingual microcirculation parameters, frequently observed in critically ill patients, are associated with development of organ failure and poor outcomes. Early detection of microcirculatory alterations can lead to prompt treatment and may potentially avoid poor outcomes. In critically ill patients, microvascular tissue perfusion can be observed directly using a handheld noninvasive sublingual videomicroscope.
- The current study was designed to investigate any correlation between CRT and microcirculatory abnormalities

STUDY DESIGN

- The study was a prospective, observational, and pilot study. This design allowed for the observation of patients over time and the collection of data on CRT and microcirculatory parameters.
- This study took place from October 2021 to January 2022 in the ICU of Zhongnan Hospital, Wuhan University, China.

POPULATION STUDIED

- Adult critically ill adult patients were enrolled in the study within 24 hours of ICU admission after initial hemodynamic stabilization was achieved defined as mean arterial pressure (MAP) >65 mm Hg, and no change in vasopressor use for 2 hours.
- The following patients were excluded from the study:
    - Patients with severe coagulopathy or bleeding disorders, and pregnancy
    - Patients with oral or maxillofacial trauma
    - Prone position, high O_2 dependency

- Patients with known sublingual pathology (e.g., tumors and cysts)
- Patients who were unable to undergo sublingual microcirculation measurements
- Recurrent ICU admission (only included first time)
- Consent not given

METHODOLOGY

- Sublingual microcirculation and CRT were assessed simultaneously using standard techniques published earlier.
- *Sublingual microcirculation:* Sublingual microcirculation was assessed using a sidestream dark field (SDF) imaging device and a video clip of ≥5 seconds was recorded for calculating microvascular flow index (MFI).
- MFI was computed as the mean of the predominant flow classification of small vessels over the four quadrants of the video screen.
    - 0 = Absent flow
    - 1 = Intermitted flow
    - 2 = Sluggish flow
    - 3 = Continuous flow
    - The abnormal microcirculatory flow was defined as MFI <2.6.
- Additionally, the total vessel density (TVD), the perfused vessel density (PVD), the proportion of perfused vessels (PPV), the heterogeneity index (HI), and DeBacker score were calculated, as described previously.
- *Capillary refill time:* CRT measurements were performed by using a standard method described in the ANDROMEDA-SHOCK study.
- A glass microscope slide was used to apply pressure to the ventral surface of the right index fingertip, until the skin turned white, then held for 10 seconds. The time taken for the return of the normal skin color after the release of pressure was CRT.
    - The CRT assessment was performed immediately after the SDF measurement.
    - Two CRT acquisitions were made in <1 minute, and CRT was recorded as the average of values.
    - CRT ≥3 seconds was defined as abnormal.

OUTCOME

- 282 patients were prospectively evaluated.
- Patients with an abnormal CRT showed a higher Sequential Organ Failure Assessment (SOFA) score, higher Acute Physiology and Chronic Health Evaluation II (APACHE II) score, higher rate of patients diagnosed with sepsis at ICU admission, higher lactate levels, and higher 28-day mortality.
- The study found a significant correlation between prolonged CRT and abnormal microcirculation (e.g., MFI, PPV, and HI).
    - Prolonged CRT was independently associated with abnormal microcirculation and increased 28-day mortality.
    - However, CRT has a poor correlation with TVD and DeBacker score.
- Increased CRT is associated with more severe organ dysfunction in terms of SOFA score.
- Abnormal microcirculation is associated with organ failure and poor outcomes.
- CRT is superior to predicting microvascular blood flow maldistribution than lactate, MAP, and blood gas indices.

AUTHORS' VIEWPOINT

- The authors suggest that CRT is a valuable and easily obtainable indicator of microcirculatory abnormalities in critically ill patients.

- The authors emphasize the critical role of microcirculation in determining outcomes in critically ill patients.
- The authors stress the importance of assessing microcirculatory function early in the course of ICU admission. They suggest that early identification of microcirculatory dysfunction can facilitate timely intervention and potentially improve outcomes.
- The authors envision a future where sublingual microcirculation parameters and CRT can be integrated into routine bedside monitoring in ICUs.

STRENGTHS OF THE STUDY

- The study explores, for the first time, the relationship between sublingual microcirculation parameters and CRT in ICU patients.
- The authors used standardized techniques for measuring sublingual microcirculation parameters and CRT, ensuring consistency and reliability.
- The study's prospective design allows for a stronger causal relationship between CRT and microcirculatory abnormalities. Also allowing for the collection of data in real-time and reducing the risk of bias.
- The simultaneous measurement of CRT and sublingual microcirculation using SDF imaging provides a comprehensive assessment of peripheral perfusion.
- A relatively large sample size of 282 patients enhances the generalizability of the findings.
- The use of multivariate analysis helps to control for confounding factors and isolate the independent effect of CRT on microcirculatory abnormalities and outcomes.
- Demonstrates the feasibility of using CRT as a surrogate for microcirculatory assessment in critically ill patients.

DRAWBACKS OF THE STUDY

- *Limited generalizability:* The study was conducted in a single ICU, which may limit the generalizability of the findings to other healthcare settings.
- Although the study included a relatively large sample size, the findings may not apply to all critically ill populations, especially those with different underlying conditions or geographic locations.
- *Observational design:* While the study provides valuable insights, an observational design cannot establish definitive causality. RCTs with a control group would be necessary to definitively prove a causal relationship between CRT and outcomes.
- External factors such as skin temperature and ambient temperature were not thoroughly controlled, which may affect CRT.
- *Single-point assessment:* The study relied on a single-point assessment of CRT and microcirculation, limiting the ability to assess changes over time and their use as a resuscitation tool.
    - It did not explore how CRT changes during treatment or after interventions
    - Assessment is done after resuscitation; on admission, assessment can be done to know the dynamics of the patient.
    - What happened to patients whose vasopressor requirement is not stable for 2 hours in the first 24 hours is not mentioned.
- *Restricted group*: Fluid boluses without criteria being fulfilled
- *Limited follow-up*: The study only assessed patients during the early phase

of ICU admission, which may not capture the full spectrum of microcirculatory changes.

- Less sick patients
- The study did not evaluate the cost-effectiveness of using CRT to assess microcirculatory dysfunction.

REVIEWERS' VIEWPOINT

- Novel study design providing a strong correlation between CRT and microcirculatory changes
- However, further studies are required to confirm the generalizability of these findings across patients' population.

Multiple Electrolytes Solution Versus Saline as Bolus Fluid for Resuscitation in Pediatric Septic Shock: A Multicenter Randomized Clinical Trial[4]

Sankar J, Muralidharan J, Lalitha AV, Rameshkumar R, Pathak M, Das RR, et al. Multiple Electrolytes Solution Versus Saline as Bolus Fluid for Resuscitation in Pediatric Septic Shock: A Multicenter Randomized Clinical Trial.

Crit Care Med. 2023;51(11):1449-60.

CLINICAL QUESTION

In pediatric septic shock, does resuscitation with a balanced crystalloid solution [e.g., multiple electrolytes solution (MES)], or normal saline (0.9% saline), affect the development of new and/or progressive AKI?

WHAT IS ALREADY KNOWN?

- Isotonic crystalloids are recommended as the resuscitation fluid of choice for both adult and pediatric patients with septic shock.
- 0.9% saline is the most widely used isotonic crystalloid in India and globally because of its wide availability, familiarity, and low cost. However, several adverse consequences of 0.9% saline are now being recognized, including hyperchloremia, nonanion gap metabolic acidosis, renal adverse effects, and a potential increase in mortality. Balanced crystalloids that more closely resemble plasma in their composition are gaining more attention as alternative resuscitation fluid.
- Evidence supporting one fluid over another is currently limited and still maintains equipoise among randomized studies and systematic reviews. This is particularly true in the pediatric patient population.

STUDY DESIGN

- This study was a blinded, parallel-group, and RCT.
- It was conducted over 3 years (April 10, 2017 to January 31, 2020) in the pediatric emergency and pediatric intensive care units (PICUs) of four tertiary care centers in India.

POPULATION STUDIED

- Children ≤15 years old with a clinical diagnosis of septic shock who were deemed by the treating clinicians to require a fluid bolus were screened for enrollment.
    - Septic shock was defined as per international consensus guidelines.

- Children were excluded from enrollment if they fulfilled any of the following criteria:
  - Received any fluid boluses before enrollment
  - Met criteria for chronic kidney disease
  - Unrepaired cyanotic congenital heart disease
  - Severe malnutrition
  - Known metabolic disorders
  - Parents declined consent.
- A patient was considered eligible only for their first episode of shock during the admission.
- All consenting subjects who fulfilled eligibility criteria were randomized to receive either a balanced crystalloid [multiple electrolyte solution (MES, PlasmaLyte A)] or 0.9% saline as resuscitation fluid.
  - Block randomization was carried out by a statistician blinded to patient identity.
  - Randomization was stratified by site.
  - The patient, the treating physician, and the outcome assessor were all blinded to the allocated fluid, which was packed by the research assistants who had no role in patient randomization or enrollment.

INTERVENTION

- All patients randomized to the MES group, received at least one fluid bolus of 20 mL/kg body weight of MES, at the time of shock recognition.
  - All subsequent boluses administered till day 7, remained the same blinded fluid, i.e., MES.
  - The maintenance fluids administered were at the discretion of the treating team.

COMPARATOR

- In the 0.9% saline group, the choice of both initial bolus of 20 mL/kg body weight and subsequent boluses till day 7, remained 0.9% saline.
  - Maintenance fluid of choice remained at the discretion of the treating team
- The primary outcome of the study was the development of new or progressive AKI in the first 7 days post-enrollment.
  - The definition of new or progressive AKI for the study was adapted from the pediatric definitions in the 2012 Kidney Disease: Improving Global Outcomes guidelines.

OUTCOME

- 714 of 1,080 patients screened initially were randomized. Written consent was refused by the parents of six patients after the initial verbal one.
  - Finally, 708 patients were included for analysis—361 in the MES group and 357 in the 0.9% saline group.
- Baseline characteristics were not different between groups.
  - Median age of patients included in the study was 5 years; 43% being girls.
- Median volume of fluid boluses received in the two groups was similar at the first hour, at 6 hours, and at 24 hours.
  - Type or the proportion of maintenance fluids administered in the first 24, 48, or 72 hours was not different between the two groups.
- *Primary outcome:* A significantly lower percentage of patients in the MES group met the criteria for new onset or worsening AKI at day 7 [21% vs. 33%; relative risk (RR) (95% confidence interval (CI): 0.62 (0.49–0.80); $p < 0.001$].

- *Secondary outcomes:*
  - Serum Na^+ and Cl^- values were lower at 24, 48, and 72 hours in the MES group. However, there were no between-group differences in values of serum K^+.
  - Groups did not defer significantly in terms of ICU mortality, time to shock resolution, vasoactive drug therapy, organ dysfunction score at 24 hours, ventilator or ICU-free days.
  - There was no between-groups difference in infusion-related adverse events such as fever, thrombophlebitis, or fluid overload.

AUTHORS' VIEWPOINT

In pediatric septic shock, fluid resuscitation with MES resulted in a significantly lower incidence of new and/or progressive AKI till day 7 after randomization compared to 0.9% saline.

STRENGTHS OF THE STUDY

- Investigator-initiated study
- Including a large number of patients from four large teaching hospitals across India confirms the generalizability of the study results
- Randomization of >66% of patients initially screened further reconfirms the generalizability of its results
- Patients, treating physicians, and outcome assessors all were blinded to the allocated fluids.
- Confounding effects of pre-enrollment fluids could be avoided by excluding patients who had received prior fluid boluses before randomization.
- Both groups received similar treatment protocols
- Good matching of baseline characteristics
- Intention-to-treat analysis
- No loss to follow-up

DRAWBACKS OF THE STUDY

- Protocol violations, if any, are not reported in the study.
- Despite blinding, treating physicians could potentially have an idea of the type of fluid prescribed from the electrolyte values.
- The results of the study may be specific to MES and cannot be extrapolated to other isotonic balanced crystalloids.
- Only resuscitation fluids were compared, not maintenance fluids.
- High cost of MES used in the study may be a potential hindrance in implementing the results of the study in clinical practice.

REVIEWERS' VIEWPOINT

- Results of this investigator-initiated, large, blinded, multicenter randomized study conducted in a low- and middle-income country, further present strength to the existing evidence on the renal adverse effects of 0.9% saline in septic shock.
- 0.9% saline should be avoided in pediatric septic shock patients, especially when used in large volumes.

Choice of Creep or Maintenance Fluid Type and Their Impact on Total Daily ICU Sodium Burden in Critically Ill Patients: A Systematic Review and Meta-analysis[5]

Waskowski J, Salvato SM, Müller M, Hofer D, van Regenmortel N, Pfortmueller CA. Choice of creep or maintenance fluid type and their impact on total daily ICU sodium burden in critically ill patients: A systematic review and meta-analysis.

J Crit Care. 2023;78:154403.

CLINICAL QUESTION

Does the use of low-sodium maintenance or creep fluids, compared to high-sodium fluids, reduce total daily sodium load, and complications such as hypernatremia, fluid overload, and hyperchloremia in critically ill ICU patients and how does it affect the outcome?

WHAT IS ALREADY KNOWN?

- Nonresuscitation fluids, such as maintenance fluids and creep fluids, used for drug administration, flushing the lines, and maintaining open lines, account for a significant portion (>65%) of total fluid intake in ICU patients.
- Sodium overload due to high-sodium nonresuscitation fluids may contribute to hypernatremia and fluid overload, which are associated with increased mortality in critically ill patients, but results of different studies have been contradictory and such association has not been proven for maintenance/creep fluids.
- There is increasing interest in exploring whether lower-sodium maintenance/creep fluids can reduce these risks without causing hyponatremia or other complications.

STUDY DESIGN

- *Design:* Systematic review and meta-analysis following PRISMA, MOOSE, and Cochrane Collaboration guidelines.
  - Protocol was registered on the PROSPERO registry.
  - PubMed, Embase, and Cochrane Library databases were searched, and a total of 7,437 articles were screened.
- *Trials:* The systematic review included five trials with a total of 1,105 patients; four were included in the meta-analysis consisting of one RCT and three observational studies.
- *Analysis:* A PRISMA flowchart, PRISMA checklist, ROBINS-I tool, and funnel plot were included in the manuscript or supplementary material. A random-effects model was used to evaluate the primary and secondary outcomes.

POPULATION STUDIED

- *Sample size:* Four observational trials and one RCT, total of 1,105 ICU patients from five different studies. Only four trials were included in the meta-analysis, and one additional trial in the systematic review.
- *Inclusion criteria:* Medical, surgical, or mixed ICU patients receiving maintenance or creep fluids.
- *Exclusion criteria:* Noncontrolled trials, trials not available in English, trials performed in ED only or those which included only pediatric patients, studies evaluating resuscitation fluids or highly selected (e.g., burns) cases only, and case reports.

INTERVENTION

Use of low-sodium maintenance or creep fluids, typically defined as solutions containing 35–54 mmol/L of sodium. Some studies used no-sodium fluids such as glucose 5% (G5%) as a maintenance fluid with minimal or no sodium content.

COMPARATOR

Use of high-sodium fluids, typically isotonic solutions with 140–154 mmol/L of sodium, such as normal saline (NaCl 0.9%).

OUTCOME

- *Primary outcome:* Meta-analysis showed a significant reduction in daily sodium intake (mean reduction of 117 mmol or approximately 2.7 g) in the low-sodium fluid group.
- *Secondary outcomes:*
  - *Hypernatremia:* No significant difference in the risk of hypernatremia between the low- and high-sodium groups [odds ratio (OR): 0.85, (CI: 0.51–1.41)], though a trend favoring low-sodium strategy
  - *Hyponatremia*: A nonsignificant trend toward higher rates of hyponatremia in the low-sodium group [OR: 2.21 (CI: 0.77–6.33)].
  - *Hyperchloremia:* A significantly lower incidence of hyperchloremia in patients receiving low-sodium fluids.
  - *Fluid balance:* A trend toward more favorable fluid balance in the low-sodium group, but not statistically significant.
  - *Delirium:* One study suggested a higher risk of delirium with low-sodium fluids, while another study showed no significant difference in neurological symptoms.

AUTHORS' VIEWPOINT

- The authors concluded that using low-sodium fluids can significantly reduce sodium burden and potentially lower the risk of hyperchloremia in critically ill ICU patients. This in turn may positively impact outcomes such as renal failure, length of stay, and mortality.
- However, they acknowledged significant gaps in knowledge regarding the safety and effect of this approach on patient outcomes.
- They call for further research, particularly large RCTs, to investigate the clinical relevance of reduced sodium nonresuscitation fluids and its effects on outcomes such as mortality, renal function, and ICU length of stay.

STRENGTHS OF THE STUDY

- The study systematically reviewed and meta-analyzed recent trials obtained from multiple databases, providing a clear picture of the impact of maintenance and creep fluid choice on sodium load. The meta-analysis established a clear association between sodium content and the risk of hyperchloremia.
- Since data on the effect of maintenance/creep fluids in critically ill is scarce, the meta-analysis and systematic review did an important job of summarizing it and tried to answer important questions related to it.
- The authors conducted a meta-analysis following high-quality methodology. They followed rigorous guidelines for systematic reviews, including PROSPERO registration, PRISMA guidelines, and risk of bias assessment. All relevant databases were searched, and the search strategy was clearly stated in the manuscript.

DRAWBACKS OF THE STUDY

- *Heterogeneity:* The included studies had high heterogeneity, which limits the generalizability of the findings. Differences in study designs, patient populations, and interventions contributed to this issue.
- *Limited sample size:* Only five studies were included in the meta-analysis, which reduced the power to detect significant differences in important outcomes including mortality, fluid overload, delirium, etc.
- Three out of four trials included in the meta-analysis were observational before and after studies.
- *Moderate risk of bias:* The majority of the included studies had a moderate risk of bias, further limiting the strength of the conclusions.

REVIEWERS' VIEWPOINT

- The study suggests that the common practice of using high-sodium or isotonic fluids as maintenance/creep fluids has a significant impact on daily sodium load in ICU patients. A significantly high risk of hyperchloremia is also reported.
- While the data suggest that low-sodium fluids can reduce sodium burden and the risk of hyperchloremia, the evidence is still limited and inconsistent.
  - The effect of low-sodium strategy on relevant clinical outcomes could not be established by this meta-analysis. There is also a potential risk of hyponatremia and delirium with low-sodium fluids, which warrants caution.
- The authors emphasize the need for more high-quality RCTs to determine the effect of sodium content in maintenance and creep fluids on outcomes such as organ failure and mortality in critically ill patients. The existing evidence, while promising, is insufficient to make definitive clinical recommendations.
- An intensivist should carefully weigh the benefits of reducing sodium intake against the potential risks of hyponatremia and other complications.
  - If sodium concentrations are carefully monitored, the use of low-sodium maintenance/creep fluids in critically ill seems reasonable.

Blood Volume and Hemodynamics During Treatment of Major Hemorrhage with Ringer Solution, 5% Albumin, and 20% Albumin: A Single-centre Randomized Controlled Trial[6]

Jardot F, Hahn RG, Engel D, Beilstein CM, Wuethrich PY. Blood volume and hemodynamics during treatment of major hemorrhage with Ringer solution, 5% albumin, and 20% albumin: a single-center randomized controlled trial.

Crit Care. 2024;28(1):39.

CLINICAL QUESTION

- Does 20% albumin have the strongest plasma volume expansion (PVE) effect during major intraoperative hemorrhage situations?
- Would adding a predefined amount of 5% or 20% albumin to crystalloids better maintain the blood volume (BV) compared to using a crystalloid alone program in a 3:1 ratio to the blood loss?

WHAT IS ALREADY KNOWN?

- In patients with uncontrolled hemorrhage (trauma patients), blood and blood products transfusion is preferred. However, hemorrhage in better-controlled environments is treated with clear fluids until a prespecified hemoglobin level is reached.
- Fluid management is more challenging during general anesthesia, as its depressive effect on lymphatics promotes hypovolemia.
- As crystalloids quickly equilibrate between intravascular and interstitial compartments, very large fluid volumes are needed which increases the risk of overfilling in patients, raising complications such as pulmonary edema, rebleeding due to dilution effect, and poor healing.
- Smaller volumes are believed to be needed when colloids are used.
- The hyperoncotic 20% albumin is known to offer strong PVE per infused volume, being approximately twice the infused volume in patients with minor hemorrhage.
- The PVE of albumin solutions has not been adequately studied during surgery associated with major hemorrhage.

STUDY DESIGN

- This study was an investigator-initiated, open-label, three-arm randomized, active controlled, single-center randomized clinical trial.
- The trial period was from May 26, 2022 to April 13, 2023, at the Department of Urology of the University Hospital Bern, Switzerland.
- The primary aim of this clinical trial was to compare the PVE properties of iso-oncotic 5% albumin, hyperoncotic 20% albumin, and Ringer lactate (RL) as the fluid therapy during major intraoperative hemorrhage situations.
- Open radical cystectomy was chosen as the study model, which is associated with blood loss of 500–1,200 mL during the 0.5–1 hour when the bladder is removed in the middle part of the operation.

POPULATION STUDIED

- Patients who were 18 years of age or older admitted for planned open radical cystectomy.
- The following patients were excluded from the study:
    - Renal dysfunction [estimated glomerular filtration rate (eGFR) <60 mL/min/1.73 m^2]
    - Heart failure
    - Hypersensitivity or allergy to exogenous albumin
    - Breastfeeding mothers
    - Pregnant patients
    - Suspected drug or alcohol abuse

INTERVENTION

- Patients were allocated to one of the three-volume replacement groups: RL group, 5% albumin group, and 20% albumin group.
    - *5% albumin group*: It was given at a volume of 12 mL/kg (ideal body weight) and continued over 30 minutes during cystectomy.
    - *20% albumin group*: It was given at a volume of 3 mL/kg (ideal body weight) and continued over 30 minutes during cystectomy. Both albumin solutions were complemented by RL matching blood loss in a 1:1 ratio.

COMPARATOR

- *RL group:* RL was administered in the control group at a 3:1 ratio of blood loss.
- The following interventions were common in both groups:
    - A baseline intravenous fluid administration was performed using 1 mL/kg/hour of RL solution during first

and second part of surgery. It was increased to 3 mL/kg/hour during the third part of surgery until its end.
- Fresh frozen plasma was administered in case of microvascular bleeding.
- Packed red blood cells (PRBCs) were transfused to maintain a hemoglobin of >80 g/L.

OUTCOME

- 64 patients were screened, and 42 underwent randomization.
  - 14 patients were included in the 20% albumin group, 14 patients were included in the 5% albumin group, and 14 patients were included in the RL group for primary analysis.
- There was no difference in baseline characteristics between the two groups.
- *Primary outcome:* RL solution group expanded the plasma volume by 0.18 times the infused volume while the corresponding power of 5% albumin and 20% albumin was 0.74 and 2.09, respectively.
  - The 5 and 20% albumin groups were more effective in filling the vascular system; this was evidenced by the BV changes of only +63 mL and –44 mL, respectively, by long-lasting PVE with a median half-time of 5.5 hours and 4.8 hours respectively and by increase in central venous pressure.
  - The RL group resulted in slight hypovolemia by –313 mL

AUTHORS' VIEWPOINT

- The authors concluded that during major surgery with an intraoperative hemorrhage of 800 mL, 20% albumin has a better PVE property compared to 5% albumin and RL.
- Both 5 and 20% albumin were potent plasma volume expanders, and the effect is long-lasting.
- RL has a limited PVE property.

STRENGTHS OF THE STUDY

- The present study is the first study to separate the PVE properties of different infusion fluids when administered simultaneously during ongoing hemorrhage.
- Randomized study design.
- This approach might contribute to effective intraoperative fluid management in the future.

DRAWBACKS OF THE STUDY

- Single-center study
- Open-label design
- This study model is focused on a controlled hemorrhage model.
- Only specific types of surgical patients were included limiting the generalizability of the findings.
- The strategy to administer fluid study arms was not fully congruent.
  - The amount of infused fluid in the RL group was titrated to match the intraoperative blood loss in a 3:1 ratio.
  - By contrast, albumin was administered as a bolus infusion over 30 minutes.

REVIEWERS' VIEWPOINT

- Albumin solution, especially hyperoncotic albumin solution, clearly shown to have volume-sparing effects compared to isotonic crystalloids.
- However, a larger multicenter study, adequately powered to show significant differences in patient-centered outcomes, is required before recommending this study results in general perioperative patients with hemorrhage.
- The study results should not be used in traumatic hemorrhage situations. In the SAFE study, albumin infusion is shown to be detrimental in this patient subgroup.

Albumin Versus Saline Infusion for Sepsis-related Peripheral Tissue Hypoperfusion: A Proof-of-concept Prospective Study[7]

Gabarre P, Desnos C, Morin A, Missri L, Urbina T, Bonny V, et al. Albumin versus saline infusion for sepsis-related peripheral tissue hypoperfusion: a proof-of-concept prospective study.

Crit Care. 2024;28(1):43.

CLINICAL QUESTION

In patients with sepsis and persistent impaired tissue hypoperfusion despite initial resuscitation, does albumin infusion improve peripheral tissue perfusion compared with saline infusion?

WHAT IS ALREADY KNOWN?

- During sepsis, endothelial responses are dysregulated because the damage to the glycocalyx layer leads to a decrease in microcirculatory blood flow.
- There is no specific available treatment to limit decreased microvascular blood flow in patients with sepsis and septic shock.
- Preliminary studies have demonstrated that albumin infusion may improve endothelial function in septic patients. A similar effect was not seen, however, with saline infusion.

STUDY DESIGN

- Prospective, nonrandomized, and comparative study
- The study was conducted in two tertiary care French teaching hospitals.

POPULATION STUDIED

- Adult (>18 years) patients with sepsis according to the 3rd International Consensus definition in the period between 6 and 48 hours after initial resuscitation, who continued to have prolonged fingertip CRT (>3 seconds).
- All patients received initial fluid expansion with crystalloids @20 mL/kg and initial antibiotics and source control
- Septic patients requiring vasopressor after stabilization, i.e., MAP >65 mm Hg with no change in vasopressor requirement in the past 2 hours
- Clinicians who were in-charge considered to infuse further fluid boluses.
- Clinicians were free to infuse saline 0.9% or 20% human albumin solution.

INTERVENTION

- At study enrollment (H0), 500 mL of 0.9% saline was infused over 15 minutes.
- After 1 hour (H1) repeat fluid therapy (0.9% saline) was guided by CRT.

COMPARATOR

- At H0, 100 mL of 20% human albumin solution was used as fluid of choice.
- Decision for repeat 20% albumin bolus at H1 was at the discretion of attending clinician guided by CRT.

COMMON MANAGEMENT

- Before inclusion, all patients were resuscitated and received antibiotics.
- CRT was measured at H0 and H1 for both the groups.
- All patients were undergoing repeated transthoracic echocardiography for assessment of left ventricular (LV) function, cardiac output as well as volume status.

- At H4 (hour 4) heart rate (HR), CRT, MAP, cardiac index, arterial lactate, and urinary output were recorded.
- Same physician did CRT measurement at H0, H1, and H4 to limit inter-rated variability.

OUTCOME

- 62 patients were included in the study.
- Groups were matched for comorbidities, clinical, and biological characteristics.
    - Baseline CRT, mottling score, and arterial lactate levels were not different in the two groups.
- *Primary endpoint:* At H1, the rate of CRT normalization was significantly more in the albumin group as compared to the saline group (63 vs. 29%, $p = 0.02$).
- *Secondary endpoints:* There was a higher decrease in mottling score in patients of albumin group as compared to saline (0.5 vs. 0, $p = 0.05$).
    - No statistically significant difference in the groups for HR, MAP, and cardiac index at H1.
    - At H4, CRT continued to be lower in albumin group (2.7 vs. 3.1, $p = 0.03$).
    - At H4, albumin group had higher urine output (1.1 vs. 0.7 mL/kg/hour, $p = 0.08$).
    - Between H1 and H4, lactate levels lowered significantly in the albumin group. Similar effect was not observed in the saline group at H4.

AUTHORS' VIEWPOINT

The authors concluded that in patients with sepsis (resuscitated), albumin infusion might lead to greater improvement of tissue hypoperfusion as compared to saline.

STRENGTHS OF STUDY

- Authors asked a clinically relevant question
- Both the groups received protocolized care

DRAWBACKS OF THE STUDY

- Constrained sample size
- No randomization of patients
- Unblinded study
- *Confounding bias:* The decision to administer saline or albumin left to the clinician's discretion

REVIEWERS' VIEWPOINT

- This small study has provided some preliminary data about some possible beneficial effects of hyperoncotic albumin infusion compared to saline in restoring peripheral perfusion.
- However, we need a larger, multicenter, randomized trial to validate the results of this study.
- Till then use of hyperoncotic albumin in this subgroup of septic patients should be left up to the discretion of clinicians.

Protocolized Reduction of Non-resuscitation Fluids Versus Usual Care in Septic Shock Patients (REDUSE): A Randomized Multicentre Feasibility Trial[8]

Lindén A, Spångfors M, Olsen MH, Fisher J, Lilja G, Sjövall F, et al. Protocolized reduction of non-resuscitation fluids versus usual care in septic shock patients (REDUSE): a randomized multicentre feasibility trial.

Crit Care. 2024;28(1):166.

CLINICAL QUESTION

To investigate the feasibility of protocolized reduction of nonresuscitation fluids and to assess fluid volume administration, outcome reporting, and protocol adherence compared with usual care in patients with septic shock.

WHAT IS ALREADY KNOWN?

- Nonresuscitation fluids are administered to patients as vehicles for nutrition and medication to correct electrolyte disturbances and ensure adequate hydration.
- Nonresuscitation fluids account for a major fluid source after the first day in the ICU and are associated with harmful effects.
- Numerous trials comparing protocolized reduction of resuscitation fluids with usual care in adult septic shock patients found no differences in clinical outcomes between groups and achieved relatively small differences in total fluid volumes.

STUDY DESIGN

REDUSE was an investigator-initiated, multicenter, parallel-group randomized trial done in six Swedish ICUs between March 7 and September 13, 2022.

POPULATION

- *Inclusion criteria:*
  - Adult patients (≥18 years of age)
  - With septic shock (suspected/confirmed infection, plasma lactate >2 mmol/L)
  - Ongoing infusion of vasopressor to maintain MAP >65 mm Hg after adequate fluid resuscitation)
- Initially, it was mandated that patients should have fulfilled the criteria for septic shock within 3 hours preceding inclusion. To promote patient inclusion, the latter criterion was dropped after the inclusion of seven patients.
- *Exclusion criteria:*
  - Confirmed or suspected pregnancy
  - Participants readmitted to the ICU after hospital discharge

INTERVENTION

- Nonresuscitation fluids were defined as fluids other than colloids, blood products, and crystalloids administered to correct hemodynamic impairment. The type of maintenance fluids was according to local practice.
- Maintenance fluids were discontinued in participants who were positive in cumulative fluid balance and were judged not to be dehydrated by the treating physician.
- Intravenous fluid and enteral water were given as needed to correct electrolyte disturbances.
- Participants who were neutral or negative in cumulative fluid balance, received fluids in a dose that ensures that the total

dose of fluids covers the daily need of water (1 mL/kg/hour) and ongoing losses.

- Enteral nutrition had an energy density of at least 2 kcal/mL and will be administered according to local practice.
- Glucose was used at a maximum dose of 1 g/kg/day, using a concentration of 20% or greater starting at 72 hours after inclusion as nutrition, if enteral feeding was not tolerated.
  - Glucose at this (or lower) dose was started earlier in participants with insulin-dependent diabetes if enteral feeding is not tolerated and if local protocol mandates this.
- Parenteral nutrition was administered according to local protocol.
- Intravenous medications were concentrated according to a trial-specific protocol.

COMPARATOR: USUAL CARE GROUP

- Participants received nonresuscitation fluids according to local routines
- Maintenance fluids (crystalloids and/or glucose solutions and/or enteral water) were given at a dose of 1 mL/kg/hour unless local protocol states otherwise.
- Glucose was used at a maximal concentration of 10% for maintenance/nutrition unless local protocol states otherwise.
- Medications were concentrated according to local protocol.
- Enteral nutrition was administered according to local routines.
- In both groups, resuscitation fluids were administered according to the Surviving Sepsis Campaign (SSC) guidelines in the salvage and optimization phase and according to local protocol in the stabilization and de-escalation phases.
- In participants who required surgery, fluids were administered at the discretion of the anesthetist.
- The assigned interventions continued for the duration of the ICU stay up to a maximum of 90 days.

OUTCOMES

- Eligibility was assessed in 142 adult patients.
- A total of 49 patients were randomized to receive a protocolized reduction of nonresuscitation fluids, and 49 patients were randomized to usual care.
  - *Feasibility outcomes:*
    - The median length of stay in the ICU was 67 (IQR 32–169) hours in the restrictive fluid group and 72 (IQR 40–145) hours in the usual care group.
    - Within the first 3 days of inclusion, participants in the restrictive fluid group received a median of 6,008 (IQR 3,960–8,123) mL of total fluids, and the usual care group received 9,765 (IQR 6,804–12,401) mL. The Hodges–Lehmann median difference between groups was -3,560 (95% HLCI -5,302 to -1,614, $p < 0.001$) mL.
    - In a sensitivity analysis of participants admitted to the ICU for 3 days or more (complete case analysis), participants in the restrictive fluid group ($n = 24$) received 7,144 (IQR 5,872–8,582) mL and participants in the usual care group ($n = 28$) received 12,237 (IQR 9,932–14,268) mL in the first 3 days—a median difference of -4,749 (95% HLCI -6,507 to -2,879, $p < 0.001$) mL.
  - *Secondary feasibility outcomes:*
    - The proportions of participants with outcome data on all-cause

mortality, days alive and free of mechanical ventilation, and any AKI or ischemic events in the ICU within 90 days of inclusion were 98/98 (100%), 95/98 (98%), and 95/98 (98%), respectively.
    - The proportion of randomized patients who survived to 6 months and were assessed by Montreal Cognitive Assessment (MoCA) was 39/52 (75%) and by EQ-5D-5L was 41/52 (79%).
    - The proportion of randomized participants experiencing at least one protocol deviation was 15/98 (15%).
- *Exploratory clinical outcomes:*
    - All-cause mortality at 90 days, days alive and free of mechanical ventilation, AKI and ischemic complications, cognitive function, and quality of life did not differ between the groups.
    - The total volume of nonresuscitation fluids on days 3 and 5 was lower in the restrictive fluid group than in the usual care group [median difference -3,316 (95% HLCI -4,833 to 1,954, $p < 0.001$) and -3,191 (95% HLCI -5,199 to -1,166, $p = 0.006$)] mL, respectively.
    - The total volume of resuscitation fluids on days 3 and 5 did not differ between groups [0 (95% HLCI: 750–627, $p = 0.77$) and 37 (95% CI: 742–680, $p = 0.96$)] mL, respectively.
    - Cumulative fluid balance on days 3 and 5 were lower in the restrictive fluid group than in the usual care group [–2,109 (95% HLCI -3,480 to –831, $p < 0.001$) and –1,812 (–3,140 to –502) mL, respectively]
    - Hypoglycemia occurred in 10 participants in the restrictive fluid group and in four participants in the usual care group.

AUTHORS' VIEWPOINT

- Study results supported the hypothesis that fluid administration in septic shock could be effectively reduced by targeting nonresuscitation fluids.
    - The protocolized reduction of nonresuscitation fluids reduced cumulative administration by approximately 3.6 L in the first 3 days compared with usual care. This is almost twice as large as the reduction observed in fluid-restrictive trials.
    - This reduction was larger (reaching 5 L) in patients who stayed in ICU beyond 3 days.
- The larger amount of resuscitation fluid received in the usual care group was consistent with that reported by other observational studies, this, however, may vary between different centers and regions.

STRENGTHS

- Randomized, multicenter trial design and the fact that a prespecified protocol and statistical analysis plan were followed.
- Few exclusion criteria increase the generalizability

LIMITATIONS

- In the usual care group, protocolling of nonresuscitation fluids administration was not strictly protocolized and may have varied from site to site, as no guidelines or definitions describe what constitutes usual care for administering nonresuscitation fluids. And it may limit the external validity of the results.
- Inclusion criteria were modified slightly after the inclusion of seven patients and

patients with lower lactate at the time of randomization were included which may have influenced the patient population.

- Baseline cognitive function and health-related quality of life were not known and baseline differences in these outcomes may have influenced results.
- Flushing volumes to flush lines after drug injection were not protocolized.
- Low flushing volumes could have resulted in under-dosing of the concentrated drugs, such as antibiotics, in the intervention group.
- Treated physicians and the participants were not blinded to the allocated treatment due to the nature of the intervention.

REVIEWER' VIEWPOINT

- This trial addressed an important practice in the ICU, which is associated with harmful effects if unregulated.
- Trial results showed that with a protocolized approach is possible to reduce the maintenance fluid therapy and to reduce the total cumulative fluid load.
  - However, the large difference in the volume of received between the two groups could be due to the Hawthorne effect, and lack of blinding of the treating physicians.
- Restricting fluids require intensive monitoring of possible side effects like over-dependence on vasopressor therapy to meet hemodynamic goals, risk of renal failure, and possible device-related effects such as clogging of central venous catheters due to insufficient flushing.
- These trial results would make clinicians more wary in planning and monitoring fluid therapy after resuscitation to avoid both under and overloading, both of which are associated with harm.

Twenty Percent Human Albumin Solution Fluid Bolus Administration Therapy in Patients after Cardiac Surgery-II: A Multicentre Randomized Controlled Trial[9]

Wigmore GJ, Deane AM, Presneill JJ, Eastwood G, Serpa Neto A, Maiden MJ, et al. Twenty percent human albumin solution fluid bolus administration therapy in patients after cardiac surgery-II: a multicentre randomised controlled trial.

Intensive Care Med. 2024;50(7):1075-85.

CLINICAL QUESTION

After cardiac surgery, does fluid bolus therapy (FBT) with 20% albumin reduce the duration of vasopressor therapy compared with crystalloid boluses?

WHAT IS ALREADY KNOWN?

- Intravenous FBT is common after cardiac surgery to optimize intravascular volume and end-organ perfusion aiming to reduce the duration of vasopressor therapy.
- Crystalloids and 4% albumin are the most commonly used fluids for bolus therapy in ICUs.
- 20% albumin is more physiological with survival benefits in liver failure and septic shock patients, with longer-lasting effects on PVE.

STUDY DESIGN

- This study was a multicentered, open-label, and randomized clinical trial conducted in 6 ICUs in Australia.

- The trial period was from August 31, 2020 to August 31, 2022.

POPULATION STUDIED

- *Inclusion criteria:* Patients 18 years of age or older admitted in ICU needing FBT after cardiac surgery requiring cardiopulmonary bypass.
  - Patients were mechanically ventilated at the time of ICU admission with arterial line and central line.
- *Following patients were excluded from the study:*
  - Previous FBT in the ICU after cardiac surgery
  - Known contraindication to the study fluid (e.g., hypersensitivity reaction)
  - Documented refusal of study fluid
  - Imminent death
  - Previous enrollment in HAS FLAIR-II
  - Pregnancy
  - Age <18 years

INTERVENTION

- For 7 days after randomization, or until vasopressor therapy was discontinued for four consecutive hours (with MAP ≥65 mm Hg), patients received all FBT in the ICU as the assigned fluid.
- Clinician determined FBT in the form of 20% albumin as a 100 mL bottle
- Maximum 400 mL of 20% albumin FBT allowed per calendar day
- If additional FBT required, it was given in the form of 4% albumin 500 mL.

COMPARATOR

- FBT was given in the form of crystalloids. Suitable crystalloid solutions included 0.9% sodium chloride solution, compound sodium lactate, or Plasma-Lyte 148.
- The group was not permitted to receive any form of albumin until cumulatively at least 1,000 mL of crystalloid fluid bolus had been received. Thereafter, the treating clinician could use 4% albumin.
- *The following interventions were common in both groups*:
  - Other treatments as per the treating clinician
  - Once the patient was discharged from the ICU, the type of fluid administered was not dictated by the trial protocol.

OUTCOME

- 480 patients underwent randomization (240 patients in each group)
  - Seven patients withdrew consent from each group
  - A total number of 233 patients from 20% albumin and 233 from the crystalloid group were included for primary analysis.
- Baseline and clinical characteristics were similar in both groups.
- *Primary outcome:* The difference in the cumulative duration of vasopressor therapy between the 20% albumin and the crystalloid group was −3.8 (95% CI −8 to 0.4; $p = 0.08$) hours.
- *Secondary outcome:* Day one fluid balance was less with 20% albumin FBT (mean difference −701 mL, 95% CI −872 to −530)
- Cumulative proportion of patients receiving any vasopressor therapy was similar
- No difference in ventilation-free days
- No difference in time to readiness for ICU discharge
- No difference in ICU or hospital length of stay

AUTHORS' VIEWPOINT

- The authors concluded that in patients after cardiac surgery, FBT with 20% albumin compared to crystalloid fluid did not significantly reduce the cumulative duration of vasopressor therapy.

- However, FBT with 20% albumin was associated with a reduced volume of fluid used for resuscitation and a less positive fluid balance.

STRENGTHS OF THE STUDY

- The fact that the trial was conducted in six ICUs with mortality and care processes similar in the global cardiac registry increases external validity.
- Good matching of baseline characteristics
- The permuted block random allocation sequence was concealed and stratified by the study center to prevent bias.
- No loss of data for primary outcome

DRAWBACKS OF THE STUDY

- Unblinded trial
- Primary outcome may have been influenced by bedside clinicians.
- The decision to administer FBT was at the discretion of the treating clinical team.
- The number of additional episodes of vasopressor requirement was not included after 4 hours of vasopressor-free time.
- 4% albumin was allowed in the comparison group which may have led to the masking of benefits of 20% albumin.
- Inclusion was not restricted to patients receiving vasopressors prior to randomization with the assumption that a proportion would go on to receive vasopressor therapy later. This proportion would be decreased if 20% albumin was a more effective therapy in improving blood pressure.
- Data regarding transfusion of nonalbumin blood products, sedation, and steroids were not recorded.

REVIEWERS' VIEWPOINT

- Looking at the results of this trial, there appears to be no significant difference between crystalloids and 20% albumin as fluid boluses in postcardiac surgery patients in terms of vasopressor duration.
- However, given the previous evidence regarding the benefits of albumin in volume expansion and decreased cumulative fluid balance which itself is associated with decreased mortality warrants further studies comparing 20% albumin to crystalloids for fluid boluses while standardizing other parameters such as concomitant steroids, use of other blood products, sedation scores which independently may affect vasopressor therapy and duration.

REFERENCES

1. Bollaert PE, Monnier A, Schneider F, Argaud L, Badie J, Charpentier C, et al. Fluid balance control in critically ill patients: results from POINCARE-2 stepped wedge cluster-randomized trial. Crit Care. 2023;27(1):66.
2. Mansouri A, Buzzi M, Gibot S, Charpentier C, Schneider F, Louis G, et al. Fluid balance control in critically ill patients: results from as-treated analyses of POINCARE-2 randomized trial. Crit Care. 2023;27(1):426.
3. Huang W, Xiang H, Hu C, Wu T, Zhang D, Ma S, et al. Association of Sublingual Microcirculation Parameters and Capillary Refill Time in the Early Phase of ICU Admission. Crit Care Med. 2023;51(7):913-23.
4. Sankar J, Muralidharan J, Lalitha AV, Rameshkumar R, Pathak M, Das RR, et al. Multiple Electrolytes Solution Versus Saline as Bolus Fluid for Resuscitation in Pediatric Septic Shock: A Multicenter Randomized Clinical Trial. Crit Care Med. 2023;51(11):1449-60.
5. Waskowski J, Salvato SM, Müller M, Hofer D, van Regenmortel N, Pfortmueller CA. Choice of creep or maintenance fluid type and their impact on total daily ICU sodium burden in

critically ill patients: A systematic review and meta-analysis. J Crit Care. 2023;78:154403.

6. Jardot F, Hahn RG, Engel D, Beilstein CM, Wuethrich PY. Blood volume and hemodynamics during treatment of major hemorrhage with Ringer solution, 5% albumin, and 20% albumin: a single-center randomized controlled trial. Crit Care. 2024;28(1):39.
7. Gabarre P, Desnos C, Morin A, Missri L, Urbina T, Bonny V, et al. Albumin versus saline infusion for sepsis-related peripheral tissue hypoperfusion: a proof-of-concept prospective study. Crit Care. 2024;28(1):43.
8. Lindén A, Spångfors M, Olsen MH, Fisher J, Lilja G, Sjövall F, et al. Protocolized reduction of non-resuscitation fluids versus usual care in septic shock patients (REDUSE): a randomized multicenter feasibility trial. Crit Care. 2024;28(1):166.
9. Wigmore GJ, Deane AM, Presneill JJ, Eastwood G, Serpa Neto A, Maiden MJ, et al. Twenty percent human albumin solution fluid bolus administration therapy in patients after cardiac surgery-II: a multicentre randomized controlled trial. Intensive Care Med. 2024;50(7):1075-85.

SECTION

2

Respiratory/Ventilation/ARDS

Section Editor: *Jaicob Varghese*

Associate Editors: *Biji Thomas Philip, Melwin George, Nilanjan Umesh*

Convalescent Plasma for COVID-19-Induced ARDS in Mechanically Ventilated Patients

Misset B, Piagnerelli M, Hoste E, Dardenne N, Grimaldi D, Michaux I, et al. Convalescent Plasma for COVID-19-Induced ARDS in Mechanically Ventilated Patients.

N Engl J Med. 2023;389:1590-600.

CLINICAL QUESTION

Does the administration of convalescent plasma to patients with COVID-19-induced acute respiratory distress syndrome (ARDS) who are on mechanical ventilation improve their survival outcomes compared to standard care?

Passive immunization with plasma collected from convalescent patients has been regularly used to treat coronavirus disease 2019 (COVID-19). But minimal data are available regarding the use of convalescent plasma in patients with COVID-19-induced ARDS.

WHAT IS ALREADY KNOWN?

Convalescent plasma is directed against the cause of COVID-19-induced ARDS. Intensive care unit (ICU) patients infected with SARS-CoV-2 can shed high titers of virus both in the upper and lower respiratory tract and tend to be prolonged shedders. Convalescent plasma may reduce the quantity of virus alive in the lungs of patients who continue to shed the virus.[1] Convalescent plasma had high neutralizing activity (median interquartile range titer 1:526) and its administration increased antibodies to SARS-CoV-2 by 14.4%.[2] It may counteract the delayed kinetics of neutralizing antibody production in these patients. Delayed seroconversion kinetics correlated with impaired viral control in deceased patients.[3]

Convalescent plasma contains both neutralizing antibodies that mediate viral elimination and non-neutralizing antibodies that can modulate inflammation.[4] Patients receiving treatment with convalescent plasma have been shown to have lower levels of serum inflammatory mediators than those not receiving treatment.

STUDY DESIGN AND POPULATION STUDIED

A randomized, open-label clinical trial was conducted at 17 Belgian sites, led by the University Hospital of Liège. Patients who recently began invasive mechanical ventilation due to COVID-19 ARDS were enrolled and divided into two groups: Early enrollment (within 48 hours) and late enrollment (48–120 hours). Patients were then randomly assigned to receive either convalescent plasma with high-titer neutralizing antibodies against SARS-CoV-2 or standard care.

Patient Eligibility

- Adult patients diagnosed with COVID-19-induced ARDS with a WHO clinical progression scale of 7–9
- Admitted to the ICU and on invasive mechanical ventilation for up to 5 days
- Not severely frail (Clinical Frailty Scale score <6)
- Not pregnant, with no history of transfusion reactions, and not enrolled in other COVID-19 trials

Donor Eligibility

- Adults who had fully recovered from COVID-19 infection 28 days to 10 months prior
- High levels of neutralizing antibodies against SARS-CoV-2 (titer ≥1:320 preferred, ≥1:160 accepted if shortage of high titer plasma)

INTERVENTION STUDIED AND COMPARATOR

Two units (400–500 mL in total) of ABO compatible convalescent plasma collected from two different donors preferably having recovered from COVID-19 with a titer ≥1/320 was administered within 24 hours of inclusion in the study to the study group in addition to standard of care therapy.

The control arm received standard of care therapy only without any convalescent plasma. Patients were followed up to 1 year.

Standard of care included restrictive fluid management, low V_t ventilation, plateau pressure <30 cm, and individualized positive end-expiratory pressure (PEEP) >5 cm minimum. Use muscle relaxants in case of ARDS with PaO_2/FiO_2 ratio <150 mm Hg, for a maximum of 48 hours, use a prone position in case of ARDS with PaO_2/FIO_2 ratio <150 mm Hg, dexamethasone 10 mg intravenously (IV) once a day for 10 days, and veno-venous extracorporeal membrane oxygenation (VV ECMO) or inhaled nitric oxide (iNO) on a case-by-case basis.

OUTCOMES EVALUATED

The primary outcome was death by Day 28 after randomization.

Secondary outcomes included adverse events (AEs) (transfusion-related acute lung injury, serious allergic transfusion reactions, and transfusion-associated circulatory overload), inflammatory and anti-SARS-CoV-2 antibody responses, the Sequential Organ Failure Assessment (SOFA) score, the use of organ support, the length of hospital stay, and death by Day 90 and 365.

RESULTS

- *Patient groups:* 237 patients received convalescent plasma, and 238 received standard care.
- *Timing of treatment:* 72% of patients started treatment within 48 hours of needing a ventilator, while 28% started >48 hours after mechanical ventilation.
- *Mortality rates:* Overall, 35.4% of patients in the plasma group died, compared to 45.0% in the standard care group (a statistically significant difference).
    - For patients treated within 48 hours, mortality was 32.7% in the plasma group and 46.8% in the standard care group.

    - For patients treated after 48 hours, mortality was 42% in both groups.
- *Survival curves:* The survival rates for the two groups started to diverge around Day 17, with the plasma group showing a better survival outcome.

SECONDARY OUTCOMES AND SUBGROUP ANALYSES

- *Adverse events:* A total of 711 AEs were observed, 209 of which were considered serious. However, none of these events were directly linked to the convalescent plasma treatment.
- *Secondary infections:* Both groups experienced similar rates of secondary bacterial infections and pneumonia.
- *Organ support and hospital stay:* The duration of organ support (such as ventilation) and the length of hospital stays were comparable between the two groups.
- *Extracorporeal membrane oxygenation (ECMO):* The need for ECMO was similar in both groups.
- *Long-term mortality:* Lower mortality rates were observed at 90 days and 365 days in the convalescent plasma group.

AUTHORS' VIEWPOINT

The authors are of the opinion that administration of convalescent plasma with high levels of neutralizing antibodies within 48 hours of starting ventilation significantly reduced mortality at 28 days. This effect was most pronounced in patients who received treatment early in their disease course, and a greater effect was seen in patients with a higher illness severity at inclusion. There were no significant safety concerns as AEs including serious AEs were similar in both groups. They conclude that the trial has a good potential for generalizability to most patients with COVID-19-induced ARDS.

STRENGTHS OF THE STUDY

The strengths of the study include:

- *Randomized controlled trial design, clear inclusion criteria:* The study included a well-defined patient population with severe COVID-19 and ARDS, requiring mechanical ventilation.
- *Convalescent plasma with high antibody titers:* The study used convalescent plasma with high levels of neutralizing antibodies, assessed for NT50, increasing the potential for a positive treatment effect.
- *Early treatment window:* The study included patients in the early treatment within 48 hours of ventilation initiation, likely contributing to the observed benefits.
- *Detailed data collection:* The study collected comprehensive data on patient outcomes, and continued follow-up till 1 year
- *Statistical significance:* The study demonstrated a statistically significant reduction in mortality at 28 days in the convalescent plasma group compared to the standard care group.
- *Large sample size:* The study included a relatively large sample size, increasing statistical power and the reliability of the findings.

WEAKNESS OF THE STUDY

- *Trial was not blinded*: They avoided placebo because it would add extra fluid volume which is against conservative fluid strategy for managing ARDS.
- A nonsubjective primary outcome, death by Day 28 was chosen to reduce the risk due to lack of blinding. The open design may have resulted in subtle differences in clinical decisions after randomization.

- The convalescent plasma was obtained between April 2020 and May 2021, when the ancestral virus and then its alpha variant were predominant in Belgium; however, the trial recruited from September 2020 to March 2022. The neutralizing antibodies might have been less active against subsequent variants which emerged after May 2021.
- Trial was terminated prematurely because of the absence of new inclusion, presumably owing to the reduced virulence of the omicron BA.2 variant. However, they ultimately included 475 patients, representing 95% of the planned inclusions, and it is unlikely that the results would have been modified by including 25 patients more.

REVIEWERS' VIEWPOINT

Well-conducted randomized study showing the benefit of convalescent plasma with sufficient neutralizing antibody titer, showing mortality reduction which was rather pronounced in the early treatment group. Convalescent plasma may be useful if future SARS-CoV-2 variants with increased virulence occur.

IMPACT ON CURRENT PRACTICE AND TAKE-HOME MESSAGE

Convalescent plasma, derived from the blood of recovered COVID-19 patients, shows promise as a potential treatment for ARDS in critically ill patients requiring mechanical ventilation.

Early administration, within the first 48 hours of ventilation, appears to be particularly beneficial. The effectiveness of this treatment may be linked to the high levels of neutralizing antibodies present in the plasma.

However, it is important to note that convalescent plasma is not a definitive cure, and further research is needed to establish optimal dosing, timing, and duration of treatment. While it offers hope, potential risks, such as allergic reactions and thrombosis, must be considered.

Five Sessions of Hyperbaric Oxygen for Critically Ill Patients with COVID-19-Induced ARDS: A Randomised, Open Label, Phase II Trial

Kjellberg A, Douglas J, Pawlik MT, Hassler A, Al-Ezerjawi S, Boström E, et al. Five sessions of hyperbaric oxygen for critically ill patients with COVID-19-induced ARDS: A randomised, open label, phase II trial.

Respir Med. 2024;232:107744.

CLINICAL QUESTION

The main goal was to assess whether hyperbaric oxygen therapy (HBOT) could lower the rate of intensive care unit (ICU) admissions compared to the current best practices for severe COVID-19 treatment. Given HBOT's known anti-inflammatory and immunomodulatory effects, the researchers hypothesized that it could decrease mortality rates, enhance oxygen tolerance, and prevent organ failure in patients with severe COVID-19 by suppressing the inflammatory response.

WHAT IS ALREADY KNOWN?

Aggressive oxygen therapy is a mainstay treatment for critically ill COVID-19 patients and has been used in various methods to reduce mortality. Refractory hypoxemia necessitates endotracheal intubation in these patients. HBOT benefits patients by intensifying the oxygen pressure in the alveoli, consequently, the diffusion rate and the diffusion distance of oxygen will increase compared to standard oxygen therapy (e.g., face mask and invasive ventilation). HBOT remains one of the most effective and safest interventions to compensate for oxygen deprivation in ARDS.[5]

Patients treated with HBOT showed improvements in their clinical factors and indexes as follows: (A) Arterial blood gas (ABG) analysis, (B) liver function tests, (C) complete blood count (CBC, differential), and (D) improvement of lung structure clearance based on computed tomography (CT scan).[6]

Mehrtak M, et al. did a systematic review of published data on HBOT in COVID-19 and included eight studies of which three were clinical trials, all studies had a small number of patients. They concluded that most of the patients recovered after receiving HBOT, and blood oxygen saturation increased after several sessions of HBOT. Of the studies, three clinical trials showed the efficacy of the HBOT on patients infected with COVID-19. The results indicated a significant effect of HBOT on patients, and it was safe and beneficial for them.[5]

Grenstein et al. did a propensity matched controlled trial including 20 patients who received HBOT at 2.0 atm up to five treatments administered daily in addition to standard care, and 60 propensity matched controls who received standard treatments. The adjusted subdistribution hazard ratios were 0.37 for inpatient mortality ($p = 0.14$) and 0.26 for mechanical ventilation ($p = 0.046$) in favor of HBOT.[7]

STUDY DESIGN AND POPULATION STUDIED

This was an investigator initiated, randomized, controlled, parallel-arms, open-label, multicenter, phase II clinical trial that was conducted at three hospitals, two in Sweden and one in Germany. Adult patients 18–90 years old, hospitalized for severe COVID-19 with moderate-to-severe ARDS, with a ratio of arterial oxygen partial pressure to fractional inspired oxygen (PaO_2/FiO_2) below 26.7 kPa (200 mm Hg), based on ABG measurement, with at least two risk factors for increased risk of ICU admission or mortality and likely to need intubation within 7 days of admission to hospital were included.

Exclusion criteria included severe chronic obstructive pulmonary disease (COPD) (GOLD class III–IV), pulmonary fibrosis >10% and contraindications for HBOT. The trial was terminated prematurely for futility by the sponsor approximately 1 year after the last inclusion in each country based on a slow inclusion rate.

INTERVENTION STUDIED

Both groups received best-practice treatment for COVID-19, including normobaric medical oxygen up to 100% administrated as needed, low-dose steroids, and low molecular weight heparin. The HBOT group received, in addition to best practice, HBOT with medical oxygen 100% at 2.4 ATA for 80–90 minutes, with two 5-minute air breaks, once a day, maximum five treatments within 7 days from randomization. The first HBOT was given within 24 hours from inclusion. All treatments in Sweden were delivered in monoplace chambers, and treatments in Germany were delivered in a multiplace chamber with attending staff inside.

COMPARATOR USED

Adult patients 18–90 years old, hospitalized in non-ICU wards for severe COVID-19 with moderate-to-severe ARDS, with ratio of arterial oxygen partial pressure to fractional inspired oxygen (PaO_2/FiO_2) below 26.7 kPa (200 mm Hg), who received standard treatment with exemption of HBOT served as controls. Eligible subjects were randomized in a 1:1 allocation, stratified by site and sex, in blocks of eight (blinded to all study personnel) to either HBOT or control.

OUTCOMES EVALUATED

The primary end point was requirement for ICU admission from Day 1 to 30, based on criteria at the discretion of the investigator.

The main secondary endpoints were:

- Proportion of subjects with 30-day mortality, all-cause mortality, from Day 1 to 30
- Time-to-intubation, i.e., cumulative days free of invasive mechanical ventilation, from Day 1 to 30
- Time-to-ICU, i.e., cumulative ICU-free days, derived as the number of days from Day 1 to ICU admission, where all ICU-free subjects are censored at Day 30.
- Mean change in inflammatory response [C-reactive protein (CRP), lactate dehydrogenase (LDH), D-dimer procalcitonin, and ferritin], from Day 1 to 30.

The safety of the treatment was assessed by monitoring AEs. The number of patients experiencing AEs and the types of AEs were recorded for each treatment group.

RESULTS OF THE STUDY

34 subjects were randomly assigned to HBOT ($N = 18$) or control ($N = 16$) at two centers in Sweden and one center in Germany. The trial was stopped for futility by the sponsor due to a slow inclusion rate with 34 randomized subjects and only primary, main secondary, and safety endpoints are reported.

Primary Endpoint: Intensive Care Unit Admission

There was no significant difference between the two groups in the proportion of patients requiring ICU admission, 5 (50%) in control vs. 13 (72.2 %) in HBOT.

Secondary Endpoints

- *Mortality:* Four patients in the HBOT group and one in the control group died within 30 days of treatment. Overall survival rates were 77.8% for the HBOT group and 93.8% for the control group, a difference that was not statistically significant.
- *Time to intubation and ICU admission:* There were no significant differences between the two groups in the number of days patients avoided invasive mechanical ventilation or ICU admission.
- *Inflammatory response:* A significant decrease in CRP levels was observed in the HBOT group compared to the control group.
    - No significant differences were found in other inflammatory markers, such as LDH, D-dimer, procalcitonin, and ferritin.
- *Safety:* The safety profile of HBOT was not fully assessed due to the small sample size and early termination of the trial. The AEs and SAEs were more commonly reported in the control group, but severe AEs were more common in the HBOT group. Four subjects expired in the HBOT group and one in the control group, but all deaths were assessed as unrelated to HBOT, pneumomediastinum and pneumothorax were more common in the control group, five versus only one in the HBOT group. Infections were also more common in the control group, seven versus three in the HBOT group.

AUTHORS' VIEWPOINT

As the trial was prematurely terminated, the study was inconclusive to meet the criteria in the power calculation. There was no statistically significant difference between the treatment arms in ICU admission. However, there was a trend toward better oxygenation and faster recovery in the HBOT group compared with control. The authors note that HBOT has an anti-inflammatory effect that improves oxygenation in individuals with severe and critical COVID-19 and that it has a favorable profile of harms and may be beneficial in the intervention strategies for ARDS regardless of underlying causative agents.

STRENGTHS OF THE STUDY

The strengths of the study include: (1) *Randomized study design,* (2) *Clear inclusion* and exclusion criteria, (3) *Multicenter design* although countries of similar geographical and economic parameters, (4) *Feasibility assessment:* The trial successfully demonstrated the feasibility of administering HBOT to critically ill COVID-19 patients with ARDS, and (5) *Favorable safety profile:* The study reported a favorable safety profile for HBOT, with no significant AEs directly attributable to the intervention.

WEAKNESS OF THE STUDY

- *Small sample size:* The relatively small sample size of the study limits its statistical power and may have contributed to the lack of statistically significant differences between the treatment and control groups.
- *Premature termination:* The trial was prematurely terminated due to futility, which means that it did not have sufficient power to detect a clinically meaningful difference between the groups, even if one existed.
- *Open-label design:* The open-label design can introduce bias, as both patients and clinicians are aware of the treatment assignment.
- *Lack of long-term follow-up:* The study did not include long-term follow-up data, which could provide insights into the potential long-term effects of HBOT on patient outcomes.

REVIEWERS' VIEWPOINT

This study provides preliminary evidence that HBOT may not be beneficial in reducing ICU admission in critically ill COVID-19 patients with ARDS. However, the limitations of the study, including the open-label design and small sample size, suggest that further research is needed to confirm these findings. A larger, double-blind, randomized controlled trial is necessary to definitively assess the efficacy and safety of HBOT in this patient population including the following aspects—the optimal dose and timing of HBOT, benefits and harms on intubated subjects with ARDS.

IMPACT ON CURRENT PRACTICE AND TAKE-HOME MESSAGE

- *No conclusive evidence:* The study did not demonstrate a significant reduction in ICU admission or mortality with HBOT compared to standard care.
- *Favorable safety profile:* HBOT was found to be feasible and had a favorable safety profile.
- *Further research needed:* Larger, well-designed trials are necessary to definitively determine the potential benefits and harms of HBOT in this patient population.
- *Individualized approach:* The decision to use HBOT should be made on a case-by-case basis, considering the patient's individual circumstances and potential risks and benefits.

ARDS Mortality Prediction Model Using Evolving Clinical Data and Chest Radiograph Analysis

Cysneiros A, Galvão T, Domingues N, Jorge P, Bento L, Martin-Loeches I. ARDS mortality prediction model using evolving clinical data and chest radiograph analysis.

Biomedicines. 2024;12:439.

CLINICAL QUESTION OR PROBLEM

Whether a combination of chest X-rays (CXRs) along with ventilatory settings and ABGs can predict ARDS mortality.

WHAT IS ALREADY KNOWN?

The Berlin criteria, widely used in defining ARDS, use ABGs, specifically the PaO_2/FiO_2 ratio, and radiological evidence in the form of either CXR or chest CT scans. However, recently the ESICM published definitions that have sparked debate and challenged the reliance on chest radiography.[8] Many alternative approaches have been suggested, such as incorporating merely unilateral opacities, mandating chest CT scans and including lung ultrasound in ARDS definition.[9]

STUDY DESIGN

Retrospective cohort study conducted on mechanically ventilated COVID-19 ARDS patients admitted to the ICUs of Hospital São José and Hospital Curry Cabral in the time period between April 2020 and January 2021.

POPULATION INCLUDED

Patients who fit into the definition of ARDS according to the Berlin definition and required invasive mechanical ventilation for at least 48 hours were included.

INTERVENTION STUDIED

A binary logistic regression (LogReg) model was developed for predicting COVID-19 ARDS mortality based on the age, PaO_2/FiO_2 ratio (P/F) on Days 1 and 3, CNN-extracted CXR features and its usefulness was studied.

COMPARATOR USED

Logistic regression models were developed and certain complex algorithms such as multilayer perceptron (MLP), support vector machine (SVM), and random forest (RndForest) were used for comparison. A model was also created using only clinical data with age and P/F d3 called model B which was used for comparison.

OUTCOMES EVALUATED

110 patients were enrolled in the study, the mean age being 63.2 ± 11.92 (26–83 years). Deep learning image features (DLFs) increased the sensitivity from 0.643 (model B) to 0.714 (model A); the specificity from 0.711 to 0.778; the positive predictive value (PPV) from 0.675 to 0.75 and the AUC from 0.701 to 0.77. Also by the Bayesian t-test results, the probability of the first model (model A) being better than model B was 0.739. The model incorporating DLFs showed an 89% probability of superior accuracy for LogReg as well as 82% for MLP compared to the clinical variables-only model (Model B).

AUTHORS' VIEWPOINT

As the research around ARDS evolves, utilizing machine techniques, particularly in analyzing chest radiographs, provides valuable information regarding mortality and severity prediction, as done here of COVID-19

ARDS. Integrating DLFs in the LogReg model showed superior prediction accuracy.

STRENGTHS OF THE STUDY

Multiple regression models were used in the study which would enhance its accuracy. Detailed assessment of the features embedded in radiography was used, which were subtle yet clinically significant.

DRAWBACKS OF THE STUDY

Only 110 patients were included in the study. Only P/F ratios on Day 1 and Day 3 were considered. Comprehensive data on ventilation parameters, such as driving pressure and plateau pressure, were not uniformly obtained during the specified timeframe.

REVIEWERS' VIEWPOINT

Larger prospective randomized controlled trials would be required to ensure the impact of DLFs and their incorporation in mortality prediction models.

IMPACT TO CURRENT PRACTICE AND TAKE-HOME MESSAGE

Recent studies using imaging patterns to optimize ventilation have shown mixed outcomes. The LIVE trial,[10] for instance, concluded that personalizing treatment using a CT-based image classification did not reduce mortality. Lung ultrasound is also being studied as an important tool for personalization of ARDS management.[11] Further prospective large trials are required to determine the accuracy of machine predictive models to predict ARDS mortality and severity and we need to gradually but cautiously imbibe them in our clinical practice.

Pressure Control Plus Spontaneous Ventilation versus Volume Assist-Control Ventilation in Acute Respiratory Distress Syndrome. A Randomised Clinical Trial

Richard JM, Beloncle FM, Béduneau G, Mortaza S, Ehrmann S, Diehl JL, et al. Pressure control plus spontaneous ventilation versus volume assist-control ventilation in acute respiratory distress syndrome. A randomised clinical trial.

Intensive Care Med. 2024;50(10):1647-56.

CLINICAL QUESTION

Whether a pressure-controlled strategy with non-synchronized unassisted spontaneous ventilation (PC-SV) was inferior to a conventional volume assist-control ventilation (ACV) on the outcome of patients with ARDS.

WHAT IS ALREADY KNOWN?

Acute respiratory distress syndrome patients exhibit high ventilatory drive which necessitates the use of deep sedation and even muscle relaxants to properly manage ventilation, at least in the early phase. The transition to a spontaneous breathing mode is difficult.[12] More recently, the concept of lung and diaphragm-protective approach is advocated where lung protective ventilation is followed as well as spontaneous diaphragmatic activity is allowed, avoiding excessive distension to prevent diaphragm atrophy. It has been shown to be associated with improved outcomes.[13]

STUDY DESIGN

It was a multi-centered open-labeled randomized clinical trial in 22 ICUs in France.

POPULATION STUDIED

Patients with moderate-to-severe ARDS (PaO_2/FiO_2 ratio ≤200 mm Hg with PEEP ≥5 cmH_2O) were taken for enrollment if the four criteria of the Berlin definition were met for no later than 48 hours.

INTERVENTION STUDIED

Patients were randomly assigned to PC-SV or ACV with similar titration of tidal volumes and PEEP. Muscle relaxants were stopped after 24 hours, and sedation was not to hinder patients' spontaneous breathing. The primary endpoint studied was in-hospital mortality from any cause at Day 60.

COMPARATOR USED

Statistical analysis was done using the *t* test or Mann–Whitney test for continuous variables and the χ^2 test or Fisher exact test for categorical variables.

OUTCOMES EVALUATED

Primary outcome was defined as in-hospital mortality from any cause at 60 days which was 34.6% in the patients treated with PC-SV versus 33.5% for those treated with ACV. There was no difference in secondary outcomes such as mortality at Day 28, numbers of ventilator-free, organ failure-free, and vasoactive drugs-free days at Day 28, and durations of ventilation and ICU stay.

AUTHOR'S VIEWPOINT

The mortality observed in the current study is similar to that in recent randomized trials in ARDS and slightly lower than the landmark LUNG SAFE study. There was a significant reduction in the need for neuromuscular blockers and sedation during the first week with spontaneous ventilation. Also, patients in the spontaneous ventilation group were significantly less proned based on the recommendation of proning for severe hypoxemia. Hence probably using this mode of ventilation should be advocated more often.

STRENGTH OF THE STUDY

It was a randomized clinical trial and the study population was large, covering over 22 ICUs in France. Baseline characteristics were well matched, and similar settings of tidal volume and PEEP were used in both groups.

DRAWBACKS OF THE STUDY

The study was unblinded in nature coupled with the use of adjunctive therapies left to the discretion of the attending physician in case of severe hypoxemia. There was a lower incidence of proning in the experimental group in spite of similar profound hypoxia in both groups, indicating the hesitance of the physician to prone patients in the experimental group. Also, the lack of experience with PC-SV in France compared to ACV, which was predominantly used before the study, could have interfered with the behavior of caregivers in spite of the protocolization of both experimental and control strategies.

REVIEWER'S VIEWPOINT

Even though the study showed a significant reduction in the need for sedation and neuromuscular blockade in the experimental group, it was an open-labeled trial, and adjunctive therapies were used as per the attending physician in severe hypoxemia.

A more comprehensive blinded study needs to be done at multiple centers across the world and mortality benefit needs to be demonstrated before we fully adopt this practice.

IMPACT ON CURRENT PRACTICES AND TAKE-HOME MESSAGE

After the ACURASYS study[14] which showed a beneficial impact of paralysis on outcome in severe ARDS, results of the ROSE trial showed no significant decrease in mortality using a neuromuscular blocking agent (NMBA), and the systematic use of NMBA at the early phase of severe ARDS is no longer recommended.[15] Hence using spontaneous modes of ventilation is feasible and the same should be cautiously tried in selected ARDS patients which would facilitate early weaning and extubation.

Effects of Early versus Delayed Application of Prone Position on Ventilation–Perfusion Mismatch in Patients with Acute Respiratory Distress Syndrome: A Prospective Observational Study

Yuan X, Zhao Z, Chao Y, Chen D, Chen H, Zhang R, et al. Effects of early versus delayed application of prone position on ventilation–perfusion mismatch in patients with acute respiratory distress syndrome: a prospective observational study.

Crit Care. 2023;27(1):462.

CLINICAL QUESTION

Is there a substantial difference in ventilation-perfusion (V/Q) mismatch and oxygenation levels between early and delayed implementation of prone positioning in patients with ARDS?

WHAT IS ALREADY KNOWN?

Acute respiratory distress syndrome begins with an early exudative phase that includes inflammation and damage to the alveolar-capillary barrier, followed by a later phase of fibroblastic growth and organization in the lung tissue.[16] Prone positioning improves oxygenation and survival in early ARDS (exudative phase) by enhancing V/Q distribution and reducing ventilator-induced lung injury (VILI). However, its effects on persistent ARDS (fibroproliferative phase) are not well-studied.[17,18]

STUDY DESIGN

This was a prospective observational study conducted from June 30, 2021 to October 1, 2022, at Zhongda Hospital, Southeast University.

POPULATION STUDIED INCLUDING DEMOGRAPHICS

Fifty-seven adult patients with moderate-to-severe ARDS were included. The study population consisted of 33 patients with early ARDS (≤7 days) and 24 with persistent ARDS (>7 days). The average age was around 71 years, with a majority being male (64.9%).

INTERVENTION STUDIED

The studied intervention involved the use of prone positioning therapy in patients with both early stages and persistent forms of ARDS.

COMPARATOR USED

The comparator was the supine position, with measurements taken before and 12 hours after the first prone session.

OUTCOMES EVALUATED

- *Primary outcome:* Change in V/Q distribution between supine and prone positions in early versus persistent ARDS.
- *Secondary outcomes:* Changes in shunt, dead space, oxygenation (PaO_2/FiO_2), respiratory mechanics, and hemodynamic variables.

AUTHORS' VIEWPOINT

The authors concluded that prone positioning significantly reduces V/Q mismatch and improves oxygenation in early ARDS but has limited benefits and may increase V/Q mismatch in persistent ARDS.[19] They emphasize the importance of early intervention.

STRENGTH OF THE STUDY

The study provides valuable insights into the timing of prone positioning and its differential effects on early versus persistent ARDS, using real-time monitoring with electrical impedance tomography (EIT).

DRAWBACKS OF THE STUDY

- Electrical impedance tomography does not provide whole lung images.
- Lack of esophageal pressure data
- Did not directly assess hemodynamic effects
- The study's findings are based on a single-center cohort, which may limit generalizability.

REVIEWERS' VIEWPOINT

The study is well-conducted and gives valuable information about the timing of prone positioning in ARDS. Prone positioning improves oxygenation in early ARDS. As a result, it should be adopted early in the ARDS management process. The study points out that, while proning may not improve oxygenation in persistent ARDS, its overall effect on mortality warrants additional investigation. However, the limitations, such as the lack of total lung imaging and hemodynamic evaluation, should be addressed in future studies.

IMPACT ON CURRENT PRACTICE AND TAKE-HOME MESSAGE

Prone positioning should be initiated early in the course of ARDS for optimal benefits. The study highlights the limited effect of proning on oxygenation in persistent ARDS, suggesting the need for early intervention to improve outcomes.

Combined Lung and Diaphragm Ultrasound Predicts Extubation Outcomes in ARDS: A Prospective Study

Liu Y, Zhou Y, Liu P, Ying W, Wu H, Dong Z. Combined lung and diaphragm ultrasound predicts extubation outcomes in ARDS: a prospective study.

Eur J Med Res. 2024;29:510.

CLINICAL QUESTION OR PROBLEM

Can the combination of lung ultrasound and diaphragmatic ultrasound predict extubation outcomes in patients with ARDS who are mechanically ventilated?

WHAT IS ALREADY KNOWN?

Mechanical ventilation is crucial for managing ARDS, but it can lead to complications, including difficult extubation in 10–20% of patients, which in turn correlates with increased mortality. Diaphragmatic dysfunction is common among these patients due to factors such as mechanical ventilation, sedation, and systemic inflammatory responses, further complicating their respiratory mechanics.[20] Lung ultrasound has been effectively used to evaluate lung aeration and can distinguish ARDS morphologies through the lung ultrasound score (LUS). Additionally, diaphragmatic function can be assessed using ultrasound metrics such as diaphragmatic displacement (DD), diaphragm thickening fraction (DTF), and the diaphragmatic-rapid shallow breathing index (D-RSBI). Despite the individual effectiveness of these techniques, there is limited research on their combined application to predict extubation outcomes in mechanically ventilated ARDS patients.

STUDY DESIGN

This was a prospective cohort study conducted from January 2019 to December 2022.

POPULATION STUDIED INCLUDING DEMOGRAPHICS

The study included 132 ARDS patients ready for extubation, admitted to the ICU of Ningbo Medical Center LiHuiLi Hospital. The median age was 66.5 years, with 73.48% male and 26.52% female participants.

INTERVENTION STUDIED

The intervention studied involves the *combined use of lung ultrasound and diaphragmatic ultrasound* to assess and predict extubation outcomes in mechanically ventilated patients with ARDS. Lung ultrasound evaluates lung aeration and classifies ARDS morphology using a scoring system, while diaphragmatic ultrasound measures DD, diaphragm thickening fraction (DTF), and the diaphragmatic–rapid shallow breathing index (D-RSBI) to assess diaphragm function. These ultrasound assessments are conducted at the end of a spontaneous breathing trial (SBT) before extubation. The primary outcome measured is *extubation success*, defined as sustained spontaneous breathing for >48 hours postextubation without mechanical ventilation

COMPARATOR USED

The study compared the predictive performance of single ultrasound indicators (LUS, DD, DTF, D-RSBI) and their combinations.

OUTCOMES EVALUATED

The primary outcome was extubation success, defined as sustained spontaneous breathing for >48 hours postextubation without mechanical ventilation. Secondary outcomes included ICU stay length, hospital stay length, reintubation rate, ICU mortality, and hospital mortality.

AUTHORS' VIEWPOINT

The authors highlight the effectiveness of combining LUS and diaphragmatic ultrasound (D-RSBI) to enhance the prediction of extubation outcomes in mechanically ventilated patients with ARDS. They found that this combination provides greater predictive accuracy than using single indicators alone, emphasizing that both lung aeration and diaphragmatic function are critical for successful extubation. The study suggests that the multifactorial nature of extubation success requires a comprehensive assessment of respiratory mechanics.[21] Ultimately, they believe that this combined ultrasound approach can aid clinicians in making informed decisions about extubation and adjusting treatment strategies effectively.[22]

STRENGTH OF THE STUDY

The strength of this study lies in several key areas:

- *Comprehensive evaluation:* The study evaluates both lung aeration and diaphragm function using ultrasound, providing a more holistic view of the factors influencing extubation outcomes in ARDS patients.
- *Combination of indicators:* By combining LUS and D-RSBI, the study enhances the accuracy of predicting extubation success, offering a more reliable tool for clinicians.
- *Quantitative analysis:* The use of specific cut-off values and statistical measures such as AUC and calibration adds robustness to the study's conclusions.

DRAWBACKS OF THE STUDY

Limitations include the single-center design, potential selection bias, and the exclusion of patients with severe chronic organ dysfunction, previous diaphragmatic paralysis, diaphragmatic hernia, pregnancy, and children. The study's findings may not be generalizable to all ICU settings and patient populations.

REVIEWERS' VIEWPOINT

The study on combining LUS and D-RSBI to predict extubation outcomes in ARDS patients is notable for its innovative approach and clinical relevance. It provides a practical tool for clinicians, backed by robust methodology, including LogReg and ROC curves. The study acknowledges limitations such as the need for further validation in diverse patient populations and potential operator-dependent variability in ultrasound measurements. Future research areas highlighted include larger, multi-center studies to validate the findings and improve generalizability. Overall, the study significantly contributes to the field with its comprehensive and insightful approach.

IMPACT ON CURRENT PRACTICE AND TAKE-HOME MESSAGE

The study suggests that combining LUS and D-RSBI can improve the accuracy of predicting extubation success in ARDS patients. This combined approach could help clinicians make more informed extubation decisions, potentially reducing extubation failure rates and improving patient outcomes.

REFERENCES

1. Saud Z, Ponsford M, Bentley K, Cole JM, Pandey M, Jolles S, et al. Mechanically ventilated patients shed high-titer live severe acute respiratory syndrome Coronavirus 2 (SARS-CoV-2) for extended periods from both the upper and lower respiratory tract. Clin Infect Dis. 2022;75(1):e82-8.
2. Bennett-Guerrero E, Romeiser JL, Talbot LR, Ahmed T, Mamone LJ, Singh SM, et al. Severe Acute Respiratory Syndrome Coronavirus 2 Convalescent Plasma Versus Standard Plasma in Coronavirus Disease 2019 Infected Hospitalized Patients in New York: A Double-Blind Randomized Trial. Crit Care Med. 2021;49(7):1015-25.
3. Lucas C, Klein J, Sundaram ME, Liu F, Wong P, Silva J, et al. Delayed production of neutralizing antibodies correlates with fatal COVID-19. Nat Med. 2021;27:1178-86.
4. Bandopadhyay P, D'Rozario R, Lahiri A, Sarif J, Ray Y, Paul SR, et al. Nature and dimensions of systemic hyperinflammation and its attenuation by convalescent plasma in severe COVID-19. J Infect Dis. 2021;224:565-74.
5. Oliaei S, Seyed Alinaghi S, Mehrtak M, Karimi A, Noori T, Mirzapour P, et al. The effects of hyperbaric oxygen therapy (HBOT) on coronavirus disease-2019 (COVID-19): a systematic review. Eur J Med Res. 2021;26:96.
6. Harch PG. Hyperbaric oxygen treatment of novel coronavirus (COVID-19) respiratory failure. Med Gas Res. 2020;10(2):61-2.
7. Gorenstein SA, Castellano ML, Slone ES, Gillette B, Liu H, Alsamarraie C, et al. Hyperbaric oxygen therapy for COVID-19 patients with respiratory distress: treated cases versus propensity-matched controls. Undersea Hyperb Med. 2020;47(3):405-13.
8. Grasselli G, Calfee CS, Camporota L, Poole D, Amato MBP, Antonelli M, et al. ESICM guidelines on acute respiratory distress syndrome: Definition, phenotyping and respiratory support strategies. Intensiv Care Med. 2023;49:727-59.
9. Matthay MA, Arabi Y, Arroliga AC, Bernard G, Bersten AD, Brochard LJ, et al. A New Global Definition of Acute Respiratory Distress Syndrome. Am J Respir Crit Care Med. 2023;209:37-47.
10. Constantin J-M, Jabaudon M, Lefrant J-Y, Jaber S, Quenot J-P, Langeron O, et al. Personalised mechanical ventilation tailored to lung morphology versus low positive end-expiratory pressure for patients with acute respiratory distress syndrome in France (the LIVE study): A multicentre, single-blind, randomised controlled trial. Lancet Respir Med. 2019;7:870-80.
11. Mongodi S, Santangelo E, Bouhemad B, Vaschetto R, Mojoli F. Personalised mechanical ventilation in acute respiratory distress syndrome: The right idea with the wrong tools? Lancet Respir Med. 2019;7:e38.
12. Dianti J, Fard S, Wong J, Chan TCY, Del Sorbo L, Fan E, et al. Strategies for lung- and diaphragm-protective ventilation in acute hypoxemic respiratory failure: a physiological trial. Crit Care Lond Engl. 2022;26:259.
13. Goligher EC, Dres M, Patel BK, Sahetya SK, Beitler JR, Telias I, et al. Lung- and diaphragm-protective ventilation. Am J Respir Crit Care Med. 2020;202:950-61.
14. Papazian L, Forel J-M, Gacouin A, Penot-Ragon C, Perrin G, Loundou A, et al. Neuromuscular blockers in early acute respiratory distress syndrome. N Engl J Med. 2010;363:1107-16.
15. Moss M, Ulysse CA, Angus DC; National Heart, Lung, and Blood Institute PETAL Clinical Trials Network. Early neuromuscular blockade in the acute respiratory distress syndrome. Reply. N Engl J Med. 2019;381:787-8.
16. Gattinoni L, Tonetti T, Quintel M. Regional physiology of ARDS. Crit Care. 2017;21(Suppl 3):312.
17. Guérin C, Reignier J, Richard JC. Prone positioning in the acute respiratory distress syndrome. N Engl J Med. 2013;369(10):980-1.
18. Henderson AC, Sá RC, Theilmann RJ, Buxton RB, Prisk GK, Hopkins SR. The gravitational distribution of ventilation-perfusion ratio is more uniform in prone than supine posture in the normal human lung. J Appl Physiol (1985). 2013;115(3):313-24.

19. Xin Y, Martin K, Morais CCA, Delvecchio P, Gerard SE, Hamedani H, et al. Diminishing Efficacy of Prone Positioning with Late Application in Evolving Lung Injury. Crit Care Med. 2021;49(10):e1015-24.
20. Goligher EC, Jonkman AH, Dianti J, Vaporidi K, Beitler JR, Patel BK, et al. Clinical strategies for implementing lung and diaphragm-protective ventilation: avoiding insufficient and excessive effort. Intensive Care Med. 2020;46(12):2314-26.
21. Schmidt GA, Girard TD, Kress JP, Morris PE, Ouellette DR, Alhazzani W, et al.; ATS/CHEST Ad Hoc Committee on Liberation from Mechanical Ventilation in Adults. Official Executive Summary of an American Thoracic Society/American College of Chest Physicians Clinical Practice Guideline: Liberation from Mechanical Ventilation in Critically Ill Adults. Am J Respir Crit Care Med. 2017;195(1):115-9.
22. Ji L, Cao C, Gao Y, Zhang W, Xie Y, Duan Y, et al. Prognostic value of bedside lung ultrasound score in patients with COVID-19. Crit Care. 2020;24:700.

SECTION

3

Neurocritical Care

Section Editor: *Sivakumar MN*

Associate Editor: *Lakshmikanth Charan S*

Desmopressin for Patients with Spontaneous Intracerebral Haemorrhage Taking Antiplatelet Drugs (DASH): a UK-based, Phase 2, Randomised, Placebo-controlled, Multicentre Feasibility Trial

Desborough MJR, Al-Shahi Salman R, Stanworth SJ, Havard D, Woodhouse LJ, Craig J, et al. Desmopressin for patients with spontaneous intracerebral haemorrhage taking antiplatelet drugs (DASH): a UK-based, phase 2, randomised, placebo-controlled, multicentre feasibility trial.

***Lancet Neurol.* 2023;22(7):557-67.**

CLINICAL QUESTION OR PROBLEM

To recruit patients taking antiplatelets who develop intracerebral hemorrhage, give them desmopressin, and follow them up for 3 months to see if it reduces mortality or disability.

WHAT IS ALREADY KNOWN?

- Intracerebral hemorrhage is a medical emergency, caused by a blood vessel bleeding directly into the brain. Outcome is directly related to the amount of bleeding that occurs. Many patients die early and others are left with significant disability.
- A quarter of all people with intracerebral hemorrhage are taking an antiplatelet drug, which is associated with larger volumes of brain hemorrhage and significantly worse outcomes. 4–5 million people are taking antiplatelet drugs in the UK and use continues to rise in an aging population. Despite advances in treatment of ischemic stroke, there is no effective drug treatment for intracerebral hemorrhage.
- Desmopressin is a drug that reverses blood thinning effects of antiplatelet drugs, by indirectly increasing platelet adhesion, which we hypothesize will minimize the devastating consequences of intracerebral hemorrhage.
- Desmopressin is commonly used in patients with inherited platelet dysfunction disorders and is an appealing treatment for antiplatelet-associated intracerebral hemorrhage.
- Desmopressin is affordable, available and could be implemented clinically across the UK and worldwide in the next 5 years with immediate benefit for stroke patients, their families and society.

- There are no randomized trials comparing desmopressin with placebo for reversing antiplatelet drug effects in spontaneous intracerebral hemorrhage.

STUDY DESIGN

- It is a Phase 2, multicenter, randomized, and placebo-controlled feasibility study.
- Patients who were 18 years of age or older, using an antiplatelet medication, and having an intracerebral hemorrhage with stroke symptoms within 24 hours after randomization were eligible to be recruited from 10 acute stroke centers in the United Kingdom.
- Participants were assigned to receive a placebo or a single intravenous dose of desmopressin (20 μg) at random (1:1).
- All study participants, including staff and patients, were blinded about treatment allocation.

POPULATION STUDIED INCLUDING DEMOGRAPHICS

Inclusion Criteria

- Adult (aged ≥18 years),
- With intracerebral hemorrhage confirmed on brain CT, and
- Prescribed and thought to be taking a daily oral antiplatelet drug in the preceding 7 days (i.e., cyclooxygenase inhibitors, phosphodiesterase inhibitors, or $P2Y_{12}$ inhibitors).

Exclusion Criteria

- Known secondary causes of intracerebral hemorrhage,
- Patients at risk of fluid retention,
- Systolic blood pressure of <90 mm Hg,
- Known drug-eluting stent in previous 3 months,
- Allergy to desmopressin,
- Pregnant or breastfeeding,
- Life expectancy of <4 hours or planned for palliative care only,
- Glasgow Coma Scale score of <5, and
- Modified Rankin Scale score of >4.

OUTCOMES EVALUATED

- Analysis was done by intention to treat, and the primary outcome was feasibility, which was determined by the proportion of eligible patients approached and the number of eligible patients randomly assigned.
- The research revealed that,
  - Patients and their relatives were happy to take part
  - Desmopressin was simple to give
  - There were no safety concerns
  - Follow-up was completed for all patients at 3 months

AUTHORS' VIEWPOINT

- Given sufficient recruiting centers and pragmatic trial methodology, it should be feasible to conduct a definitive trial to determine if desmopressin improves outcomes in patients on antiplatelet drug therapy with intracerebral hemorrhage. Although this trial could be delivered as a standalone study, it might be more efficient as part of a platform trial or to embed in an existing intracerebral hemorrhage trial.
- Given the high mortality and morbidity after intracerebral hemorrhage in patients exposed to antiplatelet drugs, and the increased frequency of patients taking antiplatelet drugs, even a small reduction in morbidity or mortality could reduce the risk of death and leave tens of thousands of patients free from disability.

STRENGTH OF THE STUDY

- Antiplatelet-induced spontaneous intracerebral hemorrhage has a significant global mortality and morbidity burden, and treatment guidelines are not universally agreed upon. Therefore, the study is extremely important.

- It offers randomized data on desmopressin usage in cases of acute intracerebral hemorrhage.
- The trial's methodology was precise, and it was shown that the strategy being studied was feasible.

DRAWBACK OF THE STUDY

- The coronavirus disease-2019 (COVID-19) pandemic caused recruitment to be halted halfway through the experiment, and recruitment rates never recovered to their pre-pandemic levels. One significant change that had a significant impact on the trial's capacity to meet its goals and exceed the recruitment target was the extended recruiting period linked to the funding extensions.
- Although the hazards of unmasking were reduced by completely blinding treatment allocation from physicians, patients, and outcome assessors, the placebo was not identical to desmopressin.
- Additionally, data supplied by each study site was included in the screening logs; the central research team was unable to validate this data because they were collected locally.
- Since arriving after hours or >24 hours after the beginning of symptoms was one of the most frequent grounds for patient exclusion, the results of this research may not be typical of all patients.
- Future trials should shorten the period between imaging confirmation of intracerebral hemorrhage and desmopressin or placebo administration by streamlining trial procedures.
- The results were skewed because all six patients receiving dual antiplatelet medication were randomly assigned to placebo.
- Minimization of other prognostic markers, such as baseline stroke severity and dual antiplatelet medication, should be taken into account in a big definitive trial.

REVIEWERS' VIEWPOINT

Currently available guidelines from the different societies on use of desmopressin for patients on antiplatelet drugs with intracerebral hemorrhage are as follows:

- The Neurocritical Care Society and Society of Critical Care Medicine recommend a single dose of 0·4 μg/kg desmopressin for patients with intracranial hemorrhage who were exposed to antiplatelet agents[1] and planned for neurosurgical procedure. These guidelines recommend that desmopressin can be used in addition to platelet transfusion.
- The American Heart Association and American Stroke Association advise that further studies are necessary to determine if there is a subgroup of patients taking antiplatelet drugs with intracerebral hemorrhage who might benefit from desmopressin.[2]
- The Intercollegiate Stroke Working Party of the Royal College of Physicians guidelines[3] and British Society for Haematology guidelines[4] make no recommendations.

Thus, there is no consensus among the different societies and hence there is a definite need for a good trial. This is the first randomized trial in patients with intracerebral hemorrhage who are taking antiplatelet drugs comparing desmopressin with placebo.

There were no safety concerns or clinically relevant hyponatremia in the study group.

IMPACT ON CURRENT PRACTICE AND TAKE-HOME MESSAGE

- For a feasibility study, this study has done justice in its good methodology and study design.
- The findings of this study support the need for a definitive, large-scale trial to determine if desmopressin could improve outcomes in patients with intracerebral hemorrhage on antiplatelet drug therapy.

Blood Pressure Management after Endovascular Therapy for Acute Ischemic Stroke: The BEST-II Randomized Clinical Trial

Mistry EA, Hart KW, Davis LT, Gao Y, Prestigiacomo CJ, Mittal S, et al. Blood pressure management after endovascular therapy for acute ischemic stroke: The BEST-II randomized clinical trial.

JAMA*. *2023;330(9):821-31.

CLINICAL QUESTION OR PROBLEM

- Are moderately low systolic blood pressure (SBP) targets (<140 and <160 mm Hg) after successful endovascular stroke treatment harmful?
- In other words, will patients in whom systolic blood pressure targets were lowered for 24 hours post-endovascular therapy in an acute ischemic stroke, have a higher volume of stroke size at 36 hours and a higher disability at 90 days.
- The objective is to determine the futility of lower SBP targets after endovascular therapy (<140 mm Hg or 160 mm Hg) compared with a higher target (≤180 mm Hg).

WHAT IS ALREADY KNOWN?

- Endovascular therapy has changed the landscape in acute stroke treatment and patients do drastically better when they receive endovascular treatment in appropriate time window.
- Despite the enormous effectiveness of endovascular treatment, about 50% of patients remain disabled or die at 90 days.
- The current American Heart Association/ American Stroke Association and European Stroke Organization guidelines recommend targeting systolic blood pressure (SBP) of 180 mm Hg or less after endovascular therapy based on prior thrombolysis trials.[5,6]
- Although higher systemic SBP is common in the setting of acute ischemic stroke due to cerebral autoregulation, observational studies have indicated that lower SBP after successful endovascular therapy may be associated with better functional outcomes.[7,8]
- A prospective multisite observational study identified that a maximal SBP of approximately 160 mm Hg in the first 24 hours after endovascular therapy delineated patients with good and poor functional outcomes.[9]
- Others showed that moderate SBP levels of between 140 and 160 mm Hg were associated with better patient outcomes.[10]
- However, a recent randomized trial among Chinese patients who had undergone successful endovascular therapy found that SBP lowered to <120 mm Hg was harmful.[11]
- In a 2017 survey of clinical practice, among 58 US sites, 69% of institutions

practiced moderate SBP lowering and only 5% of institutions practiced extreme SBP lowering to <120 mm Hg for patients successfully treated with endovascular therapy.[12]

STUDY DESIGN

- Randomized
- Open-label
- Blinded end point
- Phase 2
- Futility clinical trial

POPULATION STUDIED INCLUDING DEMOGRAPHICS

Study enrolled 120 patients (average age, 70 years; 57% female) who had an acute ischemic stroke and successful endovascular treatment at one of three urban comprehensive stroke centers (Vanderbilt University Medical Center in Nashville, Tennessee; University of Cincinnati in Cincinnati, Ohio; and Hartford Health Medical Center in Hartford, Connecticut) between January 2020 and February 2022.

The inclusion criteria:

- Adult patients (≥18 years)
- With ischemic stroke
- Who had undergone successful endovascular therapy (defined as modified thrombolysis in cerebral ischemia, ≥2b-50–89% reperfusion; 2c-90–99% reperfusion; and 3-complete reperfusion)
- For an occlusion in an anterior cerebral circulation large vessel (specifically, internal carotid artery and M1 or M2 segments of the middle cerebral artery).

The exclusion criteria:

- A diagnosis of heart failure with ejection fraction <30%;
- On left ventricular assist device; or
- On extra corporeal membrane oxygenation
- Pregnant individuals and
- Patients enrolled in other clinical trials were excluded.

A total of 40 patients were randomly assigned to have their systolic blood pressure lowered to a target of ≤180 mm Hg, 40 patients were assigned to a systolic blood pressure target of <160 mm Hg, and 40 patients were targeted to reach a systolic blood pressure of <140 mm Hg. Patients were treated with nicardipine, an antihypertensive medication administered intravenously, started within 1 hour after endovascular treatment and given for 24 hours if their systolic blood pressure was above the target they were assigned.

It was assessed whether lowering BP causes harm to brain (particularly vulnerable during the 24 hours after a stroke) and to assess disability 90 days later.

OUTCOMES EVALUATED

- The main outcomes of the study were the size of stroke at 36 hours and degree of disability at 90 days. The study did not find significant evidence of an unequivocal harm due to lower blood pressure targets in terms of worsening size of stroke or increasing disability. But the trends indicated that there may be only marginal benefit on long-term disability by lowering blood pressure after endovascular treatment. In fact, there was an indication that lowering the blood pressure after thrombectomy may worsen patients' long-term disability.
    - In ≤180 mm Hg target group, average systolic blood pressure reached 129 mm Hg.
    - In <160 mm Hg target group, average systolic blood pressure reached 130 mm Hg.
    - In <140 mm Hg target group, systolic blood pressure lowered to an average of 123 mm Hg.

- The mean follow-up infarct volume was:
  - 32.4 mL (95% CI, 18.0–46.7 mL) for the <140-mm Hg group,
  - 50.7 mL (95% CI, 33.7–67.7 mL), for the <160-mm Hg group, and
  - 46.4 mL (95% CI, 24.5–68.2 mL) for the 180-mm Hg or less group
  - Average 36-hour stroke volumes showed no conclusive evidence of harm.
- The mean utility-weighted Modified Rankin Score (mRS) was:
  - 0.51 (95% CI, 0.38–0.63) for the <140-mm Hg group,
  - 0.47 (95% CI, 0.35–0.60) for the <160-mm Hg group, and
  - 0.58 (95% CI, 0.46–0.71) for the high-target group
  - In the 90-day disability outcome, there was only a slight indication of harm.

AUTHORS' VIEWPOINT

Lower SBP targets of 140 mm Hg or 160 mm Hg following successful endovascular therapy did not meet predetermined criteria for futility as compared to an SBP target of 180 mm Hg or less in patients who had an acute ischemic stroke. However, the results indicated that, if attempted in a larger study in the future, there would be a small probability of benefit from reduced SBP targets following endovascular therapy.

STRENGTH OF THE STUDY

Robust methodology for a futility trial

The trial advances the knowledge regarding the feasibility of achieving SBP targets.

DRAWBACK OF THE STUDY

- The study is limited by enrollment at only three centers and a small sample size.
- Nicardipine was used as the first-line treatment for the majority of enrolled patients. Although nicardipine is commonly used in neurointensive care units within the US, it may not be readily available globally.
- Some baseline characteristics differed among groups. These may impact the generalizability of the results.
- Though the target SBP in the three groups were fixed (140, 160, and 180 mm Hg), the average SBP found to be reached in all the groups were between 120 and 130 mm Hg which was not the intended methodology to find out the difference between the groups.

REVIEWERS' VIEWPOINT

According to this study, patients' blood pressure should be allowed to autoregulate after endovascular treatment unless it is >180 mm Hg. However, physicians should exercise caution while aggressively lowering a patient's blood pressure because there may be chances of further worsening. Individualized decision-making is necessary in certain situations, such as when there are additional medical reasons for reducing blood pressure or when there are high possibilities of hemorrhagic transformation.

IMPACT ON CURRENT PRACTICE AND TAKE-HOME MESSAGE

If investigated in a bigger trial in the future it is thought that the results indicated that there was low probability of benefit from lower SBP objectives.

Still the criteria for futility were not met by lower SBP targets following effective endovascular therapy for acute ischemic stroke.

As of now based on the current available evidence including this trial it is better to maintain systolic BP <180 mm Hg and not aim for a further lower threshold.

Effectiveness of Lumbar Cerebrospinal Fluid Drain among Patients with Aneurysmal Subarachnoid Hemorrhage: A Randomized Clinical Trial

Wolf S, Mielke D, Barner C, Malinova V, Kerz T, Wostrack M, et al. Effectiveness of lumbar cerebrospinal fluid drain among patients with aneurysmal subarachnoid hemorrhage: A randomized clinical trial.

JAMA Neurol. 2023;80(8):833-42.

CLINICAL QUESTION OR PROBLEM

In patients with aneurysmal subarachnoid hemorrhage (aSAH), does lumbar cerebrospinal fluid (CSF) drainage compared to standard therapy improve clinical outcomes as measured by the modified Rankin Scale (mRS) score at 6 months?

WHAT IS ALREADY KNOWN?

- Aneurysmal subarachnoid hemorrhage frequently leads to death or permanent disability due to both the initial insult and delayed cerebral ischemia (DCI).
- Delayed cerebral ischemia occurs predominantly due to vasospasm in patients with SAH may be related to blood degradation products in the CSF near the basal cisterns.
- Cerebrospinal fluid drainage via a lumbar drain may preferentially remove more of the blood degradation products due the effect of gravity and thus may decrease rates of vasospasm and DCI is a hypothesis.
- Retrospective data and meta-analyses of lumbar drain use in aSAH have demonstrated lower mortality, and reduced rates of clinical vasospasm, ischemic stroke and improved neurological outcomes[13,14]

LUMAS, a prospective single center RCT, including patients with aSAH [World Federation of Neurosurgical Societies (WFNS) grade 1–3], demonstrated reduced rates of delayed ischemia and better early neurological outcome but without difference in outcome at 6 months.[15]

STUDY DESIGN

- Parallel group, multi-center, open label randomized clinical trial
- Randomization – 1:1 to standard care or additional use of lumbar drain
  - Via internet randomizer – permutated blocks of 6
  - No stratification
- Blinded end-point evaluation
- Patients followed up to their death or 6 months post randomization
- Intention to treat analysis
- Protocol and analysis plan published prior
- Power calculation:
  - 300 patients would be required to detect a decrease in unfavorable outcome from 50 to 33% with 85% power and 5% α error
- 19 hospitals in Germany, Switzerland, and Canada
  - All provided 24 hours acute neurosurgical and neurocritical care with >30 aneurysm procedures/year
- Data collected from Jan 2011 to Jan 2016
- *Inclusion:*
  - ≥18 years, acute SAH with confirmed aneurysm origin via CT-angiography or DSA
  - Aneurysm treatment within 48 hours of SAH

- *Exclusion:*
    - Presence of therapeutic anticoagulation
    - Contraindications for lumbar drain
    - Absent or compressed basal cisterns on admission CT-brain
    - Pregnancy
    - Reduced life expectancy
    - Participation in another interventional trial
    - Hemorrhage from non-aneurysmal origin
    - No hemorrhage present on initial CT-B (Fischer 1/modified Fischer grade 0)
- 307 patients randomized:
    - Lumbar drain >155 randomized (11 excluded)
    - Standard care >152 randomized (9 excluded)
- Baseline characteristics of lumbar drain versus standard care:
    - Similar between groups
    - *Median age:* 54 versus 56 years
    - *Female:* 68% versus 69%
    - *mRS score of 0 on admission:* 94 versus 93%
    - *Presence of intraventricular hemorrhage (IVH):* 63% versus 59%
    - *Presence of intracerebral hemorrhage (ICH):* 39% versus 35%
    - The World Federation of Neurosurgical Societies classification:
        - 1 = 37% versus 29%
        - 2 = 15% versus 15%
        - 3 = 5% versus 7%
        - 4 = 10% versus 11%
        - 5 = 33% versus 39%
    - *Modified Fisher score of 4:* 59 versus 55%
    - Location, size, and number of aneurysms similar

Intervention

- Insertion of lumbar drain with drainage of lumbar CSF at 5 mL/hour
- Commenced within 72 hours of aneurysmal SAH in addition to standard therapy
- Continued for least 4 days and up to 8 days
- *Safety:* If intracranial pressure (ICP) pressure >20 mm Hg or >5 mm Hg difference between ICP + lumbar drain - recommended to cease lumbar drainage
- Median CSF lumbar drainage of 108 mL in first 8 days

Control

No lumbar drainage

Management Common to Both Groups

- Treatment of aneurysmal SAH with endovascular coiling or clipping determined by local treating teams
- Local teams determined if external ventricular drain (EVD) or ICP monitor inserted
    - External ventricular drains inserted in 70.8% of lumbar drain group and 76.9% of control group
    - Median daily drainage via EVD lower in lumbar drain group (98 vs. 171 mL)
    - Total CSF drainage via both EVD +/– lumbar drains similar between groups
- *Local standard management for aSAH:*
    - Daily transcranial Doppler monitoring as per local protocol
    - Cerebral vascular imaging via computed tomographic angiography (CTA), magnetic resonance angiography (MRA), or digital subtraction angiography (DSA) for suspected vasospasm or routine day 7–10
    - Treatment for vasospasm at discretion of local investigators—not protocolized
- Rates of aneurysm treatment (53 vs. 50% coiled) and vasospasm prophylaxis (99

vs. 99% nimodipine) use similar between groups

- Mean arterial pressure (MAP), fluid intake, and fever burden similar between groups

OUTCOMES EVALUATED

- *Primary outcome (lumbar drain vs. control):*
  - Rate of unfavorable neurological outcome measured at 6 months (defined as mRS 3–6)
  - *Statistically significant lower rate of unfavorable outcome*
    - 32.6% versus 44.8%
    - RR 0.73 (95% CI: 0.51–0.98; $p = 0.04$)
  - Adjustment for age, severity via Hunt-Hess grade, and presence of ICH and IVH:
    - RR 0.76 (95% CI: 0.54–1.00, $p = 0.047$)
  - Effect consistent across prespecified subgroups (age, sex, grade, Location, IVH/ICH, treatments provided, and center size)
- *Secondary outcomes (lumbar drain vs. control):*
  - *Significant difference in:*
    - Rate of secondary infarction following discharge
      - 28.5% versus 39.9% (RR 0.71, 95% CI: 0.49–0.99, $p = 0.04$)
    - GOS-E 1–4 at 6 months and Barthel Index <80 at 6 months
  - *No significant difference in:*
    - Mortality within 6 months
      - 13.2 versus 17.5%
    - Rate of vasospasm
      - *Clinical:* 29 versus 33%
      - *TCD:* 27 versus 25%
      - *Angiographic:* 46 versus 44%
    - Infection of any cause
      - 39 versus 36%
- *Adverse outcomes*
  - *Lumbar drain group:*
    - One patient developed elevated gradient >5 mm Hg between ICP + lumbar drain prohibiting drainage
    - One patient developed local skin infection—required surgical excision
    - One patient had lumbar drain torn off, requiring surgical removal

AUTHORS' VIEWPOINT

In patients with aSAH, prophylactic lumbar CSF drainage to lessen the burden of secondary cerebral infarction and unfavorable outcome is warranted.

STRENGTH OF THE STUDY

- Pragmatic as study design relies on local standard practice allowing easy translation to routine clinical care
- Meaningful patient-centered outcome
- Functional outcomes determined by blinded evaluators minimizing detection bias
- Included poor grades of aSAH which other trials have not, therefore increasing relevance for neurocritical care population

DRAWBACK OF THE STUDY

- Majority of patients randomized from only two of the centers
  - Possibly lower risk of adverse outcomes if lumbar drains more routinely used at these sites
- Clinicians may alter their "standard" therapy based on unblinded randomization
- Selection bias possible due to limited screening data available
  - Certain patient groups may have been excluded that would have changed outcome (e.g., a patient was excluded for poor grade)

- 35 patients in lumbar drainage group were not treated as per protocol
    - 13 had no drain inserted, 22 had drain inserted but no relevant drainage performed
    - However, no difference in sensitivity analysis (per protocol and as treated)
- Potential for time-lag bias (trial enrolled from 2011 to 2016)
- A significant number of patients in the lumbar drain group did not receive the designated intervention, although the intention-to-treat analysis was consistent even when considering this discrepancy.
- The lack of blinding among patients, their relatives, and acute care clinicians introduced potential bias, though blinded assessments of outcomes tried to mitigate this.
- The study did not collect data on factors such as preexisting hypertension, initial CT scan details regarding clot thickness and blood quantity, or medical complications commonly seen in subarachnoid hemorrhage patients.
- Potential treatments such as clot thrombolysis or subarachnoid space irrigation were not explored, nor did the trial evaluate the benefits of higher drainage rates than the recommended 5 mL per hour, even though some patients exhibited higher lumbar drainage amounts.

REVIEWERS' VIEWPOINT

- In addition to standard care, use of lumbar CSF drainage may improve neurological outcomes in patients with aSAH is the basic hypothesis of the study.
- It was stated that although both groups had similar volumes of cerebrospinal fluid drainage, a striking visual difference was observed in the fluid color between the ventricular and lumbar drains. The lumbar drain's fluid appeared darker and more reddish, indicating a higher concentration of blood and its degradation products. This observation underscores the sedimentation of erythrocytes in the fluid, suggesting that lumbar drainage may be more effective at removing these components.
- But the complications associated with the intervention such as coning and infections are dreadful.
    - Hence, based on this study alone it might be difficult to change the existing practice.

IMPACT ON CURRENT PRACTICE AND TAKE-HOME MESSAGE

- Considering the high-risk nature of the intervention, it is advisable to wait for further studies to confirm the potential benefits of early lumbar drainage in aSAH.

Trial of Early Minimally Invasive Removal of Intracerebral Hemorrhage - ENRICH trial.

Pradilla G, Ratcliff JJ, Hall AJ, Saville BR, Allen JW, Paulon G, et al. Trial of early minimally invasive removal of intracerebral hemorrhage.

N Engl J Med. 2024;390(14):1277-89.

CLINICAL QUESTION OR PROBLEM

In patients with spontaneous intracranial hemorrhage (ICH), does the use of early minimally invasive surgery with standard management compared to standard management alone, result in better functional outcomes at 180 days?

WHAT IS ALREADY KNOWN?

- Spontaneous ICH is a condition with high mortality, poor functional outcomes, and high costs of care.
- The mainstay of standard medical management for ICH has been the reversal of coagulopathy, blood pressure control and best supportive care.
- While showing mortality benefit, surgical intervention with craniectomy (STITCH, STITCH II)[16,17] and minimally invasive techniques (MISTIE III)[18] has failed to show long-term benefits in functional outcomes
- Data from these trials showed a trend toward benefit with early surgical intervention in superficial lesions and with greater clot evacuation
- The ENRICH trial was designed to investigate any benefit of early minimally invasive trans-sulcal parafascicular surgery (MIPS) in superficial ICH.

STUDY DESIGN

- Multi-center, two-arm, randomized, and adaptive design
- 1:1 block randomization stratified by:
  - ICH location (anterior basal ganglia vs. lobar)
  - Index GCS (<9 or ≥9)
- Interim analysis at 150 patients and then in blocks of 25 to determine if early stopping rules are met. If accrual stopped due to futility in one site (anterior basal ganglia or lobar) then this would lead to enrichment for the other site. Pre-specified stopping rules for both futility and success.
- Primary outcome defined as mean differences in utility weighted mRS (H_1: $\Delta > 0$). To demonstrate superiority, a Bayesian model-based posterior probability of MIPS benefit (i.e., $\Delta > 0$) was set to be ≥0.975

Intervention

- Early ICH evacuation (within 24 hours, ideally <8 hours) using MIPS + standard management
  - Standardized surgical approach with training provided
  - Imaging guided
  - BrainPath and Myriad device for minimally invasive technique (manufactured by NICO)
  - Video recording and independent review of surgeries at each site
- Pre-specified futility criteria for basal ganglion hemorrhage met at the interim analysis for 175 patients
  - Following this only lobar hemorrhages enrolled

- Median time from last known well to surgery was 16.8 hours

Control

Standard management alone.

Management Common to Both Groups

Based on AHA/ASA guidelines:

- Aggressive resuscitation
- Blood pressure control
- Correction of bleeding diathesis
- Traditional surgical techniques permitted (EVD, craniectomy, etc.)

POPULATION STUDIED INCLUDING DEMOGRAPHICS

- 37 hospitals in the USA
- December 2016 – August 2022
- 59 treating neurosurgeons
- *Inclusion:*
  - Aged 18–80 years
  - Acute spontaneous, primary ICH with volume of 30–80 mL
  - Intervention within 24 hours of last known well
  - GCS 5–15
  - Previously mRS 0–1 before ICH occurred
- *Exclusion:*
  - Recurrent ICH or other underlying vascular abnormality
  - Primary thalamic or infratentorial intraparenchymal hemorrhage
  - NIHSS <5
  - Intraventricular hemorrhage (IVH) >50% of lateral ventricles
  - Uncorrected coagulopathy or a known clotting disorder
  - Anticoagulants not rapidly revisable or need for anticoagulation within 5 days of index admission
  - Not expected to recover, Do Not Resuscitate (DNR), and life expectancy <6 months
- *300 patients enrolled:*
  - 11,603 assessed for eligibility
  - 10,611 did not meet inclusion criteria/met exclusion criteria
  - 692 excluded with basal ganglion hemorrhage after adaptation of enrollment criteria
- Comparing baseline characteristics of surgery versus control group
  - *Age:* 64 versus 62 years
  - *Female sex:* 48 versus 52%
  - *Median score on NIH stroke scale:* 16 versus 18
  - *Glasgow Coma Scale (GCS) at randomization:*
    - *4 – 8:* 17% versus 19%
    - *9–14:* 83% versus 81%
  - *Median hematoma volume:* 54 versus 55 mL
  - *Intraventricular hemorrhage present:* 43% versus 39%
  - *ICH location:*
    - *Anterior basal ganglia (ABG):* 32% versus 29%
    - Lobar 68% versus 71%
  - *Median ICH score:* 2 versus 2
  - *Median APACHE II score:* 12 versus 12
  - *Medical history:*
    - *Cardiovascular disease (CVD):* 82% versus 78%
    - *Central nervous system (CNS) disease:* 30% versus 28%
    - *Endocrine or renal disorder:* 28% versus 26%
  - *Smoker (current/former):* 45% versus 40%
  - Time from last known well to randomization:
    - *≤8 hours:* 28% versus 25%
    - *≤12 hours:* 49% versus 46%

OUTCOMES EVALUATED

- *Primary outcome:*

    - Mean score on utility weighted modified Rankin scale at 180 days:
        - 0.458 (surgical group) versus 0.374 (control group)
        - Difference of 0.084 (95% Cr I 0.005–0.163) and posterior probability of superiority 0.981
    - This benefit was attributable to ICH in lobar location:
        - *Anterior basal ganglia:* 0.340 (surgery) versus 0.381 (control)
            - Difference of -0.013 (95% Cr I -0.147–0.116)
        - *Lobar:* 0.513 (surgery) versus 0.371 (control)
            - Difference of 0.127 (95% Cr I 0.035–0.219)
    - The benefit for intervention on mRS was seen at discharge/7 days, 30 days, 90 days, and 180 days
- *Secondary and safety outcomes:*
    - Comparing surgery versus control group
    - Significantly greater in surgery group:
        - *Change in hematoma volume:* –43.9 versus 4.0 mL
    - No significant difference in
        - *Score of ≤3 on mRS at 180 days:* 50.3 versus 41.0%
    - Significantly less in surgery group
        - *ICU length of stay:* 6.9 versus 9.7 days
        - *Hospital length of stay:* 14.9 versus 18.1 days
        - *One or more serious adverse events:* 63.3 versus 78.7%
- *Exploratory outcomes:*
    - *Decreased duration of mechanical ventilation in surgery group:* 5.3 versus 8.8 days
    - *Decreased decompressive hemicraniectomy in surgery group:* 3.3 versus 20%

AUTHORS' VIEWPOINT

- Among patients in whom surgery could be performed within 24 hours after an acute ICH, minimally invasive hematoma evacuation resulted in better functional outcomes at 180 days than those with guideline-based medical management.
- The effect of surgery appeared to be attributable to intervention for lobar hemorrhages.

STRENGTH OF THE STUDY

- The rationale for the study was sound, guided by evidence and trends displayed in previous trials
- Primary endpoint of functional outcome—patient-centered and meaningful outcome
- Balanced baseline characteristics for the intervention and control
- Multicenter and randomized
- Minimal loss to follow up (8/300)
- Efforts to minimize bias associated with subjective reporting of mRS by including caregivers in assessment and having blinded review of the assessment by a neuropsychologist.
- Success/safety of surgical intervention in terms of reduction in hematoma volume and low rate of rebleeding
- Statistical analysis plan was pre-published

DRAWBACK OF THE STUDY

- *Single country*
    - Strict exclusion criteria—very specific population in terms of ICH size and location. Exclusion of <30 mL and >80 mL of hematoma volume, thalamic bleed, and intraventricular extension removes substantial number of patients.
    - Recruitment of patients with anterior basal ganglia bleed was stopped due

to futility after relatively few patients have been enrolled, so inferences of potential benefits in these patients are limited.
- High rates of decompressive craniectomy in the control group—this is a procedure that has been shown to increase survival but with high rates of poor functional outcomes.
- Sponsorship by NICO, the manufacture of the devices used in the trial, although no incentives provided, no involvement in data collection, analysis, or trial design.

REVIEWERS' VIEWPOINT

- Previous studies that compared surgical interventions with medical management indicated an increase in survival rates but did not demonstrate improvement in neurological function.
- However, for the first time, ENRICH trial shows that in addition to reducing the risk of further brain damage and death, it also improves neurological function in patients with lobar ICH.
- This approach results in fewer adverse events and diminishes the necessity for emergency brain decompression surgeries.
- Lobar hemorrhage represents a fractionally small population of ICH, the benefit associated with the intervention is functionally important.
- Decisions around surgical intervention should be based on multi-disciplinary discussions with neurosurgical specialists

IMPACT ON CURRENT PRACTICE AND TAKE-HOME MESSAGE

- Rapid minimally invasive evacuation of supratentorial lobar ICH of 30–80 mL, presenting within 24 hours, improves outcomes and lowers the need for prolonged ICU stay and decompressive hemicraniectomy.
- Extrapolating this result to our practice needs further research into availability of these modern techniques and the expertise of our neurosurgeons in it.

Liberal or Restrictive Transfusion Strategy in Patients with Traumatic Brain Injury - HEMOTION trial

Turgeon AF, Fergusson DA, Clayton L, Patton MP, Neveu X, Walsh TS, et al. Liberal or restrictive transfusion strategy in patients with traumatic brain injury.

N Engl J Med. 2024;391(8):722-35.

CLINICAL QUESTION OR PROBLEM

In adult patients with moderate or severe traumatic brain injury (TBI), does a liberal transfusion strategy (transfusion if hemoglobin <10 g/dL) compared to a restrictive strategy (transfusion if hemoglobin <7 g/dL) reduce the rate of an unfavorable Glasgow Outcome Scale—Extended, at 6 months?

WHAT IS ALREADY KNOWN?

- Traumatic brain injury accounts for the most number of trauma-related deaths and has a high rate of morbidity in survivors.

- The optimal hemoglobin target in patients following TBI is unknown. A systematic review and meta-analysis of the available evidence did not find an optimal target of transfusion threshold[19]
- The TRICC trial suggested a restrictive transfusion practice was superior to a liberal strategy; however, this trial was published 15 years ago and was in the era where transfused blood was not leukodepleted. There were only small numbers of TBI patients included in the cohort.[20]
- The injured brain is vulnerable to hypoxia and anemia may exacerbate this state worsening the secondary injury.

STUDY DESIGN

- Patients were randomized 1:1 to a liberal or restrictive strategy.
- Allocation concealment and variable permuted blocks, stratified to center.
- The treating clinicians were unblinded, but the follow-up assessors were blinded.
- The transfusion target was maintained until discharge from ICU.
- An independent data and safety monitoring committee reviewed data after each 25% increment of the target enrollment. It also evaluated the results of a protocol-specified formal interim analysis that was performed when enrollment was at 50% of the target.
- Consent was obtained from the next of kin or deferred when appropriate.
- Intention to treat analysis was performed.

POPULATION STUDIED INCLUDING DEMOGRAPHICS

- A total of 34 centers in Canada, UK, France, and Brazil were included.
- Patients were randomized between September 2017 and April 2023.
- A sample size of 712 patients provided 80% power to detect an absolute difference between groups of 10% for the primary outcome.
- *Inclusion:* Adult patients with moderate or severe TBI (GCS 3–12) with anemia (Hb <10 g/dL).
  - *Exclusion:*
    - Patients who had received transfusion before randomization
    - Contraindication to transfusion or active bleeding
    - Patients who were brain dead or GCS 3 with fixed pupils
- A total of 6,188 patients were assessed for eligibility with 742 randomized. Two of these were randomized in error (had SAH) and four withdrew consent. This left 736 patients with the intention to treat analysis.
- *Baseline characteristics*
  - A total of 72.7% of patients were men, the mean age was 48.7 ± 18.9 years (+/– SD), and 73.2% had a severe TBI (GCS <8)
  - The mean injury severity score was 30.
  - Patients were assessed for chance of poor outcome using prognostic variables of the TBI-IMPACT calculator.
  - There were some imbalances between groups.

    In the restrictive-strategy group there were more:
    - Women (30% vs. 24%)
    - Patients with a GCS motor score of 1 (32.7% vs. 26%)
    - Patients with no pupillary reactivity (14.1% vs. 12.4%)
    - Patients who had an episode of hypotension (28.8% vs. 22.7%)

In the liberal-strategy group there were more:
- Episodes of low cerebral perfusion pressure (22.1% vs. 17.3%)
- Patients with a Marshall score of V or VI (indicating any lesion that was surgically evacuated or a mass lesion of >25 mL, respectively) (37.1% vs. 33.2%)
- Patients with a GCS motor score of 6 (7.9% vs. 5.4%)

- *Intervention:*
  - Liberal transfusion group
    - A total of 369 patients were analyzed in this group. Transfusion was triggered by a hemoglobin level of ≤10 g/dL
    - A total of 98.9% of patients received at least 1 unit of packed cells with the median hemoglobin being 10.8 g/dL
- *Control:*
  - Restrictive transfusion group
    - A total of 367 patients were analyzed in this group. Transfusion was triggered by a hemoglobin level of ≤7 g/dL.
    - A total of 38.4% of patients received at least 1 unit of packed cells with the median hemoglobin being 8.8 g/L
- *Management common to both groups:*
  - Transfusion was initiated within 3 hours of the trigger hemoglobin level
  - 1 unit of leukodepleted packed cells were administered at a time
  - Most patients had ICP monitoring
  - Few patients had CBO2 monitoring and decompressive craniectomy

OUTCOMES EVALUATED

- *Primary outcome:*
  - Glasgow Outcome Scale-Extended (GOS-E) score at 6 months was <4 (unfavorable) in 68.4% in the liberal-strategy group and 73.5% in the restrictive-strategy group
  - Adjusted absolute difference, restrictive strategy versus liberal strategy, 5.4 percentage points; (95% CI, –2.9–13.7)
  - Findings were consistent across subgroups and also with the worst, intermediate, and best predicted prognoses
- *Secondary outcomes:*
  - Comparing liberal versus restrictive group
    - No significant difference in death in ICU (17.1% vs. 15.3%), death in hospital (23% vs. 21.5%), and death at 6 months (26.8% vs. 26.3%)
    - No significant difference in functional independence measure or other measures of functional outcome
- *Tertiary outcomes:*
  - Median (IQR) number of red-cell units transfused was 3 (2–5) in the liberal group and 0 (0–1) in the restrictive group
- *Safety:*
  - Six patients in the liberal group and one in the restrictive group had a mild reaction to transfusion
  - Venous thrombo embolism incidence was the same in each group

AUTHORS' VIEWPOINT

In critically ill patients with TBI and anemia, a liberal transfusion strategy did not reduce the risk of an unfavorable neurologic outcome at 6 months.

STRENGTH OF THE STUDY

- Allocation concealment, intention to treat analysis, minimal loss to follow-up.
- Multicenter study in various countries gives the study good external validity.
- There was a clear separation between the groups with median daily hemoglobin levels.

- Although the bedside clinicians were unblinded, the outcome assessors of functional status were unaware of the allocation.

DRAWBACK OF THE STUDY

- The trial was powered to detect a 10% difference in unfavorable outcome.
- The result showed a 5.4% difference which may be clinically significant.
- There were baseline differences between the two groups.
- It is shown that there may be up to 13.7% absolute reduction in risk of an unfavorable outcome with a liberal transfusion strategy which looks significant.
- The statistical analysis has taken a frequentist approach. The authors are also planning a Bayesian Analysis which is pending.

REVIEWERS' VIEWPOINT

- Modern ICU practice has erred on the side of restrictive transfusion strategies based mainly on the TRICC study which was published in the age of non-leukodepleted blood component therapy. In addition, there were few patients with TBI in that landmark study.
- This study challenges the paradigm of following a restrictive transfusion regime in moderate-severe TBI patients which seemed to be an interesting research topic.
- Overall, the findings from this trial revealed that a liberal transfusion strategy did not reduce the risk of an unfavorable outcome at 6 months in critically ill patients with TBI and anemia.
- There were lot of drawbacks in the statistical values taken as significance in this trial.
- Further studies are required to understand the findings from the secondary outcomes and Bayesian analysis.

IMPACT ON CURRENT PRACTICE AND TAKE-HOME MESSAGE

With current available evidence including this trial it is advisable to continue the practice of restrictive transfusion strategy to maintain 7 g/dL Hb in patients with TBI.

Tranexamic Acid for Intracerebral Hemorrhage in Patients on Non-Vitamin K Antagonist Oral Anticoagulants (TICH-NOAC): A Multicenter, Randomized, Placebo-Controlled, Phase 2 Trial

Polymeris AA, Karwacki GM, Siepen BM, Schaedelin S, Tsakiris DA, Stippich C, et al. Tranexamic acid for intracerebral hemorrhage in patients on non-vitamin k antagonist oral anticoagulants (TICH-NOAC): A multicenter, randomized, placebo-controlled, phase 2 trial.

STROKE. 2023;54(9):2223-34.

CLINICAL QUESTION OR PROBLEM

Does tranexamic acid prevent hematoma expansion in intracerebral hemorrhage (ICH) in patients on non-vitamin K antagonist oral anticoagulants?

WHAT IS ALREADY KNOWN?

- Intracerebral hemorrhage is a devastating disease with high mortality and morbidity. Oral anticoagulation is a well-defined complicating factor of ICH, resulting in increased risk of hematoma expansion (HE), mortality, and morbidity compared with patients with ICH without anticoagulation therapy.

- Novel, non-vitamin K antagonist oral anticoagulants (NOAC) are the mainstay of oral anticoagulation and have largely replaced vitamin K antagonists over the past decade. With the increasing use of NOAC, the proportion of NOAC-associated ICH is steadily increasing, too.
- Knowledge about NOAC-associated ICH is scarce, but retrospective observational studies reported high rates of HE (40%), high rates of in-hospital mortality (25%), and substantial disability.[21-23] Currently, no evidence-based hemostatic treatment exists for NOAC-associated ICH.
- Non-vitamin K antagonist oral anticoagulant-specific reversal agents (idarucizumab for direct thrombin inhibitors and andexanet alfa for direct factor Xa inhibitors) have been approved by medical authorities but lack clear evidence from randomized controlled trials to be superior to any other standard of care.
- While guidelines recommend the use of NOAC-specific reversal agents and 4-factor prothrombin complex concentrate (4fPCC) to restore coagulation in NOAC-associated ICH, no robust evidence exists that these treatments limit HE or improve clinical outcomes.
- Tranexamic acid (TXA)—an antifibrinolytic drug—has been investigated in non–NOAC-associated ICH, most notably in the recent TICH-2 trial. Although its efficacy with regard to functional outcome has not been established, it may be modestly effective in reducing early death and limiting HE. It is true particularly when administered early in patients at high risk for HE. Considering the advantages of wide availability, ease of administration, low cost, and distinct non–NOAC-specific antifibrinolytic mechanism of action, TXA is an attractive candidate even for the treatment of NOAC-associated ICH, for which it has not been tested so far.

STUDY DESIGN

- Double-blind, randomized, placebo-controlled, investigator-led phase 2 trial at six stroke centers in Switzerland from December 2016 to September 2021.
- All participants were administered either IV TXA as an initial 1 g loading dose in 100 mL normal saline infused over 10 minutes and followed by another 1 g in 250 mL normal saline infused over 8 hours or placebo with identical administration procedure.
- The rest of the patient's care was left to standard medical practice, which included blood pressure management and use of other hemostatic agents at the discretion of the treatment team.
- Baseline computed tomography (CT) scans were done as part of routine care before randomization. A follow-up CT scan was done after 24 ± 3 hours to assess HE.

POPULATION STUDIED INCLUDING DEMOGRAPHICS

Inclusion Criteria

- Adults with acute non-traumatic ICH that could be randomized within 12 hours of symptom-onset and
- Taking any NOAC (apixaban ≥2.5 mg, dabigatran ≥110 mg, edoxaban ≥30 mg, or rivaroxaban ≥10 mg) with known last intake within 48 hours or proven persistent NOAC activity using NOAC-specific coagulation assays.

Exclusion Criteria

- Severe preexisting disability [modified Rankin Scale (mRS) score >4]
- Glasgow Coma Scale <5
- Prior treatment with vitamin K antagonists
- Intracerebral hemorrhage known or suspected to be secondary to trauma, vascular malformation, tumor, or other underlying structural abnormality
- Pregnancy
- Planned neurosurgical hematoma evacuation within 24 hours
- Pulmonary embolism or deep vein thrombosis within preceding 2 weeks.

Of note, concurrent use of other hemostatic agents (e.g., idarucizumab, andexanet alfa, and 4-factor PCC) was not an exclusion criterion.

OUTCOMES EVALUATED

Primary Outcome

- Presence of HE on follow-up imaging at 24 ± 3 hours, defined as intracerebral hematoma volume increase by at least 33% or 6 mL from baseline.
- In total, 41% (26/63) of study patients had HE, 38% (12/32) in the TXA group and 45% (14/31) in the placebo group [adjusted OR 0.63 (95% CI, 0.22–1.82), $p = 0.4$]. These results were not statistically significant.

Secondary Outcomes

- None of the following prespecified secondary outcomes differed between treatment arms
  - Symptomatic HE, defined as hematoma expansion with neurological deterioration (worsening of NIHSS score by at least 4 points or GCS score by at least 2 points) or death within 7 days
  - Absolute hematoma volume change by 24 ± 3 hours
  - Ordinal mRS score, mRS score 0–4, and mRS score 0–3 at 90 days
  - In-hospital death
  - Death within 90 days
  - Major thromboembolic events (ischemic stroke, myocardial infarction, or deep vein thrombosis/pulmonary embolism) within 90 days
  - Neurosurgical intervention up to day 2
- There were 9.5% (6/63) of patients who had major thromboembolic event within 90 days, 12.5% (4/32) of those who received TXA and 6.5% (2/31) of those who received placebo [OR 1.86 (95% CI, 0.37–9.50), $p = 0.45$].
- No difference was noted between the arms in terms of recorded seizures within 90 days, 19% (6/32) in the TXA group, and 13% (4/31) in the placebo group [adjusted OR 1.62 (0.22-1.89), $p = 0.49$]
- No difference was noted in rate of participants with any serious adverse events (including major thromboembolic events, seizures, and death) up to 90 days, and any serious adverse events up to day 7: up to 75% (24/32) in the TXA group and 65% (20/31) in the placebo group [adjusted OR 1.43 (0.45–4.47), $p = 0.54$].

AUTHORS' VIEWPOINT

Study found no evidence that TXA prevents HE in patients with NOAC-associated ICH, although there were no major safety concerns with TXA and treatment might hold potential for benefit in selected patient subgroups, particularly those treated early after ICH onset. Further trials on hemostatic treatments are urgently needed to improve outcomes in NOAC-associated ICH and should probably target an early treatment window.

STRENGTH OF THE STUDY

- This is the first randomized trial reporting on the hemostatic treatment of NOAC-associated ICH.

- Robust methodology including a double-blind placebo-controlled design, and
- Robust assessment of the primary outcome by three raters, which limit the risk of bias.

DRAWBACK OF THE STUDY

- Failure to reach its target sample size and underpowered sample size.
- A number of factors led to the premature discontinuation of TICH-NOAC, including lack of additional funding and—most notably—the negative impact of the coronavirus disease-2019 pandemic on research activities.

REVIEWERS' VIEWPOINT

In spite of robust methodology, there are major drawbacks such as low sample size. The results are not substantial enough to consider tranexamic acid as a potential treatment in this subgroup.

There were no major safety concerns noted in the use of TXA and there was a signal that it may be beneficial for preventing HE in select patients, particularly those treated within 6 hours of ICH onset.

IMPACT ON CURRENT PRACTICE AND TAKE-HOME MESSAGE

With current evidences including this trial, tranexamic acid is not advisable in ICH in patients on NOAC for reduction of hematoma expansion.

REFERENCES

1. Frontera JA, Lewin JJ 3rd, Rabinstein AA, Aisiku IP, Alexandrov AW, Cook AM, et al. Guideline for reversal of antithrombotics in intracranial hemorrhage: a statement for healthcare professionals from the Neurocritical Care Society and Society of Critical Care Medicine. Neurocrit Care. 2016;24(1):6-46.
2. Greenberg SM, Ziai WC, Cordonnier C, Dowlatshahi D, Francis B, Goldstein JN, et al. 2022 Guideline for the management of patients with spontaneous intracerebral hemorrhage: a guideline from the American Heart Association/American Stroke Association. Stroke. 2022;53:e282-e361.
3. Intercollegiate Stroke Working Party National clinical guideline for stroke. London, UK: Royal College of Physicians; 2023.
4. Makris M, Van Veen JJ, Tait CR, Mumford AD, Laffan M. Guideline on the management of bleeding in patients on antithrombotic agents. Br J Haematol. 2013;160:35-46.
5. Powers WJ, Rabinstein AA, Ackerson T, Adeoye OM, Bambakidis NC, Becker K, et al. Guidelines for the early management of patients with acute ischemicstroke: 2019 update to the 2018 guidelines for the early management of acute ischemic stroke: a guideline for healthcare professionals from the American Heart Association/American Stroke Association. Stroke. 2019;50(12):e344-e418.
6. Sandset EC, Anderson CS, Bath PM, Christensen H, Fischer U, Gąsecki D, et al. European Stroke Organisation (ESO) guidelines on blood pressure management in acute ischaemic stroke and intracerebral haemorrhage. Eur Stroke J. 2021;6(2):XLVIII-LXXXIX.
7. Goyal N, Tsivgoulis G, Pandhi A, Chang JJ, Dillard K, Ishfaq MF, et al. Blood pressure levels post mechanical thrombectomy and outcomes in large vessel occlusion strokes. Neurology. 2017;89(6):540-7.
8. Mistry EA, Mistry AM, Nakawah MO, Khattar NK, Fortuny EM, Cruz AS, et al. Systolic blood pressure within 24 hours after thrombectomy for acute ischemic stroke correlates with outcome. J Am Heart Assoc. 2017;6(5):e006167.
9. Mistry EA, Sucharew H, Mistry AM, Mehta T, Arora N, Starosciak AK, et al. Blood Pressure after Endovascular Therapy for Ischemic Stroke (BEST): a multicenter prospective cohort study. Stroke. 2019;50(12):3449-55.
10. Anadani M, Arthur AS, Tsivgoulis G, Simpson KN, Alawieh A, Orabi Y, et al. Blood pressure goals and clinical outcomes after successful

endovascular therapy: a multicenter study. Ann Neurol. 2020;87(6):830-9.

11. Yang P, Song L, Zhang Y, Zhang X, Chen X, Li Y, et al. Intensive blood pressure control after endovascular thrombectomy for acute ischaemic stroke (ENCHANTED2/MT): a multicentre, open-label, blinded-endpoint, randomised controlled trial. Lancet. 2022;400(10363):1585-96.
12. Mistry EA, Mayer SA, Khatri P. Blood pressure management after mechanical thrombectomy for acute ischemic stroke: a survey of the Stroke Net sites. J Stroke Cerebrovasc Dis. 2018;27(9):2474-8.
13. Grossen AA, Ernst GL, Bauer AM. Update on intrathecal management of cerebral vasospasm: a systematic review and meta-analysis. Neurosurg Focus. 2022;52(3):E10.
14. Hulou MM, Essibayi MA, Benet A, Lawton MT. Lumbar drainage after aneurysmal subarachnoid hemorrhage: a systematic review and meta-analysis. World Neurosurg. 2022;166:261-7.e9.
15. Al-Tamimi YZ, Bhargava D, Feltbower RG, Hall G, Goddard AJ, Quinn AC, et al. Lumbar drainage of cerebrospinal fluid after aneurysmal subarachnoid hemorrhage: a prospective, randomized, controlled trial (LUMAS). Stroke. 2012;43(3):677-82.
16. Gregson BA, Rowan EN, Francis R, McNamee P, Boyers D, Mitchell P, et al. Surgical Trial In Traumatic intraCerebral Haemorrhage (STITCH): a randomised controlled trial of Early Surgery compared with Initial Conservative Treatment. Health Technol Assess. 2015;19(70):1-138.
17. Mendelow AD, Gregson BA, Rowan EN, Murray GD, Gholkar A, Mitchell PM, et al. Early surgery versus initial conservative treatment in patients with spontaneous supratentorial lobar intracerebral haematomas (STICH II): a randomised trial. Lancet. 2013;382(9890):396. Erratum in: Lancet. 2021;398(10305):1042.
18. Hanley DF, Thompson RE, Rosenblum M, Yenokyan G, Lane K, McBee N, et al. Efficacy and safety of minimally invasive surgery with thrombolysis in intracerebral haemorrhage evacuation (MISTIE III): a randomised, controlled, open-label, blinded endpoint phase 3 trial. Lancet. 2019;393(10175):1021-1032. Erratum in: Lancet. 2019;393(10181):1596.
19. Montgomery EY, Barrie U, Kenfack YJ, Edukugho D, Caruso JP, Rail B, et al. Transfusion Guidelines in Traumatic Brain Injury: A Systematic Review and Meta-Analysis of the Currently Available Evidence. Neurotrauma Rep. 2022;3(1):554-68.
20. Hebert PC, Wells G, Blajchman MA, Marshall J, Martin C, Pagliarello G, et al. A multicenter, randomized, controlled clinical trial of transfusion requirements in critical care. Transfusion Requirements in Critical Care Investigators, Canadian Critical Care Trials Group. N Engl J Med. 1999;340(6):409-17.
21. Wilson D, Seiffge DJ, Traenka C, Basir G, Purrucker JC, Rizos T, et al. Outcome of intracerebral hemorrhage associated with different oral anticoagulants. Neurology. 2017;88:1693-700.
22. Tsivgoulis G, Wilson D, Katsanos AH, Sargento-Freitas J, Marques-Matos C, Azevedo E, et al. Neuroimaging and clinical outcomes of oral anticoagulant-associated intracerebral hemorrhage. Ann Neurol. 2018;84:694-704.
23. Inohara T, Xian Y, Liang L, Matsouaka RA, Saver JL, Smith EE, et al. Association of intracerebral hemorrhage among patients taking non-vitamin K antagonist vs vitamin K antagonist oral anticoagulants with in-hospital mortality. JAMA. 2018;319: 463-73.

SECTION 4

Gastroenterology/Hepatobiliary

Section Editor: *Lalita Gouri Mitra*

Associate Editors: *Jagdeep Sharma, Shrirang Nagorao Bamne, Harsimran Singh Walia*

Evaluating Mortality and Recovery of Extreme Hyperbilirubinemia in Critically Ill Patients by Phasing the Peak Bilirubin Level: A Retrospective Cohort Study

Han HS, Park CM, Lee DS, Sinn DH, Gil E. Evaluating mortality and recovery of extreme hyperbilirubinemia in critically ill patients by phasing the peak bilirubin level: A retrospective cohort study.

PLoS One. 2021;16:e0255230.

CLINICAL QUESTION

Does the level of bilirubin increase in patients with extreme hyperbilirubinemia (total bilirubin >12 mg/dL) affect the mortality or recovery and does it help in prognostication? There are no large-scale studies to date which have analyzed mortality in critically ill intensive care unit (ICU) patients with extreme hyperbilirubinemia and this study assesses the hospital mortality and recovery according to the subdivision of extreme hyperbilirubinemia level and has studied the causes and the relationship between factors causing extreme hyperbilirubinemia and how these high levels correlate with recovery.

WHAT IS ALREADY KNOWN?

Hepatic dysfunction is one of the most important prognostic factors in ICU patients who have multiorgan failure.[1] High level of serum bilirubin indicates liver dysfunction and also contributes to an imbalanced immune response, aggravated bacterial infections, and impaired renal or cardiac function.[2] Increased bilirubin levels are closely associated with increased mortality and the sequential organ failure assessment (SOFA) score grades liver dysfunction in the range 0–4 at respective bilirubin cut-off bilirubin levels of 1.2, 2.0, 6.0, and 12.0 mg/dL. Extreme hyperbilirubinemia (>12.0 mg/dL), which can arise due to multiple causes, is poorly understood as extreme hyperbilirubinemia is not subdivided further in the SOFA scoring system.

Brienza et al. reported that hepatic dysfunction, which is defined as a total bilirubin increase >2 mg/dL, occurs in 31% of critically ill patients and shows independent roles in clinical outcomes.[3] In comparison to other prognostic values, hepatic dysfunction is more closely related to the risk of death in critically ill patients.[4] Serum bilirubin is currently considered a stable and powerful marker of hepatic dysfunction.[5] Studies have only analyzed the prognostic value of hyperbilirubinemia between 2 and 12 mg/dL.[3,4]

STUDY DESIGN

This was a retrospective cohort study of 427 critically ill patients admitted to the ICU, who had developed a serum total bilirubin ≥12 mg/dL at least once during their ICU stay at Samsung Medical Center, Seoul, South Korea in 2011–2015. Patients who were <19 years of age, liver transplant recipients, and patients whose total serum bilirubin was already >12 mg/dL at the time of ICU admission were excluded.

All serum bilirubin levels during patients' ICU stay were collected and based on the peak serum bilirubin level, patients were classified into one of four grades: Grade 1 (>12 mg/dL and <15 mg/dL), grade 2 (>15 mg/dL and <20 mg/dL), grade 3 (>20 mg/dL and <30 mg/dL), and grade 4 (>30 mg/dL). The following tests related to liver dysfunction were also recorded: Aspartate aminotransferase (AST), alanine aminotransferase (ALT), alkaline phosphatase (ALP), γ (gamma)-glutamyl transferase (GGT), international normalized ratio (INR), albumin, c-reactive protein (CRP), and lactate.[6] The mean values of all the tests done 15 days before and after the first incidence of a total serum bilirubin >12 mg/dL after ICU admission were calculated. Then, the median values [interquartile ranges (IQRs)] were calculated for the total patient population or specific groups (e.g., survivors or recovery group).

The investigators also evaluated the major causes of extreme hyperbilirubinemia which was multifactorial and were categorized as obstructive (stone, neoplasm, and stricture) and nonobstructive (hypoxic hepatitis, infection including sepsis, primary liver disease, traumatic or surgical liver injury, pigment overload (hemolysis, massive bleeding and/or transfusion, hematoma resorption, disseminated intravascular coagulation (DIC), hemolytic uremic syndrome, and hematologic disorder-related hemolysis), drug [e.g., chemotherapy agents, antibiotics, total parenteral nutrition (TPN), herbal medicine, etc.] other organ failure–related jaundice, and long-term nil-per-os (NPO).

Other than regular demographics, comorbidities including diabetes mellitus (DM), hypertension (HTN), dyslipidemia, chronic liver disease, hepatobiliary-pancreatic (HBP) cancer, solid cancer (excluding HBP cancer), and hematologic cancer were noted. A modified SOFA score[7] (not including Glasgow Coma Scale) was applied, and the presence of sepsis and shock (septic, cardiogenic, and hypovolemic) at ICU admission was assessed. Factors[8] [hepatic encephalopathy (HE), DIC, acute on chronic liver failure (ACLF), ischemic heart disease (IHD), stroke, organ dysfunction, cardiopulmonary resuscitation (CPR), extracorporeal membrane oxygenation (ECMO), liver surgery, hypoxic hepatitis, and status of ursodeoxycholic acid (UDCA) medication] that may have influenced the development of, or recovery from, hyperbilirubinemia in the period before total bilirubin reached 12 mg/dL were clinically evaluated.

OUTCOMES EVALUATED

Hospital mortality, defined as death occurring during a hospital stay was the primary outcome variable. The secondary outcome variable was recovery from hyperbilirubinemia, defined as a decrease of the serum bilirubin level <6 mg/dL which is SOFA score of two points or below regardless of whether the patient was in the ICU, general ward, or outpatient clinic after the peak serum bilirubin level.

Baseline Characteristics and Comparison between Survivors and Nonsurvivors

427 patients with a mean age of 59.8 ± 14.0 years were included in this study of which 67% were males and 33% were females. The mortality rate for the total population was 76.1% and the median duration of ICU stays was 12.3 (7.0~22.3) days. The nonsurvivors showed a higher occurrence of hematologic cancer, DIC, sepsis, and septic shock with a higher mean score of initial SOFA, a higher mean number of dysfunctional organs, and higher levels of median values of AST, INR, and lactate.

Comparison between Recovery and Nonrecovery Group from Extreme Hyperbilirubinemia

The mean value of peak bilirubin was 20.36 ± 10.9 mg/dL and was higher in nonsurvivors than survivors (24.6 mg/dL vs. 19.4 mg/dL; $p < 0.001$). The survival rate was significantly decreased as extreme hyperbilirubinemia grades increased; 37.8%, 28.3%, 18.3%, and 9.3%, respectively for grades 1–4 ($p < 0.001$). The peak bilirubin value (per mg/dL) was significantly related to hospital mortality in model 2 analysis (OR: 1.09; 95% CI: 1.04–1.15; $p < 0.001$) with the risk of mortality gradually increased as the grade increased in model 2 analysis [OR (95% CI): 1.92 (0.70–5.28); 3.55 (1.33–9.48), and 12.47 (3.07–50.59) for grades 2–4, respectively]. As more confounding variables were adjusted, the mortality risk in each hyperbilirubinemia grade gradually increased.

Extreme hyperbilirubinemia is caused by obstructive jaundice (40 cases) and non-obstructive jaundice (814 cases) with the mortality rate being higher in the non-obstructive cases. Direct hyperbilirubinemia showed a higher rate in survivors, whereas indirect hyperbilirubinemia showed a lower rate in survivors than in nonsurvivors.

Ursodeoxycholic acid and albumin were identified as favorable factors for recovery from extreme hyperbilirubinemia, whereas peak bilirubin grade, chronic liver disease, the number of dysfunctional organs, INR, and lactate were unfavorable factors.

AUTHORS' VIEWPOINT

This study demonstrated a clear difference in patients' clinical outcomes based on novel subcategorized level of extreme hyperbilirubinemia. Multivariable analysis using the logistic regression model showed a significant trend of increasing hospital mortality with increased hyperbilirubinemia grade with an inverse relationship between recovery from hyperbilirubinemia and the grade of hyperbilirubinemia and hospital mortality. Hence, both extreme hyperbilirubinemia and recovery from extreme hyperbilirubinemia could be important prognostic factors that clinicians should follow to predict the clinical course of critically ill patients.

STRENGTH OF THE STUDY

- *Relevance:* Hyperbilirubinemia is a significant concern in critically ill patients, and understanding its impact on outcomes is important.
- *Data analysis:* The study uses real-world data from medical records, which can provide practical insights.
- *Clarity:* The study presents clear findings about the relationship between bilirubin levels and patient outcomes.

DRAWBACKS OF THE STUDY

- *Retrospective design:* As a retrospective study, it relies on existing records, which may have limitations in data accuracy and completeness.

- *Confounding factors:* There may be other variables affecting outcomes that were not controlled for or considered.
- *Generalizability:* Results from a specific cohort might not be applicable to all critically ill patients with hyperbilirubinemia.

REVIEWERS' VIEWPOINT

Studies have shown that a total bilirubin increase >2 mg/dL due to hepatic dysfunction occurs in 31% of critically ill patients and plays an independent role in clinical outcomes.[3] Canalicular bile secretion reduction and reduced biliary secretion are considered the main components of hepatic dysfunction in critically ill patients and are more closely associated with the risk of death in this subset of patients.[4,6,7] Extreme hyperbilirubinemia could be an important prognostic factor in critically ill patients, but no predictive model has been established to further grade total bilirubin >12 mg/dL.

The study suggests that monitoring and understanding the timing of peak bilirubin levels can provide valuable insights into the prognosis of critically ill patients with extreme hyperbilirubinemia (total bilirubin >12 mg/dL).

The results could help in stratifying patients based on their risk and tailoring treatment strategies accordingly.

IMPACT ON CURRENT PRACTICE AND TAKE-HOME MESSAGE

- *Clinical practice:* Understanding the timing of peak bilirubin levels can aid in predicting patient outcomes and improving management strategies.
- *Future research:* Prospective studies could validate these findings and explore underlying mechanisms.
- *Overall assessment:* The study provides valuable insights into how the timing of peak bilirubin levels influences outcomes in critically ill patients. While the retrospective design has limitations, the findings could help guide clinical practice and inform future research.

Critical Care Outcomes in Decompensated Cirrhosis: A United States National Inpatient Sample Cross-sectional Study

Goble SR, Ismail AS, Debes JD, Leventhal TM. Critical care outcomes in decompensated cirrhosis: a United States national inpatient sample cross-sectional study.

Crit Care. 2024;28:150.

INTRODUCTION

Chronic liver disease is an important cause of morbidity and mortality worldwide. Cirrhotic patients requiring hospitalization and critical care are also on the rise. Compensated cirrhosis usually does not cause any symptoms as the liver can still perform its functions. The advanced stage of liver disease usually presents as decompensation. This acute decompensation manifesting as hepatic encephalopathy and esophageal variceal bleeding are associated with high mortality rates. These complications lead to an increase in intensive care unit (ICU) admissions and extensive multidimensional critical care.[9] The mortality rate in patients with cirrhosis ranges between 30 and 70%. Some of these patients might also require renal replacement therapy (RRT) and undergo cardiopulmonary resuscitation (CPR) which has a bearing on their prognosis and critical care outcomes. Various studies done previously assessing patient outcomes have shown conflicting results.

PAST RESEARCH AND CLINICAL PROBLEM

Advanced multidisciplinary and multidimensional treatment in decompensated cirrhosis might have improved survival, though the available evidence is low. But it is important to know these decompensated patients' prognosis; it helps better patient stratification and guiding discussions with the patients or their families. Avik Majumdar et al. in 2017 studied the mortality outcomes in patients with cirrhosis admitted to the critical care unit between January 2000 and December 2015. 172 ICUs were enrolled in this study. They found a significant decline in mortality among patients with cirrhosis over time. Mortality was higher in patients with associated multiorgan failures.[10]

McPhail et al. (2018) studied the epidemiology and outcome of patients with cirrhosis admitted to critical care units in the United Kingdom. The total admissions were 11,68,650; 31,361 had cirrhosis. They found that the mortality among patients with cirrhosis was 41% in 1998 and it reduced to 31% in 2012.[11] In this study, Spencer R et al. tried to demonstrate the critical care outcomes in patients with cirrhosis objectively. They also analyzed the type of decompensation, various treatment interventions used, and in-hospital mortality.[12]

METHODS AND STUDY DESIGN

This was a retrospective cross-sectional study, where the US National Inpatient Sample (NIS) data from 2016 to 2019 was analyzed. This is a de-identified database that is publicly available, so Institutional Review Board approval was waived. This database was developed for the healthcare cost and utilization project. The patients requiring critical care with a primary diagnosis of hepatic encephalopathy, esophageal variceal hemorrhage, hepatorenal syndrome, spontaneous bacterial peritonitis, and cirrhosis as a secondary diagnosis were included for assessment. These patients received intubation, central venous catheter placement, or both interventions. The main clinical outcomes included mortality, the use of RRT, and the use of CPR.

Statistical analysis: The data from the samples was collected, and appropriate statistical tests were applied. The continuous variables were described with means and analyzed by student's t-test. The categorical variables were described as proportions and analyzed using the chi-square test. Statistical analysis was done using STATA, version 17.0.

OUTCOME ANALYSIS

12,945 patients were admitted for complications of decompensated cirrhosis. On the other hand, 37,24,744 patients were admitted without the diagnosis of cirrhosis. The hospitalizations in the decompensated cirrhosis cohort tended to occur in younger patients (mean age of 58 years vs. 62.5 years). The most common primary diagnosis for admission was hepatic encephalopathy in 7,485 patients, esophageal variceal hemorrhage was present in 3,130 admissions, 1,830 patients for hepatorenal syndrome, and 500 patients for spontaneous bacterial peritonitis.

- The mortality rate was 33.1% (4,290 deaths) in patients with complications due to decompensated cirrhosis and 26.6%

(9,90,205) in patients without cirrhosis. The patients with hepatorenal syndrome had a staggering mortality rate of 50.6%; 26.7% mortality was present in patients with esophageal variceal hemorrhage.

- RRT was required in 1,580 patients with complications arising due to decompensated cirrhosis. It was most commonly utilized in patients with hepatorenal syndrome (27.3%). 50% of patients with HRS died after RRT. Mortality rates with RRT (in the decompensated cirrhosis group was 46.5%) and in the noncirrhotic group (32.3%).
- 710 patients needed CPR out of 12,945 hospitalizations for complications of decompensated cirrhosis. In patients presenting with esophageal variceal hemorrhage, 6.4% required CPR. Overall mortality in the CPR group was 88.0%.
- This study included a large, nationwide, generalizable sample that reported stratified outcomes based on primary diagnosis on admission. Including patients receiving a liver transplant also improved the generalizability of the results.

WHAT DO REVIEWERS THINK?

Decompensated cirrhosis is an acute deterioration in hepatic dysfunction in patients with preexisting cirrhosis.[13] It is characterized by jaundice, hepatic encephalopathy, ascites, esophageal variceal hemorrhage, and hepatorenal syndrome. Proper history, physical examination, and complete investigations help in making an early diagnosis, and prompt advanced treatment help in reducing mortality. The British Society of Gastroenterology provides a care bundle for guiding treatment in the first 24 hours. Recent advances in treatment have helped in an overall reduction in mortality from complications of decompensated cirrhosis.[13]

This study included a large, nationwide, generalizable sample with complications of decompensated cirrhosis as the primary diagnosis. One-third of patients admitted to the ICU did not survive to discharge as shown in this US nationwide analysis. It also showed an increase in mortality in patients requiring RRT or CPR. This study evaluated admissions for complications of decompensated liver disease. The enrolled patients underwent respiratory intubation, central venous catheter insertion, or both as a part of the delivery of critical care. Previous studies used cirrhosis as the sole inclusion criterion for admission to ICU. The type of care provided in the ICU was also not described. Mortality due to complications of acute cirrhotic decompensation has increased compared to patients with noncirrhotic issues. Infection is usually a common trigger for decompensation in this subset of patients. In this study, spontaneous bacterial peritonitis was the only evaluated infectious complication.

Renal dysfunction is present in 20% of patients with cirrhosis. Almost 50% of patients may progress to renal failure; with 20–30% requiring RRT. CPR outcomes are even worse in cirrhotic patients, with mortality rates around 88%. In patients with hepatorenal syndrome, the mortality rate increases to 96%.

The limitations of this study included a lack of use of laboratory data in the form of a model of end-stage liver disease, SOFA score which prevented complete recognition of patients with organ failure. The second limitation was the reliance on ICD-10 codes and the lack of information about patients after they were discharged from the hospital. The ICU outcomes in patients of cirrhosis are improving overall, but patients requiring CPR still carry a poor prognosis. Almost 53% of patients who needed RRT survived and were discharged.

Growing Evidence for Survival Benefit with Plasma Exchange to Treat Liver Failure

Goel A, Zachariah U, Daniel D, Eapen CE. Growing Evidence for Survival Benefit with Plasma Exchange to Treat Liver Failure.

J Clin Exp Hepatol. 2023;13:1061-73.

INTRODUCTION

Acute liver failure (ALF) is a dynamic condition associated with an overwhelming systemic immune response triggered by the release of proinflammatory cytokines due to massive necrosis of hepatocytes, leading to multiorgan dysfunction or complete organ failure.[14] The appearance of jaundice, coagulopathy, and hepatic encephalopathy usually recognizes severe hepatic injury. The development of cerebral edema and encephalopathy is associated with high fatality. With massive destruction, the liver loses its capacity to metabolize ammonia. The neurotoxic effects of hyperammonemia include alteration in the volume regulation of astrocytes, abnormalities in cerebral energy homeostasis, alteration in protein expression that affects its structure and functions and increased oxidative stress.[15] ALF and acute-on-chronic liver failure (ACLF) have a high mortality; urgent liver transplant is needed as a lifesaving treatment. Plasma exchange (PLEX) or therapeutic plasma exchange has also been reported to be useful in treating these patients. PLEX involves the removal of plasma from a patient with liver failure and replacing this with an equal volume of fluid; fresh-frozen plasma is commonly used as a replacement fluid due to coagulopathy seen in this subset of patients. PLEX has also been used to treat conditions such as thrombotic thrombocytopenic purpura, hemolytic uremic syndrome, and Guillain-Barre syndrome.

PAST RESEARCH AND CLINICAL PROBLEM

Idiosyncratic drug reactions, viral hepatitis, and rodenticide ingestion (more in southern and eastern parts) are major causes of ALF in India. These patients need urgent liver transplants and nontransplant treatment as life-saving options. PLEX can be performed by membrane or centrifugal techniques. The membrane technique involves high rates of blood flow which can cause hemodynamic fluctuations; the centrifugal technique involves the movement of fluid at low rates, thus reducing hemodynamic fluctuations and reduced stress on an already compromised liver. Different doses of plasma volume exchange have been used in PLEX. High volume (10 L), standard volume (2.5–5 L), and low volume (1.2 L) of plasma volume have been used. High, standard, and low volumes are used for the treatment of ALF, and standard/low volume is used for ACLF.

Larsen et al. in 2016 did a trial on high-volume PLEX in patients with ALF. In this multicenter trial, 182 patients were randomized to either high-volume PLEX or standard medical treatment groups. The primary objective was to find out about liver-transplantation-free survival during the stay in the hospital. The most common cause of hepatic failure was paracetamol overdose, with a 58.7% survival in the PLEX group versus 47.8% in the standard medical treatment group. This study also highlighted the requirement of nonliver transplant treatment of the patients with ALF. After the results of this trial, the American Society of Apheresis recommends high-volume PLEX as a stand-alone treatment for ALF.[16]

Maiwall et al. in 2022, conducted an open-label randomized controlled trail in 40 ALF patients. Standard medical treatment was provided in one group of patients and another group with standard-volume PLEX and standard medical treatment. Viral hepatitis was the most common cause of acute hepatic failure. 21-day survival in the PLEX group was 75% compared to 45% in the standard medical treatment group. Increased rates of survival was 30% with PLEX and SMT which a significant decrease in levels of pro-inflammatory an increase in anti-inflammatory cytokines along with a decrease in endotoxin and DAMPs.[17]

Pawaria et al. (2021) studied patients with Wilson's disease manifesting as ALF. They assessed the efficacy and safety of high-volume PLEX in these patients. The high-volume PLEX helped improve 90-day survival by 30%, in the PLEX group (47%) and SMT group (17%). High-volume PLEX not only acted as a bridge therapy to the liver transplant but also improved transplant-free survival.[18]

Kumar et al. studied the use of low-dose plasma volume exchange along with low-dose steroids in patients with ACLF and severe alcoholic hepatitis. 38% of patients in the PLEX group versus 14% of patients undergoing standard treatment had 3-month survival, with also an improved survival at 1 year.[19]

Ramakrishnan et al. in 2022 studied 28 alcohol-related ACLF (grade II) patients (14 cases and 14 controls). The patients underwent standard volume therapeutic PLEX along with standard medical treatment while the controls were treated on SMT alone. The change (baseline to day 10) in laboratory parameters, cytokine concentrations, and clinical severity scores, 30 and 90-day mortality rates were noted along with associated adverse events. Therapeutic PLEX was effective in reducing mortality at 3 months compared to standard medical treatment.[20]

Swaroop et al. published in 2023, that for patients with ACLF, therapeutic PLEX improves short-term survival but has no significant impact on long-term outcomes.[21]

SALIENT FEATURES

Indications of Plasma Exchange to Treat Liver Failure Patients

Acute liver failure patients meeting the King's College criteria for urgent liver transplant are being treated with PLEX as a bridge therapy or a stand-alone treatment. American College of Apheresis recommends high-volume PLEX as primary therapy for ALF. TN-ISG and NHM-TAEI guidelines recommend any patient with rodenticidal ALF (with INR ≥4, serial increase in INR, or hepatic encephalopathy) be treated with PLEX (preferable choice low-volume exchange).[22,23] Some ALF and ACLF patients are characterized by increased innate immune response; PLEX provides survival benefit in the same.

How Plasma Exchange Acts?

It helps by ameliorating the inflammatory immune response. It filters out large >60 kDa-sized inflammatory macro-molecules such as Von Willebrand factor (VWF); which helps to restore perfusion in hepatic microcirculation and thus helps restore liver function in these patients.[19,24] A few relative contraindications to the use of PLEX include hemodynamic instability, active sepsis, and recent gastrointestinal bleeding.

Due to the rapidly changing course of illness dynamic scores are needed to assess prognosis after PLEX. It is recommended that all blood samples be drawn at least 12 hours after the session of PLEX. If the dynamic scores improve, the patient may not need a transplant. Plex can also be used in children and pregnant women for the treatment of ALF. In the future, there might be a combined use of PLEX and continuous venovenous hemofiltration (CVVH). Algorithms need to evolve over future studies.

What is the Vellore Protocol?

Admission → USG guided PLEX port insertion into the femoral vein → Oral Prednisolone 10 mg once daily started a day before starting PLEX → Centrifugal PLEX preferred, done daily for 3 days → Cefoperazone sulbactam given as prophylactic antibiotics → Enteral nutrition preferred → Follow up (steroids given with clinical assessment balancing between its anti-inflammatory action and risk of sepsis) with OPD assessment once weekly for 4 weeks and once a month for 3 months.

What not to Do? Avoid sedatives, prophylactic blood transfusion, and potentially hepatotoxic drugs and defer invasive tests.[25]

Complications of Plasma Exchange

The various PLEX-reported complications include thrombophlebitis, bleeding, port-related infection, inadvertent arterial puncture, sepsis, citrate toxicity (as citrate is a preferred choice of regional anticoagulation for extra-corporeal circuit), and transfusion-associated circulatory overload (TACO) and transfusion-related acute lung injury (TRALI) more commonly seen in patients on mechanical ventilation.

KNOWLEDGE GAPS AND FUTURE RESEARCH

The data on outcomes of PLEX treatment for specific etiologies is scarce. There are multiple definitions to define ACLF, with different doses of PLEX being used for their treatment. This challenges the interpretation of treatment outcomes. More randomized controlled studies should be done comparing survival outcomes with PLEX and other modalities of treatment. There needs to be improvement in treatment protocols for better outcomes as short-term mortality is still very high. Way forward, studying patients with single etiology, with preferable reporting of survival at 1 month in ALF patients and 3 months or 1 year in ACLF patients with dynamic scores to predict survival should be the focus of future research.

Timely Albumin Infusion May Improve Resource Utilization in Patients with Cirrhosis and Spontaneous Bacterial Peritonitis

Kim WR, Raghunathan K, Martin GS, Davis EA, Sindhwani NS, Telang S, et al. Timely Albumin Infusion May Improve Resource Utilization in Patients with Cirrhosis and Spontaneous Bacterial Peritonitis.

Biomed Res Int. 2024;2024:6673823.

CLINICAL QUESTION OR PROBLEM

Does early starting of injection albumin infusion in the subgroup of patients of cirrhosis with spontaneous bacterial peritonitis (SBP) benefit in early recovery versus just starting injection albumin infusion in every patient of cirrhosis with SBP? In other words, does an albumin infusion timing/early administration on the presentation of SBP influence early improvement, thus reducing the length of hospital stay?

WHAT IS ALREADY KNOWN?

Administration of antibiotics and albumin in SBP improves overall outcome (resolution of infections and other organ dysfunction).[26,27] Cirrhosis patients with ascites have low oncotic pressure, and an added budding infection worsens organ perfusion including renal perfusion, thus adversely affecting outcome of the patient. Albumin is not just a fluid but is a medicine such as antimicrobials, which takes care of perfusion in the presence of low oncotic pressure. Early administration of antimicrobials in patients with sepsis and septic shock has proven mortality benefit.[28,29]

STUDY DESIGN AND POPULATION STUDIED INCLUDING DEMOGRAPHICS

This observational study was conducted from January 2009 to April 2018. Patients included in this trial were cirrhotic patients above 18 years of age who had now presented with SBP and had received more than 1 antimicrobial and fluid resuscitation in the form of crystalloids (at least 250 mL), during their stay in hospital.[30]

A total of 1,308 patients with the diagnosis of SBP were included in the final analysis as they all survived till discharge and fulfilled other criteria of inclusion, diagnosis, and resuscitation. From a total of 1,308 patients of SBP (eligible for data analysis of hospital length of stay) only 301 were eligible for a secondary outcome to measure the cost of the stay in the hospital; the remaining patients were not included in cost analysis as there was incomplete data about cost at some timepoint of stay in hospital. So to avoid the development of erroneous data analysis, 1,007 patients were excluded from secondary analysis.

Many of the hospital admissions were emergency based. More than 50% of the hospital's admitted population age was between 50 and 64 years. Of the total population included in the study, 40% were of female gender.

The majority of this population were Caucasians, comprising around 74% of the total population in each group. Other than this, African American, Asian-pacific, and Hispanics were in equal proportion in each group. Overall, <50% of patients received timely albumin.

The commercial payer group received injection albumin unknowingly more promptly.

A significant number of patients in the timely albumin group had hepatic encephalopathy (HE) in both subgroups.

Gastrointestinal bleeding was in significant proportion in the nontimely albumin group compared to timely albumin group, 18.8% versus 12% in the SBP (LOS) group, while it was not the same for another subgroup, SBP (cost), where 9.2% versus 7.6% in timely versus nontimely albumin infusion group.

Moderate to severe grade of acute kidney injury (AKI) was seen in the timely albumin group, compared to the nontimely albumin group 25.4% versus 20.7% in respective groups of SBP (LOS), this difference was further profounded in SBP (cost) subgroup analysis, showing timely albumin group was always at a higher risk of adverse outcome whereas mild grade of AKI was in equal proportion in either group.

MELD-Na was higher in the timely albumin group compared to the nontimely albumin group. A significant number of patients with SBP maintained euglycemia, while a few patients in both groups developed blood glucose level disturbances. Data showed that a total of 173 out of 1,308 patients required, i.e., 13.2% of the total study population for the SBP (LOS) group, mechanical ventilation whereas only 18 patients out of 301 SBP patients from the cost analysis subgroup required mechanical ventilation. So, comparing timely and nontimely albumin infusion among SBP (cost) subgroups may not reflect the true difference on its impact on outcome. More patients from the timely albumin group received mechanical ventilation compared to the nontimely albumin group. A total of 331 patients, i.e., around 25% of the total included SBP patients, received beta-blocker therapy as primary/secondary prophylaxis for gastrointestinal bleeding. Hypotensive, hyponatremic, refractory ascites and patients with hepatorenal syndrome-1 were not given beta-blocker therapy. Further this beta-blocker therapy even though in small groups of patients of ongoing SBP might have contributed to the development of hypotension and required vasopressor therapy, which could have had a significant impact on the overall outcome of this study. Around 20% of the total study population required vasopressor therapy. Vasopressor therapy includes dopamine, dobutamine, norepinephrine, epinephrine, phenylephrine, and vasopressin. A significant number of patients from the timely albumin group required vasopressor therapy. Near about 10% of patients of SBP (LOS) in the timely albumin group versus 7.3% of patients from the nontimely albumin group received renal replacement therapy (RRT), and a similar difference was seen in the SBP (cost) subgroup.

ICD code 9/10 was applied for SBP. ICD-10-CM code Y95 was used for a suspected nosocomial infection found in SBP, where multidrug-resistant organism (MDRO) was recovered from culture. In the final analysis of data, only those patients were included within 24 hours of the diagnosis of SBP and had received antimicrobials within 24 hours of diagnosis.

INTERVENTION(S) STUDIED

Timely versus nontimely administration of albumin infusion in cirrhosis patients having decompensation in the form of ascites, and diagnosed to have SBP within 24 hours of admission, and have received antimicrobial/s within 24 hours of admission along with fluid resuscitation.

COMPARATOR USED

COX regression with a generalized linear model were adjusted using baseline patient characteristics, viz, gender, ethnicity, age, admission of emergency, urgency or elective type, payment method, urban versus rural hospital, acute versus nonacute conditions, etc.

OUTCOMES EVALUATED

Baseline patients were sicker in timely albumin group as shown by more severe MELD-Na, serum creatinine, international normalized ratio (INR) value, Charlson Comorbidity Index (CCI), a greater number of patients on mechanical ventilator, and vasopressor therapy group.

Two outcomes were evaluated considering the timing of albumin administration:

1. Hospital length of stay, measured by time to discharge from hospital using Kaplan-Meier analysis
2. Total hospital cost of stay

AUTHORS' VIEWPOINT

Kaplan-Meier and multivariable models show that after adjusting for variables such as disease severity and comorbidity, timely albumin was associated with a 31% higher rate of discharge, reduced length of hospital stay, and a 16% reduction in hospital costs. These data suggest that albumin may be underutilized in patients with cirrhosis and SBP. Early albumin administration during SBP (in patients with less acuity than observed in this study) may decrease hospital resource utilization. Timely albumin infusion in patients with decompensated cirrhosis and SBP is associated with shorter hospital stays and reduced total hospital costs. Optimal administration of albumin may improve patient outcomes and reduce the burden of these conditions on the healthcare system, especially in patients with advanced complications of end-stage liver disease.

STRENGTH OF THE STUDY

- It might be the first study to evaluate the time of starting injection albumin infusion in SBP cases to look for its probable impact on outcome in the form of a length of stay.
- Mortality at end of 1 year, following an episode of SBP reaches up to 70%, thus focusing on length of hospital stay following resuscitative measures along with antimicrobials turns to be more practical rather than any virtual things. This can help in future to make more prospective randomized trials to pick up even small benefit of early/timely injection albumin infusion on clinical improvement in SBP.
- Patients who's data was absent or incomplete were excluded from analysis.

DRAWBACKS OF THE STUDY

- Observational study, prospective randomized study required.
- Dosages of injection albumin utilized have not been mentioned.
- Ascitic fluid or other relevant culture reports including organism and their sensitivity pattern not displayed.
- Amount of total volume of fluid resuscitation done has not been mentioned.
- There can be interinstitutional variability in patient assessment of cirrhosis with suspected SBP.
- No data about possible albumin or albumin overload-related complications, viz, pulmonary edema, renal injury/failure.
- Not mentioned about those with persistent SBP despite being on antimicrobials and other resuscitative measures.

REVIEWERS' VIEWPOINT

Albumin is a medicine just like an antimicrobial, and timely/early administration in patients with SBs, probably need to be considered, i.e., within 1–6 hours of presentation to the hospital. Probably ICU admitted/sicker patients, received albumin infusion earlier, this was considered timely (within 24 hours) in this observational study. In view of more sickness, the nature of underlying decompensated liver disease and continuous monitoring in the ICU could have aided in the decision to start injection albumin timely/early. The number of sicker patients was more in the timely injection albumin group, also a greater number of patients in the timely albumin group received mechanical ventilation, and vasopressor therapy. The same group encountered severe AKI patients.

The sicker patients would have obviously got admitted to the ICU, hence they would have received more attention and would have been subjected to many invasive/noninvasive therapies for organ support which would have been initiated promptly and timely including timely albumin infusion, which maintained not only the perfusion, but organ function. The decision for steroids and beta-blockers was balanced rather than just blanket coverage as part of practice/protocol.

As these were cases of cirrhosis of the liver with ascites, the MELD-Na score was calculated, which objectively unmasked more sick patients in different groups. Patients with MELD-Na score of 25 and above have a high risk of persistence of SBP despite being on antimicrobials.[31] MELD-Na score in the timely albumin group was 25.2 ± 8.8 versus 20.2 ± 8.8 in the nontimely albumin group of SBP (LOS) group still it remained higher as 23.3 ± 8.4 in SBP (cost) [subgroup of SBP (LOS)]. They missed to look at the number of patients who had persistent SBP.

Even though overall MDRO was not that commonly found, there were more patients of MDRO in the nontimely albumin infusion group compared to the timely albumin infusion group, with 8 patients versus 5 patients. These MDROs required targeted antimicrobials in combinations for a longer duration. This could have prolonged the course of the hospital length of stay as well as the cost increased not only from stay but from a combination of antimicrobial drug requirements for a prolonged period of time. So, to have unbiased data on LOS and cost in two groups, one needs to exclude data/adjusted analysis for such multidrug-resistant (MDR)/extensively drug-resistant (XDR) organism-isolated SBP patients. Duration of antimicrobial treatment was 131 ± 227.9 hours compared to 128.2 ± 181.4 hours in the timely versus nontimely albumin group; this makes us think whether timely albumin group patients received antimicrobials for longer duration as it can be the appropriate or optimal duration for patient with underlying immunocompromised status (as cirrhosis), similarly noticeable thing in SBP (cost) subgroup.

It is quite possible that timely starting of hemodynamic support in the form of vasopressor therapy and timely securing of the airway in these SBP patients (many of them were encephalopathic) could have prevented from development of aspiration pneumonia, thus prevented from worsening of the clinical scenarios from further waiting for intubation and mechanical ventilation. Causes for requirements of mechanical ventilation could have been worsening GCS (Glasgow Coma Scale), hypoxemia (from a lung infection, portopulmonary syndrome, and pulmonary edema). Positive pressure ventilation in the form of intubation + mechanical ventilation could worsen the clinical condition of patient by worsening pulmonary hypertension, which few patients in the given observational study could have had (pulmonary hypertension reflected as hepatopulmonary/portopulmonary syndrome). The effect of positive pressure ventilation on hepatic venous-portal gradient (HVPG) and splanchnic circulation in the setting of decompensated cirrhosis of the liver needs to be studied further. Mechanical ventilation itself has its own inherent complications as it gets prolonged in the form of ventilatory-associated pneumonia (VAP), thus contributing to mortality and delayed discharge.

Acute kidney injury is independently associated with death in liver cirrhosis patients.[32] Similar correlation was found in this study, stating that higher AKI severity, mechanical ventilation, hyperglycemia, and higher quick sepsis-related organ failure assessment (qSOFA), significantly decreased the rate of discharge.

In view of more organ dysfunction parameters in the timely albumin group compared to the nontimely albumin group, which should have reflected as delayed discharge, prolonged length of stay, and more cost of a stay, rather there were more improved outcomes in LOS and cost in timely albumin group, so it makes us think that resuscitative approach, including timely, i.e., within 24 hours of admission have increased the pace of recovery near desired rate to show these outcomes. To make the pace of recovery at the desired level in the nontimely albumin group, we should come up with care-bundle therapy with inclusive of injection albumin infusion as early as the time of diagnosis of SBP.

So, this makes us think that if injection albumin is one of the definitive medicines for maintaining perfusion in decompensated cirrhosis patients, then why should one not give injection albumin in SBP patients of any grade of illness as early as possible within 1–6 hours of hospital admission.

So, we should come up with bundle therapy in the management of hospitalized patients of SBP which includes:

- Antimicrobials
- Albumin
- Vasopressor therapy in appropriate conditions
- Judicious use of beta-blockers and steroids

Probably timely albumin infusion was given in more sicker patients as we can know from CCI score and MELD-Na score, so it is possible that more attention was given to these patients, as injection albumin and other measures were started early in these patients. If we make a protocolized care bundle in patients of SBP, which will be a care of excellence, it would avoid further progression of SBP and it will turn the corner of care and survival to discharge.

IMPACT ON CURRENT PRACTICE AND TAKE-HOME MESSAGE

So foremost importance should be given to early diagnosis, followed by bundle-care therapy for SBP for early recovery. This can be generalized following prospective randomized trials.

Aggressive or Moderate Fluid Resuscitation in Acute Pancreatitis

de-Madaria E, Buxbaum JL, Maisonneuve P, García García de Paredes A, Zapater P, Guilabert L, et al. Aggressive or Moderate Fluid Resuscitation in Acute Pancreatitis.

N Engl J Med. 2022;387:989-1000.

CLINICAL QUESTION OR PROBLEM

Is early aggressive goal-directed fluid resuscitation required in the early phase of acute pancreatitis?

WHAT IS ALREADY KNOWN?

Acute pancreatitis is typically characterized by a sterile inflammation of the pancreas that can cause systemic inflammatory response syndrome (SIRS) with a wide range of severity. Acute pancreatitis can lead to significant mortality and morbidity. About 80% of patients with acute pancreatitis who are admitted have a benign clinical course; the other patients, whose mortality rate is roughly 20%, develop significant illness. The outcome of acute pancreatitis is determined by severity, which to a large extent is determined by the amount of pancreatic necrosis. About 35% of patients with acute pancreatitis develop moderately severe or severe illness, which is linked to worse outcomes.[33] The cornerstone of treating acute pancreatitis is goal-directed fluid resuscitation, even though this approach is based on relatively little data. In animal models, necrosis is spatially linked with regional hypoperfusion of the pancreas, which can be treated by fluid resuscitation.[34-37] Preliminary observational research suggested a link between pancreatic necrosis and hemoconcentration, an indicator of systemic hypovolemia.[38,39] However, subsequent studies revealed that administering more fluid resuscitation during the first 24 hours might not enhance the results and may have detrimental effects on various organs.[40,41]

Various randomized control trials comparing different volumes of intravenous fluid have shown conflicting results restricted by small sample sizes and inclusion criteria that are too stringent.[42] Rapid fluid expansion was linked to a worse chance of survival, according to two studies including patients with severe pancreatitis.[43,44] A systematic analysis revealed that moderate hydration was associated with a reduced incidence of adverse events and a lower death rate than aggressive hydration, despite the review being constrained by the heterogeneity and quality of the source data.[45]

Hence, this WATERFALL trial (the Early Weight-Based Aggressive vs. Nonaggressive Goal-Directed Fluid Resuscitation in the Early Phase of Acute Pancreatitis: An Open-Label Multicenter Randomized Controlled Trial) was conducted to study and evaluate the safety and efficacy of aggressive fluid resuscitation compared with moderate fluid resuscitation in a wide range of acute pancreatitis patients with varying degrees of disease severity.

STUDY DESIGN, INTERVENTION(S) STUDIED, AND OUTCOMES EVALUATED

A computer-based central randomization system integrated into an online electronic case-report form (REDCap) was used to randomly assign patients in a 1:1 ratio to receive aggressive fluid resuscitation (aggressive resuscitation group) or moderate fluid resuscitation (moderate resuscitation group).[46] The trial team was not informed of the random assignment sequence beforehand. The trial center, the existence or lack of SIRS, and the existence or absence of baseline hypovolemia were used to stratify the randomization. The patients and investigators were aware of the assigned trial groups.

The aggressive-resuscitation group received an infusion at a rate of 3 mL/kg/h after receiving a bolus of lactated Ringer's solution at a dose of 20 mL/kg of body weight over 2 hours. Patients in the moderate-resuscitation group received 1.5 mL of lactate Ringer's solution per kilogram per hour (without a bolus in hypovolemia-free patients, or after receiving a bolus of 10 mL/kg given over 2 hours in hypovolemia-free patients). The fluid quantities and rates were determined using data from an earlier randomized study on hydration strategies for acute pancreatitis.[47]

A physical examination was conducted in both trial groups for 3 hours to check for fluid overload. Then biochemical and physical examinations were done after 12, 24, 48, and 72 hours. Goal-directed resuscitation was altered at these checkpoints based on the suspicion of fluid overload, the presence of hypovolemia, or normovolemia. If there was a suspicion of fluid overload, hydration was either reduced or halted in both groups; this method was according to the patient's characteristics and the level of excess fluid.

The Patient-Reported Outcome Scale in Acute Pancreatitis (PAN-PROMISE) was used to quantify the level of stomach discomfort.[48] If the score was <5 (with higher scores indicating higher symptom intensity overall; the scale ranges from 0 to 10 for each symptom). Oral feeding was initiated at 12 hours. After 8 hours of oral eating tolerance, the patient could no longer require fluid resuscitation; in the aggressive-resuscitation group, this could happen 48 hours after randomization, and as early as 20 hours in the moderate-resuscitation group.

POPULATION STUDIED INCLUDING DEMOGRAPHICS

The following patients (≥18 years old) were evaluated for eligibility if they had been diagnosed with acute pancreatitis by the Revised Atlanta Classification, which requires meeting two of the following three criteria: Typical abdominal pain, serum lipase or amylase level higher than three times the upper limit of the normal range, or signs of acute pancreatitis on imaging.[49] Patients in the research study had to have presented to the ER no later than 24 hours following the start of their pain and diagnosis should have been made no later than 8 hours before participation in this trial. Patients who were estimated to have a life expectancy of <1 year had uncontrolled arterial hypertension, hypernatremia, hyponatremia, hyperkalemia, hypercalcemia, shock, respiratory failure, renal failure, or decompensated cirrhosis as baseline criteria for moderately severe or severe disease were excluded from this study.

NEW ISSUES ADDRESSED

This trial demonstrated that the risk of volume overload increased with vigorous fluid resuscitation. The safety monitoring board and data both unanimously recommended ending the trial because of the evidence of increased harm without improvement in the primary endpoint.

The current clinical guidelines, which advocate early vigorous resuscitation for the treatment of acute pancreatitis, are not supported by these data.[50,51] The general patient population as well as subgroups of patients without SIRS at baseline, patients with SIRS at baseline (therefore carrying a higher risk of developing severe pancreatitis), and patients with hypovolemia were found to have an elevated risk of fluid overload.

AUTHORS' VIEWPOINT

The administration of aggressive fluid resuscitation increased the risk of volume overload and did not demonstrate the anticipated benefit in disease-specific outcomes in our randomized assessment of aggressive fluid resuscitation versus moderate fluid resuscitation for the treatment of acute pancreatitis.

DRAWBACKS OF THE STUDY

There were many restrictions to take into account. This trial was stopped at the first interim analysis, so there is insufficient data to provide a firm assessment of the efficacy results. The data and safety monitoring board, however, were concerned that a much larger sample size would be required for the trial to show superiority in either group, which would expose many patients to a much higher risk of fluid overload, given the small between-group difference in the risk of moderately severe or severe acute pancreatitis.[52] The Fluid Expansion as Supportive Therapy (FEAST) trial, in which intravenous fluid boluses were linked to adverse outcomes in children with serious illnesses, was affected by the same ethical challenges and decision-making.[53,54]

This randomized, controlled trial also had the drawback of being open-label, which could have led to bias. However, double blinding was not possible owing to the trial physicians' need to assess patients in turn and modify the fluid rate in response to hypovolemia or volume overload. A liberal amount of fluid was administered to patients in the moderate-resuscitation group as well, with a median of 5.5 liters over 48 hours. The aggressive-resuscitation group's hydration regimen was probably overly severe, thus more research examining more restrained techniques needs to be encouraged.

REVIEWERS' VIEWPOINT

For patients with acute pancreatitis of any severity, intravenous hydration, or resuscitation is the conventional treatment. This is done to correct hypovolemia and maintain intravascular volume for better tissue perfusion, which helps to prevent pancreatic microcirculation ischemia and lessen local consequences. In the early stages, fluid hydration must be maintained to stop the series of events that lead to pancreatic necrosis.

However, there has been a recent shift toward a more cautious strategy with fewer fluids. This WATERFALL trial, randomizing patients with acute pancreatitis between aggressive goal-directed and moderate resuscitation was halted because patients in the aggressive group experienced more fluid overload (20.5% vs. 6.3%), while not preventing progression to moderate or severe acute pancreatitis, thus indicating the need toward more conservative approach using less fluids in acute pancreatitis.

Based on current evidence, a moderate fluid resuscitation strategy, beginning with Ringer's lactate IV rate of 1.5 mL/kg/h in the first 24–48 hours, preceded by a bolus of 10–20 mL/kg in 1–2 hours if patients have moderately severe to severe pancreatitis, hypovolemia, signs of dehydration, or acute kidney injury. There is still insufficient evidence to establish the best strategy for fluid resuscitation in patients who have severe pancreatitis. Hence, still more randomized control trials on fluid management in acute pancreatitis are needed to ascertain this hypothesis.

IMPACT ON CURRENT PRACTICE AND TAKE-HOME MESSAGE

Fluid therapy/resuscitation is a cornerstone in patients with acute pancreatitis due to the pathophysiology of fluid loss as a consequence of the inflammatory process. The other aspect is that the use of aggressive fluid resuscitation led to a higher risk of volume overload and did not show the hypothesized benefit in disease-specific outcomes. Recent trials are toward a more conservative approach using less fluids in acute pancreatitis. It has been observed that administering too much fluid resuscitation results in increased vascular leakage, which exacerbates local pancreatic problems and raises the risk of infection and pulmonary complications.

Hence, fluids should be used with caution and as a drug even in patients with acute pancreatitis.

APASL Clinical Practice Guidelines on the Management of Acute Kidney Injury in Acute-on-Chronic Liver Failure

Maiwall R, Singh SP, Angeli P, Moreau R, Krag A, Singh V, et al. APASL clinical practice guidelines on the management of acute kidney injury in acute-on-chronic liver failure.

Hepatol Int. 2024;18:833-69.

INTRODUCTION

Acute and severe hepatic abnormalities characterize acute-on-chronic liver failure (ACLF) due to different types of insults in patients with chronic liver disease (CLD) and have a high short-term mortality.[55] This syndrome is associated with the rapid development of organ failures, which is precipitated most commonly by infections, with severe systemic inflammation. The kidney is the most common extrahepatic organ involved; with acute kidney injury (AKI) reported in 22.8–34% of patients. The precise approach to prevention, early diagnosis, and management can potentially improve patient outcomes.

PAST RESEARCH AND CLINICAL PROBLEM

Asian Pacific Association for the Study of the Liver (APASL) provided the first consensus statement of international experts for the definition of ACLF in 2009 and updated the same in 2014. Although inconsistent, four major societies/organizations have also provided working definitions for clinical use, laying the ground for future research. EASL-CLIF definition was based on the prospective observational study of 1,343 patients with cirrhosis admitted to 29 liver units in 12 European countries. Bacterial infections and systemic inflammation are the leading causes of multiorgan failure in these patients.

American Association for the Study of Liver Diseases (AASLD) practice guidance statement regarding the definition of ACLF includes the following criteria: Acute onset with rapid deterioration in clinical condition, the presence of liver failure defined by hyperbilirubinemia and raised international normalized ratio (INR) in patients with CLD with, or without cirrhosis, and the presence of at least one extrahepatic organ failure.[56] Kidneys are one of the most common extrahepatic organs affected in patients with ACLF, and frequently it is stage 3 AKI which responds poorly to the current treatment modalities. So, they decided to research and develop an understanding regarding early diagnosis, pathophysiology, prevention, and management of AKI in these strata of patients.

METHODS

The experts met in New Delhi in 2023, to build consensus guidelines. Three rounds of the Delphi Survey were done. The final recommendations were graded according to the Oxford Centre for Evidence-Based Medicine System and categorized as weak or strong based on the consensus agreement of the experts. The level of evidence was decided from the source of information such as meta-analysis, high-quality randomized controlled trials, or case reports. The recommendation was strong if the expert's consensus was >80% and weak if it was <80%.

RECOMMENDATIONS

The important recommendations are described here.

Recommendations for the Definition and Pathophysiological Basis of AKI in ACLF

Amathieu et al. did a retrospective study with a large sample size and explained the significance of oliguria in critically ill patients with CLD. The incorporation of urine output increased the sensitivity to the diagnosis of AKI.[57] The experts have made strong recommendations with 100% consensus for the following: AKI in ACLF patients is defined as either a fall in urine output to <0.5 mL/kg in 6 hours or a rise of >0.3 mg/dL of sCr within 48 hours or a 50% increase in creatinine levels from the baseline within 7 days. Urine output criteria must be incorporated in the staging of AKI in patients of ACLF. Patients with decompensated cirrhosis have a higher incidence of AKI.

These patients with ACLF have a distinct spectrum of structural AKI compared to patients with decompensated cirrhosis. The pathophysiology for the development of AKI includes overwhelming systemic inflammation, hyperbilirubinemia, endotoxemia, and circulatory dysfunction. Patients with stage 2 or 3 AKI are more likely to develop acute kidney disease with chances of transitioning to chronic kidney disease. The various causative risk factors include liver-specific risk factors [severity of liver failure, paracentesis-induced circulatory dysfunction (PICD), tense ascites, infection, variceal bleeding, and shock], kidney-related factors (previous AKI, underlying CKD, intrinsic kidney disease, and obstructive uropathy), and drugs (ACE inhibitors, aminoglycosides, amphotericin B, radiographic contrast).

Prevention of Acute Kidney Injury and Role of Biomarkers of AKI in ACLF

Intravenous albumin should be used to prevent renal dysfunction in the context of spontaneous bacterial peritonitis (SBP). It should also be used to prevent PICD. The dose needs to be customized based on the volume status of the patient. No data suggests that granulocyte colony-stimulating factor (G-CSF), pentoxifylline, antioxidants, beta-blockers, or prophylactic antibiotics such as norfloxacin use can prevent AKI. Prophylactic antibiotics reduce the chances of bacterial infection.

Cystatin C and other biomarkers such as neutrophil gelatinase-associated lipocalin (NGAL), IL-18, and Kim-1 are of interest in predicting AKI in decompensated cirrhosis patients, but studies are required to ascertain their role in ACLF patients. NGAL can help differentiate acute tubular necrosis (ATN) from hepatorenal syndrome (HRS)-AKI in patients with decompensated cirrhosis. Data is inadequate on the use of biomarkers to decide on starting Terlipressin therapy for HRS-AKI.[58]

Management of AKI in These Patients

Intravenous albumin should be given for volume expansion in the stage 1 AKI along with close monitoring to prevent volume overload. 4% or 5% albumin should be administered within 3 hours of hospitalization. Additionally, balanced crystalloids can also be used if a greater volume of fluid is needed. 20–25% albumin should be used for volume expansion in the absence of shock. The measurement of intra-abdominal pressures in patients with tense ascites may improve outcomes. The dose of albumin for volume expansion must be individualized and guided by dynamic indices of fluid responsiveness. A thorough cardiopulmonary assessment helps reduce the incidence of adverse events to 20% albumin.

Terlipressin is the vasoconstrictor of choice. Continuous infusion of terlipressin has been shown to be superior in reversing hepatorenal syndrome associated with AKI than norepinephrine. It also provides survival benefits to the patients of ACLF. It is given as an infusion of 2 mg/h; dose can be escalated to a maximum of 6 mg/h. Target mean arterial pressure (MAP) of 65–70 mm Hg is to be maintained. Even after achieving a target MAP of 80–85 mm Hg with the maximum recommended; if there is no improvement in AKI, such patients are nonresponders of terlipressin, and alternative treatment strategies must be sought.

Renal Replacement Therapy and Liver Transplant

They have provided a weak recommendation with the level of evidence 5, that patients of ACLF with stage 3 AKI, with progression or no response to vasoconstrictors should be considered for renal replacement therapy. The recommendation is strong for the dose and mode of replacement therapy. A lower dialysis dose of 20–25 mL/kg/h can be started initially, and if not responding can be customized to higher doses. Continuous renal replacement therapy may be preferred over the intermittent modes of dialysis in patients with stage 3 AKI. These patients once recovered from AKI or not a candidate for liver transplant must be actively weaned from the dialysis.

Expedited liver transplant can be done even in the presence of nonresolving stage 1 or 2 AKI. The patients with ACLF and AKI with a diagnosis of acute tubular necrosis or oliguria and on renal replacement therapy should undergo liver transplant or liver and kidney transplant both, be individualized according to the patients. All these patients must be closely monitored with their renal functions after discharge.

WHAT DO REVIEWERS THINK?

In-field experts have developed these guidelines from all over the world. The kidney is the most frequently involved extrahepatic organ, following a rapidly progressive course. It involves structural damage secondary to severe systemic inflammation, PICD, or acute worsening of portal hypertension. Prevention is better than cure. Avoid nephrotoxic drugs, maintenance of MAP, and regular monitoring of renal functions. The major limitation of this study includes a lack of robust data supporting various recommendations. There is a need to do high-quality randomized controlled trials and multicentric studies to generate high-quality evidence for better preparation and execution of recommendations in the management of these patients.

Way forward there needs to be more research on finding noninvasive biomarkers to diagnose cholemic nephropathy (CN) caused by injury secondary to bile acids, and to distinguish it from ATN. Further studies exploring the role of biomarkers in the diagnosis of subclinical AKI, predicting the course, and recovery from renal replacement therapy. Developing fluid management protocols is based on dynamic indices. Identifying a better mode for replacement therapy and whether the outcomes of ACLF patients on Dialysis with or without oliguria are different must be ascertained. High-quality studies will help build evidence to fill the vacuum in the management of AKI in ACLF patients.

Effect of Prophylactic Antibiotics on Mortality in Severe Alcohol-Related Hepatitis: A Randomized Clinical Trial

Louvet A, Labreuche J, Dao T, Thévenot T, Oberti F, Bureau C, et al. Effect of Prophylactic Antibiotics on Mortality in Severe Alcohol-Related Hepatitis: A Randomized Clinical Trial.

JAMA. 2023;329:1558-66.

CLINICAL QUESTION OR PROBLEM

Alcoholic hepatitis can be an acute condition or an acute on chronic condition following heavy alcohol consumption. It is characterized by rapid onset of jaundice, malaise, tender hepatomegaly, and unnoticeable features of systemic inflammatory response. Alcoholic hepatitis patients are more prone to infections and one of the causes of repeated hospital visits or admissions.[59,60] As we know the liver is a reticuloendothelial organ, involved in the body's immunity. Steroid use in patients with severe alcoholic hepatitis causes infective complications occurring in 50% of these patients and is the main cause of death, even in those who benefit from steroids.[59] Impaired functioning of this reticuloendothelial system (RES) is exaggerated by ongoing corticosteroid treatment in severe alcoholic hepatitis (steroids initiated in patients with Maddrey Functional Discriminatory Score of 32 or above). Previous studies have shown that steroids in severe alcoholic hepatitis have improved 28 days survival but not improved 90 days survival. Is this because of infective complications arising over time with ongoing steroids?

So, could starting antimicrobials in these groups of patients help in preventing infective complication, hospitalization, and mortality?

WHAT IS ALREADY KNOWN?

In alcoholic hepatitis, there are steatohepatitis, necroinflammation, and fibrosis. Corticosteroids help in alcoholic hepatitis by improving cell repair and promoting protein synthesis by its anabolic effect, and improving nutrition through its appetite-stimulating effect. The combination of steroids with underlying severe alcoholic hepatitis is a predisposed factor for infective complication and death.[59,60]

STUDY DESIGN

This was a randomized, placebo-controlled, and double-blind study with patients allocated to two groups. Enrollment occurred from June 13, 2015 to May 24, 2019.[61]

POPULATION STUDIED INCLUDING DEMOGRAPHICS

Patients of severe alcoholic hepatitis defined by transjugular hepatic biopsy in those with Maddrey functional score of 32 or more and model for end-stage liver disease (MELD) score of 21 or more were included from 2015 to 2019, in the age of 18–75 years with a history of heavy alcohol drinking (defined as 40 g/day for females and >50 g/day for males), with a recent onset of raised bilirubin which could be appreciated clinically. Patients included were from 25 centers from France and Belgium. In view of severe alcohol-related hepatitis, patients received tablet prednisolone 40 mg/day for at least 30 days.

INTERVENTION(S) STUDIED

Randomization was done in two groups amoxicillin-clavulanate group versus placebo.

In the antimicrobial group, participants received amoxicillin 1 g + clavulanate 125 mg, three times a day for 30 days, whereas in the placebo group one placebo packet for oral suspension three times daily.

After enrollment, patients were evaluated weekly thereafter for the first 4 weeks, then followed up on 45th day, 60th day, 90th day, and 180th day. Details of medication and follow-up were maintained.

COMPARATOR USED

Log-rank test was used to compare 60-day all-cause mortality between participants randomized to antibiotics and those randomized to placebo by treating patients who were lost to follow-up whose vital status information was not known and patients who underwent liver transplant as censored at the last available follow-up. Hazard ratios of all-cause mortality were estimated from the univariable Cox proportional hazards model.

Schoenfeld residual plots and the Grambsch and Therneau test were used to assess the proportional hazards assumption.

A sensitivity analysis was performed for all-cause mortality outcomes among patients treated who were treated without major deviation from study protocol including those who had received the nonallocated intervention, had received steroids within the last 6 months, did not receive any treatment, failed transjugular liver biopsy procedure, lack of confirmation of alcohol-related hepatitis by liver biopsy, and ongoing candidiasis at the time of inclusion in this study.

A comparison of secondary outcomes between the two groups was performed using the log-rank test for 90- and 180-day mortality and the Gray test (considering death as a competing event) for 60-day cumulative incidences of infection and hepatorenal syndrome considering patients who withdrew from the trial, underwent liver transplant, or were lost to follow-up before the 60-day time point as censored.

χ^2 tests were performed, for comparisons between the two groups of therapeutic response (Lille score <0.45 at 7 days) and substantial improvement in liver function rates (MELD score <17 at 60 days).

OUTCOMES EVALUATED

The primary outcome was 60 days of all-cause mortality.

Secondary outcomes:

- All-cause mortality at 90 days follow-up
- All-cause mortality at 180 days follow-up
- Incidences of infection at 60 days follow-up
- Lille score <0.45 at 7 days
- Hepatorenal syndrome incidences as per criteria at 60 days
- Percentage/number of patients at 60 days with MELD score <17

AUTHOR'S VIEWPOINT

Amoxicillin-clavulanate combined with prednisolone did not improve 2-month survival compared with prednisolone alone in patients hospitalized with severe alcohol-related hepatitis. These results do not support prophylactic antibiotics to improve survival in patients hospitalized with severe alcohol-related hepatitis.

STRENGTH OF THE STUDY

- Multicenter, randomized, and double-blind trial
- Maybe one of the first trials to look into long-term mortality outcome, particularly with antibiotics association

DRAWBACKS OF THE STUDY

- Only the population of two European countries were involved.
- No discontinuation of corticosteroids despite Lille score of >0.45 at day 7 of starting corticosteroid
- Lack of statistical power to calculate a 75% reduction of mortality compared to placebo
- Different durations of antimicrobials will have different outcomes, which might not have been taken into account.
- Details of culture reports and any supporting evidence of infection are not available.
- The cause of shock in severe alcohol-related hepatitis can be other than septic, such as cardiac dysfunction related to alcoholic cardiomyopathy.
- Bias of once mental acceptance of giving antibiotics as good practice
- Missing data
- Interruption in study drug treatment
- No data whether ruled out infection at the time of randomization while ongoing steroids.

REVIEWERS' VIEWPOINT

Though statistically primary outcome of mortality at 60 days was not significant, looking at the numbers (24 deaths out of 142 patients in amoxicillin-clavulanate group + prednisolone compared to 31 deaths out of 142 patients in placebo + prednisolone group), definitively there is a difference, which can become significant with further involvement of eligible patients. There was an absolute difference of 4.6% in 60 days mortality, favoring the antibiotic group. Similarly, there was a mortality benefit at 90 days and at 180 days, which was not statistically significant. Infection rates at 60 days were definitively lower in the antibiotic group compared to the placebo group, which was also statistically significant, supporting the role of antibiotics in patients with severe alcohol-related hepatitis. In view of underlying immune compromised status in severe alcohol-related hepatitis (in view of the loss of parenchyma, in addition to being on steroids, further can affect body's self-defense), these groups will always be at risk of catching infections from the gut, environment etc., also it is difficult to notice infective sign/symptoms (fever) in view of underlying defective immunity.

In the secondary outcome, improvement in MELD score at 60 days in both the groups (cut off of <17 as target), it reflects >30% decrease in MELD score from baseline (which was around 25). The analysis showed that at 60 days, 48 patients out of 100 patients in the amoxicillin-clavulanate group and 50 patients out of 91 patients in the placebo group had a MELD score <17. We can see that initially there were a total of 142 patients in each group with a loss of patient data collection in MELD scoring at 60 days more prominently. The explanation could be that for calculating the MELD score we require laboratory values, viz, serum bilirubin, serum Na, INR, serum creatinine, and serum albumin; however, it may not have been possible for all patients to get laboratory investigations done at this distant time, when most of these patients are not in a hospital. Percentage wise, MELD score <17 was seen in 48% of patients from antibiotic group compared to 55% patients from placebo group. Here we can see that it was possible for total 100 patients to get the calculated MELD score in the antibiotic group at the end of 60 days, whereas only 91 patients from placebo group were able to participate in the calculation of the MELD score at this distant time point. Suggesting that 9% of patients could have their MELD score calculated, one cannot have a head-to-head comparison. This shows spurious improvement in MELD score at 60 days in the placebo group, because of missing patients or data.

Improvement in survival following steroid therapy for those responders as seen with Lille's score of <0.45 at the 4th or 7th day of starting steroids has been proven, while the expected survival is similar in nonresponders and responders.[62] One can consider whether to continue steroids in selected subgroups of no-responders after infective surveillance/cultures and treating them.

Steroids may have beneficial effects because of its positive response on hemodynamics. Maddrey's Discriminant Function score threshold for starting of steroids in alcoholic hepatitis of 32 is itself low performing compared to other scoring systems as MELD, age-bilirubin-International Normalized Ratio-Creatinine score (ABIC) and Glasgow alcoholic hepatitis scores (GAHS).[63-68]

Studies have found that Lille's score has low specificity, though very good sensitivity, so all responders to steroids have a Lille's score ≤0.16.[62,69] This can avoid inadvertent use of steroids, selecting precise group of patients, thus avoid risk of infections in already immune compromised patient.

To improve the beneficial effects of antimicrobials in severe alcoholic hepatitis, we need to avoid blanket steroid therapy by early identifying nonresponders before starting steroid therapy by features of liver biopsy, those with rapidly rising bilirubin, urinary acetylcarnitine >2,500 ng/mL.

Granulocyte colony-stimulating factor (G-CSF) supporting hepatic regeneration and intrahepatic immune milieu. Thus, G-CSF may improve the prognosis of patients with severe AH.[70] Further trials need to be conducted to establish its undisputed role in AH.

One of the major factors for infective complications in AH is from gut translocation of bacteria/fungi from an altered gut microbial environment. Fecal microbiota has a role in treating, preventing infective complication in alcoholic hepatitis as well as alcoholic liver disease per se.[71,72] Plasma exchange can support those with coagulation factor deficiency and rising bilirubin or high bilirubin.

These supportive methods along with a nutritious diet will help to further improve outcomes in patients of severe alcoholic hepatitis who are already getting antimicrobials along with steroid therapy.

IMPACT ON CURRENT PRACTICE AND TAKE-HOME MESSAGE

As severe alcoholic liver disease shows wide manifestation and multiorgan involvements, antimicrobials/antifungals should be prescribed appropriately in severe grade of alcoholic liver disease, whether or not they are on steroids with other risk factors, along with other all possible supportive measures (fecal microbiota, nutrition, G-CSF, and plasma exchange) to improve the overall outcome. Here, the benefit of starting antimicrobials/antifungals in these groups of patients will be definitively more compared to the risk of development of antimicrobial resistance. There should be a meticulous selection of patients for steroid therapy in alcoholic hepatitis considering lower cut-off values of Lille's score at day 4 or day 7, considering lower specificity of cut-off of 0.45.

Controversies in Terlipressin and Transplantation in the United States: How do We MELD the two?

Przybyszewski EM, Wilechansky RM, McLean Diaz P, Allegretti AS, VanWagner LB, Cullaro G, et al.; from the HRS-Harmony Consortium. Controversies in terlipressin and transplantation in the United States: How do we MELD the two?

Liver Transpl. 2024;30:753-9.

CLINICAL QUESTION OR PROBLEM

Whether terlipressin treatment for hepatorenal syndrome-acute kidney injury (HRS-AKI) should qualify for MELD score "lock" in the United States in those who respond to vasoactive therapy?

WHAT IS ALREADY KNOWN?

- Cirrhosis can result in complications such as hepatorenal syndrome (HRS).[73] Depending on increases in serum creatinine, HRS is categorized as type 1 or type 2.[73] Type 1 HRS is frequently fatal with a median duration of survival of weeks to months; however, type 2 HRS has a more insidious onset with the highest risk of death in the weeks after diagnosis. HRS causes refractory renal failure and indicates a dismal prognosis in cirrhotic individuals.
- Around 20% of patients with decompensated cirrhosis will experience HRS-AKI, a severe, late-stage complication.[74] The development of HRS-AKI is a result of the vasodilatory physiology of decompensated cirrhosis, which leads to a reduction in the effective circulatory volume.[74] Patients with HRS-AKI are eligible for Model for End-Stage Liver Disease (MELD) exemption or MELD score "lock" in a number of European nations, including Italy, Spain, and Switzerland, due to their poor prognosis. Patients are not eligible for a MELD exception or lock in the United States under HRS-AKI.
- Terlipressin is a synthetic vasopressin analog with vasoconstrictor activity in both splanchnic as well as systemic vasculature.[75] This activity results in reduced portal hypertension and decreased portal blood flow, which is the main culprit of hemodynamic abnormalities associated with advanced cirrhosis. Terlipressin increases splanchnic and systemic vascular resistance, reduces the effects of portal hypertension and the hepatic venous pressure gradient, and enhances kidney perfusion in patients with HRS-AKI.[73] Terlipressin has been a standard of care for HRS-AKI in more than 20 countries since the first proof-of-concept study and a randomized controlled trial that showed its benefits in 2000.[76] Regardless of the status of a liver transplantation (LT) listing, terlipressin medication is generally best initiated early in the course of the disease to prevent HRS-AKI progression.[77,78] This is especially true for individuals whose serum creatinine is <5 mg/dL.[79]
- In September 2022, terlipressin became the first medication approved by the US Food and Drug Administration (FDA)[80] for the treatment of HRS-AKI, marking a revolution in the management of advanced cirrhosis in the country. The official indication for terlipressin, according to

FDA prescribing information, is to improve kidney function in adults with HRS-AKI with a rapid reduction in kidney function.[80] The FDA also places restrictions on the use of terlipressin, stating that patients with serum creatinine levels >5 mg/dL are unlikely to benefit from therapy and that there is a boxed warning regarding the risk of serious or fatal respiratory failure.[80] As a result, hypoxia (SpO_2 <90%) and active coronary, peripheral, or mesenteric ischemia are absolute contraindications for terlipressin use.[80]

- It is critical to take into account how terlipressin would impact waitlist priorities and results both before and after LT in the US transplant landscape. This review article examines the terlipressin experience in Europe and addresses the debate over whether or not responders to terlipressin treatment for HRS-AKI should be eligible for MELD score lock.

STUDY DESIGN

The experience of European nations with terlipressin was compiled, together with peer center observations and arguments in favor and against the use of terlipressin treatment response for HRS-AKI as a MELD score lock criteria.

POPULATION STUDIED, INCLUDING DEMOGRAPHICS

In this article, we review the European experience with terlipressin use and discuss the controversy of whether responders to terlipressin treatment for HRS-AKI should or should not qualify for MELD score lock.

OUTCOMES EVALUATED/NEW ISSUE ADDRESSED

The European Association for the Study of the Liver (EASL) guidelines support early treatment of HRS-AKI after diagnosis to maximize the opportunity for reversal as the availability of terlipressin has widely increased.[81] While there is no single European policy for organ transplantation since 2006 European nations have largely embraced the MELD score to prioritize liver allocation by clinical urgency.[82] The organ exchange process in Europe is also heterogeneous. Organs can be distributed nationally, globally (within continental Europe), or regionally, and "opt-out" liver donation laws are common, which reduces waiting times and maximizes the supply of organs.

Justifications exist for using the HRS-AKI terlipressin treatment response as the MELD score lock criteria. Patients who do not respond to terlipressin have an inferior prognosis, and patients with HRS-AKI have lower survival rates than patients with equivalent MELD scores who do not have renal damage.[83] The CONFIRM trial was the largest and most recent randomized trial examining terlipressin plus albumin compared to albumin alone for the treatment of HRS-AKI 32% of patients in the terlipressin group experienced HRS-AKI reversal (compared to 17% in the albumin alone group) and were half as likely to require kidney replacement therapy (KRT) at 30 days or to experience a recurrence of HRS-AKI.[84] For patients who are eligible for and respond to terlipressin therapy, a MELD score lock should be implemented because HRS-AKI is an indicator of death independent of MELD and overall results in this patient population are still dismal even in responders to the medication. Successful terlipressin treatment is anticipated to improve kidney function (along with serum creatinine), increase serum sodium levels, and subsequently lower the MELD score for patients with HRS-AKI who are classified for LT and eligible for terlipressin. This may lengthen the waitlist period for patients with HRS-AKI if there is no MELD score lock.[83] The most extreme condition could occur in patients experiencing a recurrence of HRS-AKI after any attempt to withdraw terlipressin, which may require long-lasting treatment before LT. This may lead to unwanted consequences for patients being considered for LT. Lastly, better pre- and post-transplant outcomes have been linked to terlipressin medication response; hence, utilizing a MELD score lock may present a chance to maximize organ allocation to the most benefiting recipients.

There are justifications against using terlipressin treatment response for HRS-AKI as MELD score lock criteria. Positive reactions to terlipressin may prevent the need for an immediate liver transplant. For patients with HRS-AKI, improvements in MELD are correlated with higher overall survival at 3 and 12 months.[83] Terlipressin plus albumin decreases HRS-AKI mortality by around 25% with effective renal injury reversal. Additionally, linked to better 30- and 90-day transplant-free survival is the response to terlipressin.[85] These findings bolster the theory that patients taking terlipressin, particularly those who respond, might not need to be given transplant priority.

AUTHORS' VIEWPOINT

Better patient outcomes should be expected as terlipressin use expands in the United States; this will benefit the transplant community as a whole. Previous experiences suggest that when terlipressin becomes readily available, there may be both positive and negative effects to its use. We need to be prepared to modify our care models as new therapies become available, keeping equity and evidence-based practice in mind. To improve the future LT environment, data-driven discourse can be facilitated by developing early infrastructure to evaluate its impact.

STRENGTH OF THE STUDY

This manuscript outlines the possible advantages and disadvantages of a MELD lock for US HRS-AKI terlipressin responders, and this evaluation is the first of its kind. This study discusses steps for studying terlipressin implementation in the United States which can be very beneficial if implemented. It also outlines European experience with terlipressin use with points both in favor of and against MELD score lock and are discussed in detail.

REVIEWERS' VIEWPOINT

The United States must speak with other nations that have terlipressin responders' policies in place to gain insight into how such policies were put into practice and overseen. Evidence-based practice should be utilized to determine whether patients with HRS-AKI should receive enhanced priority care or MELD score lock, as well as how objective criteria—that is, uniform diagnostic criteria for the condition—might be applied to meet the requirements for MELD score lock. However, protecting waitlist priority for terlipressin responders or partial responders should be the main priority which justifies the MELD lock.

IMPACT ON CURRENT PRACTICE AND TAKE-HOME MESSAGE

The potential positive and negative aspects of a MELD lock for HRS-AKI terlipressin responders in the United States are highlighted in this study. Protecting waitlist priority for terlipressin responders or partial responders who might miss offers owing to MELD lowering during the terlipressin treatment window is one of the main justifications for the MELD lock. The possibility that terlipressin will result in a persistent response and increase overall survival, as well as the fact that cost and availability may prevent equitable access to terlipressin, are some of the arguments made against MELD lock.

It would be premature to propose policy changes for HRS-AKI terlipressin responders without first comprehending its practical implications on organ allocation in the United States, as these arguments are well-balanced.

FUTURE DIRECTIONS

Establishing a potential multicenter HRS-AKI registry will be beneficial in the future. To comprehend the effects of the terlipressin response on organ distribution, the transplant community must use statistics to guide evidence-based policy.

There is currently a paucity of published evidence on how changes in European policy may affect the terlipressin response in HRS-AKI.[86] We have an exceptional opportunity to evaluate the use of terlipressin in the United States prospectively and modify policies to fit the US allocation system. A prospective US registry from a multicenter research collaboration would be beneficial to the transplant community in tracking patients who are prescribed terlipressin and patients who are candidates for terlipressin but do not receive it.

Making use of the Scientific Registry of Transplant Recipients and the United Network for Organ Sharing, the Scientific Registry of Transplant Recipients should be leveraged to evaluate the effect of HRS-AKI-directed treatment on waitlist morality and post-transplant outcomes. To avoid center-to-center heterogeneity in national policy discussions and to address the potential paradoxical effect of terlipressin on waitlist priority status, joint data gathering will be essential.

Gaining knowledge from other nations will be crucial. Along with understanding how other nations' policies for terlipressin responses were put into place and overseen, the United States should also interact with them. The question of whether patients with HRS-AKI should receive extra priority treatment or MELD score lock, as well as how objective criteria—that is, standardized diagnostic criteria for the condition—might be applied to meet the requirements for MELD score lock—should be examined using evidence-based practice.

REFERENCES

1. Sakr Y, Lobo SM, Moreno RP, Gerlach H, Ranieri VM, Michalopoulos A, et al. Patterns and early evolution of organ failure in the intensive care unit and their relation to outcome. Crit Care. 2012; 16:R222.
2. Horvatits T, Trauner M, Fuhrmann V. Hypoxic liver injury and cholestasis in critically ill patients. Curr Opin Crit Care. 2013;19:128-32.
3. Brienza N, Dalfino L, Cinnella G, Diele C, Bruno F, Fiore T. Jaundice in critical illness: promoting factors of a concealed reality. Intensive Care Med. 2006;32:267-74.
4. Kramer L, Jordan B, Druml W, Bauer P, Metnitz PG. Austrian Epidemiologic Study on Intensive Care ASG. Incidence and prognosis of early hepatic dysfunction in critically ill patients—a prospective multicenter study. Crit Care Med. 2007;35:1099-104.
5. Horvatits T, Drolz A, Rutter K, Roedl K, Langouche L, Van den Berghe G, et al. Circulating bile acids predict outcome in critically ill patients. Ann Intensive Care. 2017;7:48.
6. Fargo MV, Grogan SP, Saguil A. Evaluation of Jaundice in Adults. Am Fam Physician. 2017;95:164-8.
7. Namendys-Silva SA, Silva-Medina MA, Vasquez-Barahona GM, Baltazar-Torres JA, Rivero-Sigarroa E, Fonseca-Lazcano JA, et al.

Application of a modified sequential organ failure assessment score to critically ill patients. Braz J Med Biol Res. 2013;46:186-93.
8. Sarin SK, Choudhury A, Sharma MK, Maiwall R, Al Mahtab M, Rahman S, et al. Acute-on-chronic liver failure: consensus recommendations of the Asian Pacific Association for the study of the liver (APASL): an update. Hepatol Int. 2019;13:353-90.
9. Perez Ruiz de Garibay A, Kortgen A, Leonhardt J, Zipprich A, Bauer M. Critical care hepatology: definitions, incidence, prognosis, and role of liver failure in critically ill patients. Crit Care. 2022;26:289.
10. Majumdar A, Bailey M, Kemp WM, Bellomo R, Roberts SK, Pilcher D. Declining mortality in critically ill patients with cirrhosis in Australia and New Zealand between 2000 and 2015. J Hepatol. 2017;67(6):1185-93.
11. McPhail MJW, Parrott F, Wendon JA, Harrison DA, Rowan KA, Bernal W. Incidence and Outcomes for Patients with Cirrhosis Admitted to the United Kingdom Critical Care Units. Crit Care Med. 2018;46(5):705-12.
12. Goble SR, Ismail AS, Debes JD, Leventhal TM. Critical care outcomes in decompensated cirrhosis: a United States national inpatient sample cross-sectional study. Crit Care. 2024;28:150.
13. Mansour D, McPherson S. Management of decompensated cirrhosis. Clin Med (Lond). 2018;18(Suppl 2):s60-5.
14. Bernal W, Wendon J. Acute liver failure. N Engl J Med. 2013;369:2525-34.
15. Strauss GI, Knudsen GM, Kondrup J, Moller K, Larsen FS. Cerebral metabolism of ammonia and amino acids in patients with fulminant hepatic failure. Gastroenterology. 2001;121:1109-19.
16. Larsen FS, Schmidt LE, Bernsmeier C, Rasmussen A, Isoniemi H, Patel VC, et al. High-volume plasma exchange in patients with acute liver failure: An open randomized controlled trial. J Hepatol. 2016;64(1):69-78.
17. Maiwall R, Bajpai M, Singh A, Agarwal T, Kumar G, Bharadwaj A, et al. Standard-Volume Plasma Exchange Improves Outcomes in Patients With Acute Liver Failure: A Randomized Controlled Trial. Clin Gastroenterol Hepatol. 2022;20(4):e831-54.
18. Pawaria A, Sood V, Lal BB, Khanna R, Bajpai M, Alam S. Ninety days transplant-free survival with high volume plasma exchange in Wilson disease presenting as acute liver failure. J Clin Apher. 2021;36(1):109-17.
19. Kumar SE, Goel A, Zachariah U, Nair SC, David VG, Varughese S, et al. Low Volume Plasma Exchange and Low Dose Steroid Improve Survival in Patients with Alcohol-Related Acute on Chronic Liver Failure and Severe Alcoholic Hepatitis - Preliminary Experience. J Clin Exp Hepatol. 2022;12(2):372-8.
20. Ramakrishnan S, Hans R, Duseja A, Sharma RR. Therapeutic plasma exchange is a safe and effective bridge therapy in patients with alcohol-associated ACLF not having immediate prospects for liver transplantation-A case-control, pilot study. J Clin Apher. 2022;37(6):553-62.
21. Swaroop S, Arora U, Biswas S, Vaishnav M, Pathak P, Agarwal A, et al. Therapeutic plasma-exchange improves short-term, but not long-term, outcomes in patients with acute-on-chronic liver failure: A propensity score-matched analysis. J Clin Apher. 2023;38(4):376-89.
22. Eapen CE, Balasubramanian V, Ramamoorthy G, Jayanthi V, Sathiyasekaran M, Murugan N, et al. Management of Rodenticide Poisoning: Tamil Nadu Chapter of Indian Society of Gastroenterology Guidelines. Gastroenterol Hepatol Endosc Pract. 2022;2(1):1-6.
23. National Health Mission, Tamil Nadu. Handbook of Poisoning Management: Primary Care to Tertiary Care. Tamil Nadu: Tamil Nadu Accident & Emergency Care; 2023.
24. Prasanna KS, Goel A, Amirtharaj GJ, Ramachandran A, Balasubramanian KA, Mackie I, et al. Plasma Von Willebrand factor levels predict in-hospital survival in patients with acute-on-chronic liver failure. Indian J Gastroenterol. 2016;35:432-40.
25. Goel A, Zachariah U, Daniel D, Eapen CE. Growing Evidence for Survival Benefit with

Plasma Exchange to Treat Liver Failure. J Clin Exp Hepatol. 2023;13(6):1061-73.

26. Batool S, Waheed MD, Vuthaluru K, Jaffar T, Garlapati SKP, Bseiso O, et al. Efficacy of Intravenous Albumin for Spontaneous Bacterial Peritonitis Infection Among Patients With Cirrhosis: A Meta-Analysis of Randomized Control Trials. Cureus. 2022; 14(12):e33124.
27. Alaniz C, Regal RE. Spontaneous bacterial peritonitis: a review of treatment options. Pharmacy and Therapeutics. 2009;34(4): 204-10.
28. Arulappen AL, Danial M, Ng LW, Teoh JC. The impact of antibiotics administration on mortality for time in sepsis and septic shock patients including possible reasons for delayed Administration in Malaysia. Antibiotics. 2022;11(9):1202.
29. Kumar A. Early antimicrobial therapy in severe sepsis and septic shock. Curr Infect Dis Rep. 2010;12:336-44.
30. Kim WR, Raghunathan K, Martin GS, Davis EA, Sindhwani NS, Telang S, et al. Timely Albumin Infusion May Improve Resource Utilization in Patients with Cirrhosis and Spontaneous Bacterial Peritonitis. Biomed Res Int. 2024;2024:6673823.
31. Desai AP, Reau N, Reddy KG, Te HS, Mohanty S, Satoskar R, et al. Persistent spontaneous bacterial peritonitis: a common complication in patients with spontaneous bacterial peritonitis and a high score in the model for end-stage liver disease. Therap Adv Gastroenterol. 2012;5(5):275-83.
32. Scott RA, Austin AS, Kolhe NV, McIntyre CW, Selby NM. Acute kidney injury is independently associated with death in patients with cirrhosis. Frontline Gastroenterol. 2013;4(3):191-7.
33. Sternby H, Bolado F, Canaval-Zuleta HJ, Marra-López C, Hernando-Alonso AI, Del-Val-Antoñana A, et al. Determinants of severity in acute pancreatitis: a nation-wide multicenter prospective cohort study. Ann Surg. 2019;270:348-55.
34. Kinnala PJ, Kuttila KT, Gronroos JM, Havia TV, Nevalainen TJ, Niinikoski JH. Splanchnic an pancreatic tissue perfusion in experimental acute pancreatitis. Scand J Gastroenterol. 2002;37:845-9.
35. Kusterer K, Enghofer M, Zendler S, Blochle C, Usadel KH. Microcirculatory changes in sodium taurocholate-induced pancreatitis in rats. Am J Physiol. 1991;260:G346-51.
36. Juvonen PO, Tenhunen JJ, Heino AA, Merasto M, Paajanen HE, Alhava EM, et al. Splanchnic tissue perfusion in acute experimental pancreatitis. Scand J Gastroenterol. 1999;34: 308-14.
37. Niederau C, Crass RA, Silver G, Ferrell LD, Grendell JH. Therapeutic regimens in acute experimental hemorrhagic pancreatitis: effects of hydration, oxygenation, peritoneal lavage, and a potent protease inhibitor. Gastroenterology. 1988;95:1648-57.
38. Baillargeon JD, Orav J, Ramagopal V, Tenner SM, Banks PA. Hemoconcentration as an early risk factor for necrotizing pancreatitis. Am J Gastroenterol. 1998;93:2130-4.
39. Brown A, Orav J, Banks PA. Hemoconcentration is an early marker for organ failure and necrotizing pancreatitis. Pancreas. 2000;20:367-72.
40. Singh VK, Gardner TB, Papachristou GI, Rey-Riveiro M, Faghih M, Koutroumpakis E, et al. An international multicenter study of early intravenous fluid administration and outcome in acute pancreatitis. United European Gastroenterol J. 2017;5:491-8.
41. de-Madaria E, Soler-Sala G, Sanchez-Paya J, Lopez-Font I, Martínez J, Gómez-Escolar L, et al. Influence of fluid therapy on the prognosis of acute pancreatitis: a prospective cohort study. Am J Gastroenterol. 2011;106: 1843-50.
42. Vege SS, DiMagno MJ, Forsmark CE, Martel M, Barkun AN. Initial medical treatment of acute pancreatitis: American Gastroenterological Association Institute technical review. Gastroenterology. 2018;154:1103-39.
43. Mao EQ, Tang Y-Q, Fei J, Qin S, Wu J, Li L, et al. Fluid therapy for severe acute pancreatitis in acute response stage. Chin Med J (Engl). 2009;122:169-73.
44. Mao E-Q, Fei J, Peng Y-B, Huang J, Tang Y-Q, Zhang S-D. Rapid hemodilution is associated with increased sepsis and mortality among

patients with severe acute pancreatitis. Chin Med J (Engl). 2010;123:1639-44.
45. Di Martino M, Van Laarhoven S, Ielpo B, Ramia JM, Manuel-Vázquez A, Martínez-Pérez A, et al. Systematic review and meta-analysis of fluid therapy protocols in acute pancreatitis: type, rate and route. HPB (Oxford). 2021;23:1629-38.
46. Harris PA, Taylor R, Minor BL, Elliott V, Fernandez M, O'Neal L, et al. The REDCap consortium: building an international community of software platform partners. J Biomed Inform. 2019;95:103208.
47. Buxbaum JL, Quezada M, Da B, Jani N, Lane C, Mwengela D, et al. Early aggressive hydration hastens clinical improvement in mild acute pancreatitis. Am J Gastroenterol. 2017;112:797-803.
48. de-Madaria E, Sanchez-Marin C, Carrillo I, Vege SS, Chooklin S, Bilyak A, et al. Design and validation of a patient-reported outcome measure scale in acute pancreatitis: the PAN-PROMISE study. Gut. 2021;70:139-47.
49. Banks PA, Bollen TL, Dervenis C, Gooszen HG, Johnson CD, Sarr MG, et al. Classification of acute pancreatitis—2012: revision of the Atlanta classification and definitions by international consensus. Gut. 2013;62:102-11.
50. Tenner S, Baillie J, DeWitt J, Vege SS; American College of Gastroenterology. American College of Gastroenterology guideline: management of acute pancreatitis. Am J Gastroenterol. 2013;108:1400-16.
51. Working Group IAP/APA Acute Pancreatitis Guidelines. IAP/APA evidence based guidelines for the management of acute pancreatitis. Pancreatology. 2013;13(Suppl 2):e1-5.
52. Johnson CD, Abu-Hilal M. Persistent organ failure during the first week as a marker of fatal outcome in acute pancreatitis. Gut. 2004;53:1340-4.
53. Maitland K, Kiguli S, Opoka RO, Engoru C, Olupot-Olupot P, Akech SO, et al. Mortality after fluid bolus in African children with severe infection. N Engl J Med. 2011;364:2483-95.
54. Todd J, Heyderman RS, Musoke P, Peto T. When enough is enough: how the decision was made to stop the FEAST trial: data and safety monitoring in an African trial of fluid expansion as supportive therapy (FEAST) for critically ill children. Trials. 2013;14:85.
55. Zaccherini G, Weiss E, Moreau R. Acute-on-chronic liver failure: Definitions, pathophysiology and principles of treatment. JHEP Rep. 2020;3(1):100176.
56. Karvellas CJ, Bajaj JS, Kamath PS, Napolitano L, O'Leary JG, Solà E, et al. AASLD Practice Guidance on Acute-on-chronic liver failure and the Management of critically ill patients with cirrhosis. Hepatology. 2024;79(6):1463-502.
57. Amathieu R, Al-Khafaji A, Sileanu FE, Foldes E, DeSensi R, Hilmi I, et al. Significance of oliguria in critically ill patients with chronic liver disease. Hepatology. 2017;66(5):1592-600.
58. Maiwall R, Singh SP, Angeli P, Moreau R, Krag A, Singh V, et al. APASL clinical practice guidelines on the management of acute kidney injury in acute-on-chronic liver failure. Hepatol Int. 2024;18(3):833-69.
59. Karakike E, Moreno C, Gustot T. Infections in severe alcoholic hepatitis. Ann Gastroenterol. 2017;30(2):152-60.
60. Otero Sanchez L, Karakike E, Njimi H, Putignano A, Degré D, Hites M, et al. Clinical Course and Risk Factors for Infection in Severe Forms of Alcohol-Associated Liver Disease. Hepatology. 2021;74(5):2714-24.
61. Louvet A, Labreuche J, Dao T, Thévenot T, Oberti F, Bureau C, et al. Effect of prophylactic antibiotics on mortality in severe alcohol-related hepatitis: a randomized clinical trial. JAMA. 2023;329(18):1558-66.
62. Healey MA, Ramalingam G, Hang Y, Smirnova E, Asgharpour A, Patel V, et al. Utility of Lille Score in Predicting 30-Day Survival in Steroid-Treated Alcohol-Associated Hepatitis. Dig Dis Sci. 2024;69(8):3043-50.
63. Healey M, Sterling RK. Outnumbered: control prothrombin time in Maddrey's discriminant function impacts steroid use but not mortality in alcoholic hepatitis. Biology. 2022;11:1833.

64. Morales-Arraez D, Ventura-Cots M, Altamirano J, Abraldes JG, Cruz-Lemini M, Thursz MR, et al. The MELD score is superior to the Maddrey discriminant function score to predict short-term mortality in alcohol-associated hepatitis: a global study. Am J Gastroenterol. 2022;117:301-10.
65. Louvet A, Labreuche J, Artru F, Boursier J, Kim DJ, O'Grady J, et al. Combining data from liver disease scoring systems better predicts outcomes of patients with alcoholic hepatitis. Gastroenterology. 2015;149:398-406.e8.
66. Kamath PS, Therneau T, Shah VH. MELDing the Lille score to more accurately predict mortality in alcoholic hepatitis. Gastroenterology. 2015;149:281-3.
67. Forrest EH, Evans CD, Stewart S, Phillips M, Oo YH, McAvoy NC, et al. Analysis of factors predictive of mortality in alcoholic hepatitis and derivation and validation of the Glasgow alcoholic hepatitis score. Gut. 2005;54:1174-9.
68. Božin T, Rob Z, Lucijanić M, Čmarec Buhin L, Grgurević I. Comparison of prognostic scores for alcoholic hepatitis: a retrospective study. Croat Med J. 2021;62:17-24.
69. Sarin SK, Sharma S. Predictors of steroid non-response and new approaches in severe alcoholic hepatitis. Clin Mol Hepatol. 2020;26:639-51.
70. Marot A, Singal AK, Moreno C, Deltenre P. Granulocyte colony-stimulating factor for alcoholic hepatitis: a systematic review and meta-analysis of randomised controlled trials. JHEP Rep. 2020;2(5):100139.
71. Chi X, Pan CQ, Liu S, Cheng D, Cao Z, Xing H. Regulating Intestinal Microbiota in the Prevention and Treatment of Alcohol-Related Liver Disease. Can J Gastroenterol Hepatol. 2020;2020:6629196.
72. Philips CA, Ahamed R, Rajesh S, Abduljaleel JKP, Augustine P. Long-term outcomes of stool transplant in alcohol-associated hepatitis—analysis of clinical outcomes, relapse, gut microbiota and comparisons with standard care. J Clin Exp Hepatol. 2022;12(4):1124-32.
73. Frances C, Durand F, Kahn JA, Genyk YS, Nadim MK. Hepatorenal syndrome. Clin J Am Soc Nephrol. 2019;14:774-81.
74. Gines P, Schrier RW. Renal failure in cirrhosis. N Engl J Med. 2009;361:1279-90.
75. Arora V, Maiwall R, Rajan V, Jindal A, Muralikrishna Shasthry S, Kumar G, et al. Terlipressin is superior to noradrenaline in the management of acute kidney injury in acute on chronic liver failure. Hepatology. 2020;71:600-10.
76. Ortega R, Ginès P, Uris J, Cárdenas A, Calahorra B, De Las Heras D, et al. Terlipressin therapy with and without albumin for patients with hepatorenal syndrome: results of a prospective, nonrandomized study. Hepatology. 2002;36:941-8.
77. European Association for the Study of the Liver. Electronic address epee, European Association for the Study of the L. EASL Clinical Practice Guidelines for the management of patients with decompensated cirrhosis. J Hepatol. 2018;69:406-60.
78. Moore K, Jamil K, Verleger K, Luo L, Kebede N, Heisen M, et al. Real-world treatment patterns and outcomes using terlipressin in 203 patients with hepatorenal syndrome. Aliment Pharmacol Ther. 2020;52:351-8.
79. Curry MP, Vargas HE, Befeler AS, Pyrsopoulos NT, Patwardhan VR, Jamil K. Early treatment with terlipressin in patients with hepatorenal syndrome yields improved clinical outcomes in North American studies. Hepatol Commun. 2023;7:e1307.
80. Administration USF, Drug. (2023). Highlights of Prescribing Information. [online] Available from https://www.accessdata.fda.gov/drugsatfda_docs/label/2023/216718Orig1s000lbl.pdf [Last accessed January, 2023].
81. European Association for the Study of the Liver. EASL clinical practice guidelines on the management of ascites, spontaneous bacterial peritonitis, and hepatorenal syndrome in cirrhosis. J Hepatol. 2010;53:397-417.
82. Tschuor C, Ferrarese A, Kuemmerli C, Dutkowski P, Burra P, Clavien PA.; Liver

Allocation Study Group. Allocation of liver grafts worldwide - Is there a best system? J Hepatol. 2019;71:707-18.

83. Sharma P, Moore K, Ganger D, Grewal P, Brown RS, Jr. Role of Terlipressin and Albumin for Hepatorenal Syndrome in Liver Transplantation. Liver Transp. 2020;26: 1328-36.
84. Piano S, Morando F, Fasolato S, Cavallin M, Boscato N, Boccagni P, et al. Continuous recurrence of type 1 hepatorenal syndrome and long-term treatment with terlipressin and albumin: a new exception to MELD score in the allocation system to liver transplantation? J Hepatol. 2011;55:491-6.
85. Piano S, Gambino C, Vettore E, Calvino V, Tonon M, Boccagni P, et al. Response to Terlipressin and Albumin Is Associated With Improved Liver Transplant Outcomes in Patients With Hepatorenal Syndrome. Hepatology. 2021;73:1909-19.
86. Cillo U, Burra P, Mazzaferro V, Belli L, Pinna AD, Spada M, et al. A Multistep, Consensus-Based Approach to Organ Allocation in Liver Transplantation: Toward a "Blended Principle Model". Am J Transplant. 2015;15: 2552-61.

SECTION

5

Nephrology Section

Section Editor: *Kanwalpreet Sodhi*

Associate Editors: *Manu Gupta, Atul Phillips*

Continuous Renal Replacement Therapy and Survival in Acute Liver Failure: A Systematic Review and Meta-analysis.[1]

Dong V, Robinson AM, Dionne JC, Cardoso FS, Rewa OG, Karvellas CJ. Continuous renal replacement therapy and survival in acute liver failure: A systematic review and meta-analysis.

J Crit Care. 2024;81:154513.

BACKGROUND: WHAT IS KNOWN?

Acute liver failure (ALF) is marked by a swift decline in liver function and is defined as the occurrence of hepatic encephalopathy (HE) within 26 weeks of the initial appearance of jaundice in individuals without preexisting chronic liver disease. It manifests with jaundice, coagulopathy, HE, and may progress to multiorgan failure (MOF). Without emergency, liver transplantation (LT) the mortality is almost 50%. Cerebral edema driven by hyperammonemia is the key contributor to developing cerebral edema which is main mechanism of death in ALF.

Among the several strategies that are available for reduction of ammonia, more recently continuous renal replacement therapy (CRRT) has been shown to improve ammonia levels in critically ill adult patients.[2] Specifically in the ALF population, CRRT is associated with a decline in serum ammonia and improvement in transplant-free survival.[3,4] However, the role of CRRT in ALF is still not well established and further data is needed.

CLINICAL QUESTION

Does the use of CRRT in ALF patients associated with lower mortality and transplant-free survival?

STUDY DESIGN

This systematic review and meta-analysis are reported in accordance with the Preferred Reporting Items for Systematic Reviews and Meta-analysis (PRISMA) and Meta-analysis of Observational Studies in Epidemiology (MOOSE) (PROSPERO ID: CRD42019122520)

Search strategy: Studies were searched from electronic databases from 1990 to 2023: MEDLINE, EMBASE, Cochrane Library, and Web of Science. Additional searches through ClinicalTrials.gov and the Conference Proceedings Citation Index were undertaken for gray literature citations.

MATERIAL/METHODS

- *Inclusion criteria*: Adult patients (aged 18 years or older) admitted to an intensive care unit (ICU) with a diagnosis of ALF.
- *Exclusion criteria:* Studies were excluded if they:
    - Involved patients with chronic liver disease
    - Used another form of ammonia lowering therapy such as Molecular adsorbent recirculating system (MARS) or plasma exchange
- *Methods:* Intervention was the use of any form of CRRT for one or more indications such as acute kidney injury (AKI) or hyperammonemia with the comparator being standard care without the use of renal replacement therapy (RRT).

STUDY ENDPOINTS

The outcomes of interest were:

- Overall survival
- Transplant-free survival
- Reduction in serum ammonia levels

RESULTS

The initial search resulted in 1,702 citations with 55 potentially eligible studies undergoing full-text review leading to ultimately 11 eligible studies being included. All studies were observational cohort studies: seven studies were retrospective cohort studies and four were prospective cohort studies. Mortality was either a primary or secondary outcome in eight of the studies, ammonia reduction was either a primary or secondary outcome in eight of the studies, and reversal of HE was an outcome in one of the studies.

- Overall, patients who underwent CRRT had higher severity of illness with higher rates of organ support (mechanical ventilation and vasopressor use), higher severity scores (APACHE III), higher rates of high-grade encephalopathy (grade 3 or 4), higher rates of AKI, and higher levels of different biochemical markers (creatinine, lactate, and ammonia).
- *Overall survival:*
    - Based on the pooled results, CRRT may improve overall survival [risk ratio (RR): 0.83, 95% confidence interval (CI): 0.73–0.93, *p*-value <0.001, I^2 = 18.77%]
- *ALF patients receiving CRRT had a 17% (95% CI: 7–27%)* increase in overall survival compared to those who did not receive CRRT.
- *Transplant-free survival:* Based on the pooled results, CRRT may improve transplant-free survival (RR: 0.73, 95% CI: 0.57–0.94, *p*-value 0.01, I^2 = 54.74%)
- *Overall mortality:* Based on the pooled results, standard medical therapy without CRRT may increase overall mortality (RR: 1.32, 95% CI: 0.93–1.86, *p*-value 0.12, I^2 = 23.28%). Standard medical therapy without CRRT may still increase overall mortality (RR: 1.69, 95% CI: 0.34–8.43, *p*-value 0.52, I^2 = 46.60%) with lack of CRRT leading to a 69% increase in mortality.
- *Ammonia clearance:* Ammonia clearance data was not able to be pooled and not analyzable via meta-analysis due to variation in its being reported as mean and median.

AUTHORS' VIEWPOINT

- Overall, low certainty evidence of overall survival benefit and transplant-free survival benefit with the use of CRRT compared to standard medical care without the use of CRRT
- CRRT is the RRT of choice in critically ill patients as these patients are often hemodynamically unstable or have increased intracranial pressures and

are safer as compared to intermittent hemodialysis (IHD).
- CRRT is not without complications and is associated with higher rates of high-grade encephalopathy, mechanical ventilation, and vasopressor support compared to patients not started on CRRT. However, when adjusting for degree of illness, CRRT was associated with a significant decrease in mortality.

STRENGTHS

- Inclusion of a preregistered protocol, ensuring transparency and adherence to planned methodology
- A thorough literature search that incorporates the most recent studies, including both published articles and abstracts
- Rigorous methodology with duplicate and independent screening, data collection, and a formal quality assessment of the included studies and evidence
- A large patient population, enhancing the robustness and generalizability of the findings

LIMITATIONS

- The absence of randomized controlled trials (RCTs), with the review relying solely on cohort studies
- High risk of bias across all included studies, leading to an overall low quality of evidence
- Most studies are from the US, UK, and Australia, where acetaminophen toxicity is a predominant cause of ALF, resulting in the majority of included patients exhibiting a hyperacute phenotype.
- The hyperacute phenotype is more likely to require intensive care and organ support and to survive without transplantation, introducing a bias toward better survival outcomes with CRRT and reducing the certainty of the findings.
- Two studies have overlapping time periods, potentially causing duplication of patients in the meta-analysis of transplant-free survival.
- Inability to pool and analyze data on ammonia reduction, limiting evidence on the impact of CRRT on ammonia levels
- Moderate heterogeneity in the pooled data for overall survival
- Lack of analysis comparing different CRRT effluent rates for ammonia clearance and outcomes in ALF patients.

REVIEWERS' VIEWPOINT

- Hyperammonemia (defined as arterial ammonia levels ≥85 μmol/L for 3 days) is associated with greater risk of cerebral edema.
- Hyperammonemia also appears to affect posttransplant survival in patients with ALF.
- CRRT may remove several mediators involved in the formation of cerebral edema.
- Ammonia is the only readily measured solute in ALF patients and is therefore emphasized clinically as a major driver in cerebral edema.
- Studies were mostly observational with retrospective data, with high degree of heterogeneity.

TAKE HOME MESSAGE

This study highlights the use of CRRT in rightly selected patient population can be an important bridge to definitive therapy such as LT and hence can be considered in patients with ALF and ammonia levels >85 mg/dL being planned for LT.

Doppler-based Evaluation of Intrarenal Venous Flow as a New Tool to Predict Acute Kidney Injury: A Systematic Review and Meta-analysis.[5]

Bianchi Bosisio NSM, Romero-González G, De Silvestri A, Husain-Syad F, Ferrari F. Doppler-based evaluation of intrarenal venous flow as a new tool to predict acute kidney injury: A systematic review and meta-analysis.

Nefrologia (Engl Ed). 2023;43(Suppl 2):57-66.

BACKGROUND: WHAT IS KNOWN?

While renal hypoperfusion has been long known as a mechanism of renal failure, congestive nephropathy (CN) which occurs due to transmission of increased central venous pressure to low-resistance renal vessels, increases renal afterload and intra-renal pressure, resulting in renal dysfunction. An increase in pressure reduces renal perfusion and intra-tubular flow, resulting in decreased glomerular filtration rate (GFR), increased sodium and water retention through activation of the renin-angiotensin-aldosterone system, and tubular damage due to inflammatory mechanisms.[6] In the ICU, factors such as fluid overload, positive pressure mechanical ventilation, right ventricular failure, and pulmonary hypertension contribute to elevated central venous pressures. Congestion, a frequent complication in critical care, increases the risk of AKI in these patients. Recently, CN has been identified as a mechanism for worsening renal function, with pulsed Doppler (PD) evaluation of renal venous flow proving to be a valuable tool for detecting renal vein congestion.[7]

Doppler imaging enables the detection of increased renal venous congestion by analysing renal venous waveforms. Discontinuous intrarenal venous flow (IRVF) patterns indicate increased compliance of the renal parenchyma and venous vessels due to elevated venous pressure within the encapsulated kidney.[8] Doppler-based ultrasonography indices offer a noninvasive approach with high clinical feasibility and acceptable reproducibility for assessing IRVF.[9]

Renal resistive index (RRI) and IRVF are key parameters used to evaluate renal perfusion and congestion. In the kidneys, which are encapsulated organs, interstitial edema resulting from renal insult increases subcapsular pressure, leading to reduced renal perfusion, decreased vascular compliance, and elevated RRI. Furthermore, the kidneys may also be impacted by increased intra-abdominal pressure, which can arise from abdominal abnormalities or the transmission of raised airway pressure from stiffened lungs through the diaphragm.[8] In such cases, IRVF can be particularly useful, as it reflects increased pressure within a closed compartment such as Gerota's capsule. Ultrasound waveforms not only help to identify kidney injury but can also provide insights into the severity of congestion.

CLINICAL QUESTION

Does assessment of renal hemodynamics using Doppler ultrasonography predict AKI?

STUDY DESIGN

This is a systematic review and meta-analysis that was performed according to the general principles of the MOOSE statement.

There are public-domain databases which include PubMed, MEDLINE, Scopus, Embase, and the Cochrane Library. For the search, medical subject headings (MeSH) terms and text words were used with the Boolean strategy, and cross-searches were performed with the following three categories:

1. Disease ("acute renal failure", "acute kidney injury", etc.)
2. Tools ("renal Doppler", "renal vascular Doppler", etc.)
3. Setting ("ICU", "critical care", etc.)

They evaluated the association between Doppler-based IRVF demodulation and AKI. CN was defined as the presence of a pulsatile pattern (biphasic or monophasic) in the PD.

The study design included prospective and retrospective observational studies and randomized clinical trials, restricted to articles published in English and studies on humans published between the 1st of January 2000 and the 31st of December 2021.

The literature search yielded 1,143 potentially relevant articles, 182 were removed as duplicates, 848 were excluded because they were irrelevant based on the scope of this review, 109 were excluded because they did not include Doppler-based IRVF evaluation. Finally, 4 articles were analyzed.

POPULATION

The study focused on critically ill adult patients aged >18 years admitted to any type of ICU. Patients with end-stage chronic kidney disease (CKD) or a history of renal transplantation were excluded. The "intervention" involved performing renal pulsed Doppler (RPD) to assess venous patterns at the time of ICU admission, with the comparison being the relationship between IRVF patterns and the occurrence of AKI.

RESULTS

- All the four included studies were single-center prospective cohort studies, conducted between 2016 and 2020 and enrolled a total of 660 patients.
- Two studies done in Europe included 60.75% of patients and two studies done in North America included rest 39.25% of patients.
- 67.72% were males and ethnicity wise Caucasians were the most common (50.90%), followed by Africans (42.90%) and Asians (1.8%).
- 275 (41.67%) were scheduled for surgery of whom 145 underwent elective cardiac surgery.
- Severity score was determined in two studies; both studies reported the sequential organ failure assessment (SOFA) score to range from 7 to 8.
- Majority of patients were in mixed ICU, and 21.97% were in postcardiac surgery ICU.
- Three studies defined AKI according to Kidney Disease: Improving Global Outcomes (KDIGO) guidelines without introducing any definition of the baseline serum creatinine (SCr) level and one study used estimated glomerular filtration rate (eGFR) with the Modification of Diet in Renal Disease (MDRD) formula.
- Due to better accessibility, hemodynamics of the right kidney was assessed in all studies.
- RPD examination was performed by investigators trained in RPD.
- Three studies reported that the venous renal RPD signal was inadequate. This meant that 162 (24.54%) of the patients did not have an IRVF evaluation. The timing of RPD assessment was between 13 and 24 hours.
- AKI occurrence and Doppler-based evaluation of IRVF for the prediction of AKI.
- The Youden index analysis showed that RRI >0.71 was the best cut-off value to predict AKI (sensitivity 90% and specificity 100%). The RRI was also a predictor for

RRT (best cut-off 0.77; sensitivity 80% and specificity 92%).

- One study demonstrated an association between monophasic venous flow and any AKI stage [hazard ratio (HR): 2.81; 95% CI: 1.42–5.56; $p = 0.003$], while a second study described a higher percentage of an impaired IRVF (13/13 in AKI group vs. 1/17 in no AKI group; $p < 0.001$) in the patients who developed AKI.
- A significant difference between patients who had RPD continuous flow and demodulated IRVF (RR: 0.46; 95% CI: 0.28–0.76). Further, results revealed significant heterogeneity across the studies ($I^2 = 68.7\%$; 95% CI: 0–90, $p = 0.04$).
- No study analyzed the association between the IRVF patterns and the etiology of AKI or with the renal recovery.

AUTHORS' VIEWPOINTS

- Serum creatinine, which is a marker of AKI, does not rise till considerable nephron damage has occurred and has poor specificity and does not have prognostic significance.
- Ultrasound-detected waveforms hold prognostic value and can serve as a noninvasive tool to monitor the effectiveness of therapeutic interventions.
- Additionally, point-of-care ultrasonography (POCUS), performed by experts at the patient's bedside, allows for the immediate clinical integration of imaging data, facilitating prompt decision-making.
- Patients with continuous IRVF demonstrated less than half the risk of developing AKI compared to those with demodulated IRVF.

STRENGTHS

Interobserver reproducibility between a senior and inexperienced operator is good and the measures seem accurate (as indicated by the absence of systematic bias in the reviewed studies), although a lack of precision was found (based on an interobserver 95% CI of ± 0.1).

LIMITATIONS

- *Heterogeneous results:* Nonuniformity in target population: older age group (55–67 years), male preponderance, difference in severity of illness based on SOFA score.
- Diagnosis for which the patient was admitted to the ICU was not clearly defined in 241 cases (36.52%) and there was no diagnosis at admission in 92 (13.94%) patients.
- RPD examination could not be performed in 24.54% of the patients, but the authors did not clearly explain the reason—lists the feasibility and generalizability of the review.

REVIEWERS' VIEWPOINTS

It has been given that available biomarkers are only able to diagnose AKI and not predict progression of AKI, measuring renal hemodynamics can be a valuable bedside tool in monitoring the progression of AKI and also to titrate therapy to prevent or delay the onset of AKI.

This systematic review provides some insights into yet another use of POCUS in the ICU, however, the results need to be validated in larger trials. Nonetheless, it will not stop me from learning and using this technique to screen my at-risk patients.

TAKE HOME MESSAGE

Renal ultrasonography assessment of renal hemodynamics is useful for detecting venous congestion and predicting AKI. IRVF is easy to use, reproducible, feasible, and modality requiring minimum training.

Automated Electronic Alert for the Care and Outcomes of Adults with Acute Kidney Injury: A Randomized Clinical Trial.[10]

li T, Wu B, Li L, Bian A, Ni J, Liu K, et al. Automated electronic alert for the care and outcomes of adults with acute kidney injury: a randomized clinical trial.

JAMA Netw Open. 2024;7:e2351710.

BACKGROUND: WHAT IS KNOWN?

The occurrence of AKI increases the risk of in-hospital mortality and the development of cardiovascular disease and CKD, with substantial resource and economic implications. Early detection and prompt intervention are critical for improved patient outcomes.

The electronic AKI alert is a computerized algorithm that uses changes in SCr to identify AKI early. The AKI alert notifies clinicians of an AKI episode, allowing for prompt interventions. Nonrandomized trials reported improved patient-centered outcomes including AKI recovery, reduced mortality, and dialysis rate while randomized trials have suggested contrasting results.[11-14]

Medical education and practice patterns vary worldwide and it is unknown whether AKI alerts can benefit hospitalized patients, so this study was done with the objective to study whether early warning system for AKI in hospitals is expected to significantly improve the rate of timely diagnosis of AKI, reduce the use of nephrotoxic drugs, take early intervention measures such as blood volume supplementation, reduce the degree of kidney injury, and benefit the majority of hospitalized patients conducted in Chinese hospitalized patients.

CLINICAL QUESTION

Can an AKI alert combined with a care bundle improve the care and clinical outcomes of hospitalized patients with AKI?

STUDY DESIGN

Single-center, double-blind, and parallel-group RCT conducted from August 1, 2019, to December 31, 2021, in a tertiary teaching hospital in Nanjing, China.

POPULATION

- *Inclusion criteria:* Inpatient adults aged ≥18 years with AKI, defined according to the KDIGO creatinine criteria.
- *Exclusion criteria:*
    - Baseline eGFR lower than 15 mL/min/1.73 m^2
    - Admission diagnosed with end-stage kidney disease defined by the International Classification of Disease Coding 9 (ICD-9) and ICD-10
    - History of kidney transplantation
    - AKI occurring outside the hospital
    - Hospitalization for <24 hours
    - Baseline SCr lower than 0.5 mg/dL

INTERVENTION

Acute kidney injury alert was generated by comparing real-time SCr test results with historic SCr measurements.

- *AKI alert:* An AKI alert will send to the doctor in charge. The team of nephrologists would give suggestions if the doctor in charge needs a renal consultation.
- *Usual care:* Patients will receive standard clinical care by the doctor in charge.

The care bundle comprised general, nonindividualized, and nonmandatory AKI management measures. If a patient triggered multiple alerts of AKI, the message was sent up to a maximum of three times to prevent alert fatigue.

RESULTS

A total of 2,208 patients [median (IQR) age, 65 (54–72) years; 1,560 males (70.7%)] were randomized to the alert group ($n = 1{,}123$) or the usual care group ($n = 1{,}085$) and analyzed.

- *Primary outcome*:
  - Median [interquartile range (IQR)] maximum absolute changes in eGFR within 7 days after randomization were 3.7 (–6.4 to 19.3) mL/min/1.73 m^2 in the alert group and 2.9 (–9.2 to 16.9) mL/min/1.73 m^2 in the usual care group ($p = 0.24$).
  - No difference in the median (IQR) maximum relative changes in eGFR within 7 days after randomization between the alert and usual care groups [9.4% (–14.8 to 47.0%) vs. 7.7% (–18.6 to 44.0%); $p = 0.26$].
- *Secondary outcome*:
  - No significant differences between the two groups in the median (IQR) maximum absolute changes in SCr level [0.0 (–0.5 to 0.2) mg/dL for both groups; $p = 0.59$] and maximum relative changes in SCr level [–1.9% (–33.5 to 15.0%) vs. –0.7% (–31.8 to 17.1%); $p = 0.40$) within 7 days after randomization.
  - No statistically significant differences between the two groups in other patient-centered secondary outcomes, including in-hospital death, in-hospital dialysis, dialysis within 7 days, death within 7 days, death within 28 days, death within 90 days, in-hospital AKI progression, highest AKI stage achieved, AKI recovery at discharge, and incidence of being alive with dialysis dependency at 90 days.
- *Effect of AKI alerts on patient care outcomes:* Within 2 days after randomization, there was:
  - Significantly higher number of patients receiving intravenous fluids in the alert group compared with the usual care group [927 patients (82.6%) vs. 670 patients (61.8%); $p < 0.001$].
  - Higher number of patients with urinalysis [407 (36.2%) vs. 141 (13.0%); $p < 0.001$], fluid intake and output measurements [995 (88.6%) vs. 743 (68.5%); $p < 0.001$], subsequent SCr level measurement [1039 (92.5%) vs. 814 (75.0%); $p < 0.001$], kidney ultrasonography [59 (5.3%) vs. 6 (0.6%); $p < 0.001$], and correcting anemia by reaching hemoglobin level over 9.0 g/dL [517 (46.0%) vs. 252 (23.2%); $p < 0.001$] in the alert group compared with the usual care group.
  - No significant difference was found between the groups in terms of nephrologist consultation rates overall.
  - More patients in the usual care group than in the alert group were exposed to nonsteroidal anti-inflammatory drugs within 3 days [119 (11.0%) vs. 56 (5.0%); $p < 0.001$] or 7 days [134 (12.4%) vs. 72 (6.4%); $p < 0.001$] after randomization.
  - No significant differences were noted between the two groups in terms of the other nephrotoxins, including contrast, aminoglycoside, vancomycin, chemotherapy, and angiotensin-converting enzyme inhibitor and angiotensin receptor blocker at 3 and 7 days after randomization.
  - Compared with the usual care group, the alert group had more AKI documentation at discharge [560

patients (49.9%) vs. 296 patients (27.3%); $p < 0.001$].
- No significant differences in length of stay (LOS) and hospital total costs were observed between the groups.

- *Posthoc analysis*:
  - Patients with baseline eGFR of 60 mL/min/1.73 m^2 or higher [odds ratio (OR): 1.37; 95% CI: 1.05–1.78; $p = 0.02$] or patients in the surgical ICU (OR: 1.54; 95% CI: 1.08–2.20; $p = 0.02$) had a significantly higher risk of in-hospital dialysis in the alert group compared with the usual care group.
  - There was no difference in median hospital total cost, LOS, and nephrologist consultation between the alert group and the usual care group according to the AKI stage at randomization.

AUTHORS' VIEWPOINTS

Largest RCT conducted in Chinese population that showed that AKI alert combined with clinical care increased the proportion of patients receiving multiple interventions and diagnostic rate of AKI. The AKI alert was associated with increased fluid resuscitation, discontinuation of nephrotoxic medications, optimization of hemodynamic parameters, and timely nephrologist's consultation. This led to consistently increased rate of dialysis in surgical ICUs. Fluid resuscitation might have contributed to an elevated dialysis rate due to excessive fluid accumulation.

LIMITATIONS

- This was a single-center trial, and the findings may be influenced by the specific characteristics of the population and hospital, limiting their generalizability.
- The care bundle included general, nonindividualized, and nonmandatory measures, potentially reducing the effectiveness of the AKI alert system
- Despite some efforts, measures taken may not have been sufficient to prevent warning fatigue among healthcare providers.
- Urine output was not recorded for most patients during hospitalization, and the AKI alerts were based solely on the KDIGO creatinine criteria, which may have led to an underestimation of the true incidence of AKI.
- Due to the absence of universally accepted markers for kidney function in AKI, the study used the maximum change in eGFR or SCr levels within 7 days postrandomization, along with secondary outcomes, to minimize errors in assessing kidney function.

REVIEWERS' COMMENTS

This was a well-conducted study, which found that AKI alert was associated with a higher rate of dialysis. This was mainly due to excessive fluid resuscitation and seen in patients in surgical ICUs while the rate of dialysis was similar in medical ICUs. The surgical patients are at a higher risk of developing AKI and the type of surgery they underwent (cardiac vs. noncardiac), particularly cardiac surgery poses a higher risk of AKI, was not specified in the trial. Also, more patients with risk factors (diabetic and hypertension) were seen in the alert AKI group. These unmatched findings could have potentially confounded the results.

TAKE HOME MESSAGE

Although electronic AKI alerts do not directly improve kidney function or other patient-centered outcomes, they can influence care behaviors, potentially affecting short-term outcomes. These findings highlight the need for future research to combine high-quality interventions with AKI alerts to optimize their effectiveness before integrating them into routine clinical practice.

A Randomized Trial of Intravenous Amino Acids for Kidney Protection[15]

Iandoni G, Monaco F, Ti LK, Baiardo Redaelli M, Bradic N, Comis M, et al. A randomized trial of intravenous amino acids for kidney protection.

N Engl J Med. 2024;391:687-98.

BACKGROUND: WHAT IS ALREADY KNOWN?

In healthy adults, a high-protein meal enhances GFR by increasing renal blood flow through afferent arteriolar dilation. While a prolonged high-protein diet can accelerate CKD progression, short-term amino acid infusion in animal models has shown protective effects against acute ischemic kidney injuries, potentially preserving nephroprotection even during critical illness. Amino acids, especially glycine and arginine, have significant physiological effects on the kidneys, including increasing nephron blood flow by reducing afferent arteriolar resistance, decreasing tubuloglomerular feedback activation, and enhancing cortical nitric oxide synthase activity. In animal studies, amino acid infusions have been shown to boost renal perfusion, oxygenation, and GFR.

A 1973 clinical trial with 53 critically ill patients found that short-term amino acid infusion accelerated recovery from acute renal failure. A 2007 trial involving 14 critically ill patients with low creatinine clearance showed that higher doses of amino acids preserved diuresis and reduced the need for furosemide. Additionally, a subgroup analysis from a cluster RCT indicated that critically ill patients with high renal dysfunction risk who received higher protein intake were less likely to require RRT.[15-18]

Acute kidney injury is a frequent complication following cardiovascular surgery, occurring in over 40% of cases, a rate comparable to that in ICU patients. Both groups share similar risk factors for developing AKI. Hence, it was decided to include this multicenter randomized trial for this series of critical care reviews.

CLINICAL QUESTION

In adult patients undergoing elective cardiac surgery with cardiopulmonary bypass, does the administration of intravenous amino acids reduce the incidence and severity of AKI compared to a placebo (Ringer's solution)? This study aims to evaluate the efficacy of intravenous amino acid therapy in preventing AKI following cardiac surgery.

METHODS

- *Trial design*:
  - Multinational, double-blind, randomized, and placebo-controlled trial
  - Conducted at 22 centers across three countries
  - Ethics approval obtained from each participating center
  - Funded by the Italian Ministry of Health
- *Participants*: Adult patients scheduled for elective cardiac surgery with cardiopulmonary bypass.
- *Inclusion criteria:*
  - Aged 18 years or older
  - Expected to stay in the ICU for at least one night postsurgery
- *Exclusion criteria:*
  - Preoperative dialysis dependence or planned treatment with intermittent

  or continuous kidney replacement therapy (CKRT)
- Stage IV or greater CKD (eGFR <30 mL/min/1.73 m^2)
- Patients not expected to survive
- Patients with renal transplant

- *Randomization and blinding:*
  - *Patients were randomly assigned to receive either:*
    - Intravenous infusion of amino acids (2 g/kg ideal body weight/day)
    - Placebo (Ringer's solution)
    - Randomization was web-based with computer-generated sequences.
    - *Double-blind setup:* Patients, clinicians, and outcome assessors were unaware of group assignments.
- *Intervention:*
  - *The amino acid group:* Continuous infusion of a balanced mixture of amino acids at a dose of 2 g/kg/day (up to a maximum of 100 g/day) from the time of central venous catheter (CVC) insertion in the operating room. The infusion ran for up to 72 hours, or until discharge from the ICU, initiation of kidney-replacement therapy, or death (whichever occurred first).
  - The formulation was Isopuramin 10% (Baxter).
  - The median duration of the infusion was 30 hours with a median dose of 126 g of amino acids. The median infusion rate was 40 mL/hour.
- *Control:* The placebo group—continuous infusion of Ringer's solution at the same rate as the intervention group such that fluid input was identical, with the median infusion rate of 40 mL/hour.

OUTCOMES

- *Primary outcome:* Occurrence of AKI within the first week of postsurgery, defined by KDIGO creatinine criteria.
- *Secondary outcomes:* Severity of AKI, use and duration of RRT, ICU/hospital stay duration, and mortality at 30, 90, and 180 days.
- *Data collection and follow-up:*
  - Data on baseline characteristics, surgical procedures, and postoperative outcomes were collected.
  - SCr levels measured for up to 7 days postsurgery.
  - Follow-up conducted at 30, 90, and 180 days postrandomization to assess vital status.

RESULTS

- *Patient enrollment and baseline characteristics:*
  - *Total enrolled:* 3,511 patients across 22 centers
  - *Randomization:*
    - 1,759 patients assigned to the amino acid group
    - 1,752 patients assigned to the placebo group
  - *Baseline characteristics:*
    - Similar demographic and clinical characteristics between both groups
    - *Median age:* 66 years (amino acid group) and 67 years (placebo group)
    - Balanced distribution of sex, body mass index (BMI), and preoperative conditions
- *Primary outcome:*
  - *Occurrence of AKI:*
    - AKI occurred in 26.9% of the amino acid group and 31.7% of the placebo group, with relative risk (RR): 0.85 (95% CI: 0.77–0.94; $p = 0.002$).
    - *Stage 1 AKI:* 430 (24.4%) versus 492 (28.1%), RR: 0.87 (0.78–0.97)
    - *Stage 2 AKI:* 15 (0.9%) versus 11 (0.6%), RR: 1.36 (0.63–2.95)
    - *Stage 3 AKI:* 29 (1.6%) versus 52 (3.0%), RR: 0.56 (0.35–0.87)

- *Secondary outcomes:* There were no substantial differences between the two groups in other secondary outcomes
  - *Kidney replacement therapy (KRT):*
    - It is used in 1.4% of the amino acid group and 1.9% of the placebo group ($p > 0.05$).
    - Median duration of therapy: 64 hours in both groups ($p > 0.05$)
  - *ICU and hospital stay:*
    - *Median ICU stay:* 30 hours (amino acid group) versus 34 hours (placebo group) ($p > 0.05$).
    - *Median hospital stay:* 7 nights in both groups ($p > 0.05$).
  - *Mechanical ventilation: Median duration:* 11 hours for both groups ($p > 0.05$).
  - *Mortality:*
    - *30-day mortality:* 2.8% in both groups ($p > 0.05$).
    - *90-day mortality:* 3.2% (amino acid group) versus 3.0% (placebo group) ($p > 0.05$).
    - *180-day mortality:* 3.9% in both groups ($p > 0.05$).
- *Subgroup and sensitivity analyses:*
  - *Subgroup analyses:* Consistent results across age, heart failure class, and baseline eGFR.
  - *Sensitivity analyses:*
    - Results remained consistent in per-protocol and as-treated analyses
    - No significant differences in AKI incidence between trial centers
- *Safety and adverse events:* No significant differences in adverse events between the groups.
  - Similar rates of sepsis, surgical revision for bleeding, and ICU readmission.

AUTHORS' CONCLUSION

The authors concluded that in adult patients undergoing elective cardiac surgery with cardiopulmonary bypass, the continuous infusion of amino acids significantly reduced the overall occurrence of AKI compared to a placebo. This reduction in AKI was observed without an increase in adverse events, indicating that amino acid infusion is a safe and effective intervention for kidney protection in this high-risk population. The findings are particularly relevant given the high incidence of AKI following cardiac surgery and the associated risks of long-term kidney damage and mortality. The authors suggest that these results could have significant clinical implications for improving postoperative outcomes in cardiac surgery patients.

STRENGTHS

- *Large sample size:* The study enrolled 3,511 patients, providing sufficient power to detect significant differences between groups.
- *Multinational design:* It was conducted across 22 centers in three countries, enhancing the generalizability of the findings.
- *Double-blind and randomized design:* The rigorous design reduces the risk of bias in the results, ensuring a reliable comparison between the amino acid and placebo groups.
- *Broad inclusion criteria:* The study included a representative population of adult patients undergoing cardiac surgery, making the findings applicable to a wide range of patients.
- *Consistency of results:* The primary outcome and secondary outcomes were consistent across various subgroup analyses, supporting the robustness of the findings.
- *Well-controlled interventions:* Both the amino acid and placebo infusions were closely monitored, with adjustments made for nutritional intake to ensure consistent dosing.

LIMITATIONS

- *Single primary outcome measure:* The study relied solely on SCr levels to diagnose AKI, and details of glomerular filtration rate or urine output were not analyzed.
- *Lack of biomarker data:* Newly identified biomarkers of kidney injury were not included, which could have provided additional insights into subclinical AKI.
- *No strict protocol for AKI management:* While KDIGO guidelines were recommended, the absence of a strict protocol for managing AKI may have introduced variability in care across centers.
- *Protocol deviations:* Some patients experienced protocol deviations, such as undergoing off-pump surgery, which may have influenced the results.
- *Short follow-up period for long-term outcomes:* The study's follow-up period may not have been long enough to fully assess the long-term effects of amino acid infusion on kidney function and overall mortality.

REVIEWERS' VIEWPOINTS

The onset of AKI is linked to an extended stay in intensive care, a higher likelihood of developing CKD post-ICU, faster progression to end-stage kidney disease, and an increased risk of both short- and long-term mortality. Despite these serious implications, effective prevention strategies for AKI are still limited, highlighting the urgent need for more effective preventative measures.

This study presents a well-executed and methodologically sound investigation into the potential nephroprotective effects of amino acid infusion in patients undergoing cardiac surgery. The large sample size, rigorous double-blind randomized design, and inclusion of multiple centers across different countries lend considerable strength to the findings, making them robust and broadly applicable. However, most of the observed benefit was derived from a reduction in stage 1 AKI, raising questions about whether the amino acids genuinely protect kidney function or merely improve short-term SCr levels. This concern is further supported by the supplementary data showing no significant difference between groups in SCr levels at 30, 90, and 180 days, suggesting that the amino acid infusion may not confer long-term renal protection. Additionally, the absence of a more sensitive biomarker for renal injury and a lack of strict protocol for AKI management introduce potential variability in care across centers, which could influence outcomes. An economic analysis would also be valuable to assess the cost-effectiveness of this intervention. While the study contributes significantly to the field, future research should address these limitations to fully validate the benefits of amino acid infusion and explore its potential long-term impact and economic viability in diverse clinical settings.

TAKE HOME MESSAGE

While amino acid infusion shows promise in reducing AKI, its long-term benefits on renal function remain uncertain. The study highlights the need for further research to clarify whether the observed short-term improvements translate into genuine kidney protection and to assess the economic feasibility of widespread use. Careful consideration of these factors is essential before adopting amino acid infusion as a standard preventive measure for AKI in cardiac surgery patients.

Standard vs. Carbone Dioxide Adapted Kidney Replacement Therapy in Hypercapnic Ards Patients: A Randomized Controlled Pilot Trial (BigBIC).[19]

Kunz JV, Hansmann H, Fähndrich M, Pigorsch M, Bethke N, Peters H, et al. Standard vs. carbone dioxide adapted kidney replacement therapy in hypercapnic ARDS patients: a randomized controlled pilot trial (BigBIC).

Crit Care. 2024;28:198.

BACKGROUND: WHAT IS ALREADY KNOWN?

Permissive hypercapnia is an accompaniment of lung protective ventilation for acute respiratory distress syndrome (ARDS). But, the deleterious effects of this hypercapnia can be both pulmonary and/or extrapulmonary consequences including on the brain. In the lung, hypercapnia leads to lower pH, pulmonary vasoconstriction, increases in right ventricular afterload, acute cor pulmonale, and hypercapnic acidosis may further damage the lungs by increasing both nitric oxide production and inflammation and altering alveolar epithelial cells.[20] To relieve the native lungs of at least a portion of the carbon dioxide (CO_2), attempts have been made to mechanically increase alveolar ventilation with ventilatory support or direct CO_2 removal with the use of extracorporeal carbon dioxide removal (ECCO2R). Existing reviews suggest a potential advantage of CKRT-based buffering over intravenous drug buffering due to its slow and continuous regulation of acid-base balance while controlling fluid balance.[21]

CURRENT DILEMMA

More recent concept that has come up is to modify the acidosis by pCO_2-adapted-CKRT targeting the serum bicarbonate to physiological renal compensation for hypercapnia. Current CKRT protocols do not account for the physiological renal compensation of respiratory acidosis with no known clinical trial investigating the buffering of respiratory acidosis in ARDS patients on KRT.

CLINICAL QUESTION

A pilot study aimed to explore the feasibility, safety, and clinical benefits of pCO_2-adapted CKRT for hypercapnic ARDS patients with indication for CKRT.

STUDY DESIGN

A prospective, single-center, open-label, and randomized controlled pilot study.

MATERIAL AND METHODS

The study was conducted in five ICUs at three sites of the university hospital Charité in Berlin, Germany.

1. *Inclusion criteria*: The study population included patients aged ≥18 years with ARDS of any cause, on invasive mechanical ventilation with tidal volumes >4 mL/kg and respiratory rate ≥12/min, having hypercapnia with pCO_2 >7.33 kPa, on CKRT performed with regional citrate anticoagulation (RCA).
2. *Exclusion criteria*:
    - Patients on extracorporeal membrane oxygenation (ECMO)
    - Patients receiving TRIS-buffering
    - Patients with lactate acidosis (lactate >80 mg/dL) or liver failure, defined as bilirubin >8 mg/dL and INR >2.

3. *Methods*: 40 patients were enrolled and randomly assigned 1:1 of which:
   - 19 patients were randomized to the control group.
   - 21 patients were randomized to receive pCO_2-adapted CKRT.

Patients received either conventional care with bicarbonate targeted to 24 mmol/L or the study intervention with bicarbonate targeted to (1.33 kPa) × 4 mmol/L + 24 mmol/L according to the physiological renal compensation. Study duration was 6 days.

4. *Study endpoints*:
   - *Primary endpoint:* Bicarbonate after 72 hours
   - *Secondary outcomes:*
     - *Efficacy endpoint:* Kinetics of HCO_3^- concentrations measured every 12 hours
     - *Safety endpoints:*
       - Mortality during the intervention period of 6 days
       - Mortality until ICU discharge
       - 30-day mortality
       - Severe acidosis/alkalosis
       - Severe hypernatremia, severe hypo- or hypercalcemia, severe hypo- or hyperkalemia, and severe hypophosphatemia
       - Filter clotting
       - Citrate accumulation during the time of intervention of 6 days
     - *Clinical endpoints:* Median of the following parameters over the intervention period of 6 days:
       - pH
       - Tidal volumes, driving pressure, peak pressure, and respiratory minute volume
       - Catecholamine dose
       - Duration of mechanical ventilation
       - SOFA score
       - Daily blood flow and dialysate flow in RCA-CKRT
5. *Statistical analysis*: Sample size calculation was done using the Wilcoxon–Mann–Whitney rank sum test for continuous outcomes and the nQuery version 8.7.2 program. To demonstrate the effect with a power of 80% at a significance level of 5%, a sample size of 20 per group was calculated.

RESULTS

Among the 40 patients enrolled, 19 were randomized to the control group, and 21 to the pCO_2-adapted-CKRT group. Five patients were excluded prior to receiving treatment: three from the control group (one due to consent withdrawal and two for not meeting inclusion criteria) and two from the intervention group (one for not meeting inclusion criteria and one due to sudden unexpected death). These patients were not included in the final analysis.

The median plasma bicarbonate level 72 hours after randomization was significantly higher in the intervention group (30.70 mmol/L) compared to the control group (26.40 mmol/L; $p < 0.0001$). From day 3 onward, the survival rate was consistently higher in the intervention group throughout the 6-day study period and the 30-day observation period. By the end of the 6-day study period, 79% of individuals in the intervention group were alive compared to 69% in the control group. After 30 days, the survival rate remained higher in the intervention group, with 58% surviving versus 37% in the control group.

The log-rank test showed no significant difference in 30-day mortality between the groups, with 63% (10/16) mortality in the control group compared to 42% (8/19) in the intervention group ($p = 0.26$). However, a higher proportion of patients in the intervention group received lung-protective ventilation, and defined as a tidal volume <8 mL/kg of predicted body weight.

In the intervention group, tidal volumes were lower, and lung-protective ventilation was implemented more frequently. Additionally, there were no significant differences in safety endpoints between the two groups.

STRENGTHS

This study is the first to evaluate the effects of pCO_2-adapted CKRT, providing valuable insights into a simple and promising clinical approach, particularly for patients without the need for extracorporeal lung support. Given its potential benefits for patients with ARDS, future research could explore extending this intervention to a broader population with hypercapnia, including those with chronic obstructive pulmonary disease (COPD).

LIMITATIONS

- As a pilot trial, the study was primarily designed to assess feasibility and safety, and it was not powered to evaluate clinical endpoints.
- Being unblinded, the trial is subject to potential performance and detection biases.
- As an open-label study, the possibility of cointervention bias, particularly regarding lung-protective ventilation strategies, cannot be ruled out.
- The predominantly male composition of study participants limits the generalizability of the findings to female patients, as subgroup analyses were not performed.

AUTHORS' CONCLUSION

This randomized controlled pilot trial in hypercapnic ARDS patients undergoing RCA-CKRT demonstrated that targeting a pCO_2-tailored plasma bicarbonate concentration resulted in higher systemic bicarbonate levels, effectively simulating metabolic compensation for respiratory acidosis. The intervention group had lower tidal volumes and more frequent application of lung-protective ventilation. No significant differences in adverse events were observed. Mortality was higher in the control group compared to the intervention group. These findings indicate that pCO_2-adapted CKRT is both feasible and safe in this patient population.

REVIEWERS' COMMENTS

Existing literature suggests a potential advantage of CKRT-based buffering over intravenous drug buffering due to its slow and continuous regulation of acid–base balance while controlling fluid balance. Metabolic buffering via the RCA-CKRT might be a simple, cost-effective, and promising alternative as compared to ECCO2R being an expensive modality with potential complications.

TAKE HOME MESSAGE

pCO_2-adapted CKRT is a potentially feasible modality for better control of pH in ARDS patients with significant increase in bicarbonate. Further randomized control studies should be planned.

Initiation of Continuous Renal Replacement Therapy versus Intermittent Hemodialysis in Critically Ill Patients with Severe Acute Kidney Injury: A Secondary Analysis of STARRT-AKI Trial[22]

Wald R, Gaudry S, da Costa BR, Adhikari NKJ, Bellomo R, Du B, et al. Initiation of continuous renal replacement therapy versus intermittent hemodialysis in critically ill patients with severe acute kidney injury: a secondary analysis of STARRT-AKI trial.

Intensive Care Med. 2023;49:1305-16.

BACKGROUND: WHAT IS ALREADY KNOWN?

Renal replacement therapy remains a cornerstone in managing critically ill patients with AKI, which is a common and severe complication with a mortality rate exceeding 50%. Approximately 5–10% of these critically ill patients require RRT as a primary intervention. RRT substitutes kidney function in both acute and chronic renal failure, stabilizing mean arterial pressure, cerebrovascular, and renal perfusion, thus creating a conducive hemodynamic environment. Most patients who survive the critical phase are RRT-free at discharge.[24]

In critically ill patients with impaired renal filtration and resulting volume overload, daily fluid and electrolyte removal is essential. This is usually achieved via IHD or CRRT. While IHD can exacerbate hemodynamic instability due to rapid fluid and solute removal, CRRT offers a more gradual and continuous process, making it preferable for unstable patients. CRRT has demonstrated better renal recovery outcomes compared to IHD in AKI patients, though its superiority remains unproven. CRRT's limitations include prolonged immobilization, higher costs, resource needs, and the requirement for anticoagulation, all of which must be considered when choosing the appropriate RRT modality.[25,26]

CLINICAL QUESTION

Whether the initiation of CRRT versus IHD affects the outcomes in critically ill patients with severe AKI, specifically focusing on survival rates and dependence on RRT at 90 days.

METHODS

Study Design

- Post-hoc secondary analysis of the STARRT-AKI trial, a large, multinational, and RCT
- *Objective:* Evaluate the impact of timing in the initiation of CRRT-IHD on clinical outcomes in critically ill patients with severe AKI.

Participants

- *Population:* Critically ill patients with severe AKI who were enrolled in the STARRT-AKI trial.
- *Inclusion criteria:*
  - Adults aged 18 years or older
  - Patients admitted to the ICU with severe AKI defined by a doubling of SCr from baseline, a SCr level of ≥4 mg/dL, or urine output of <6 mL/kg over the preceding 12 hours
  - Initial RRT modality defined as either CRRT or IHD

- *Exclusion criteria:*
    - Patients with emergency indications for RRT
    - Prior RRT
    - Advanced CKD (GFR <20 mL/min/ 1.73 m^2)
    - Uncommon causes of AKI (e.g., renal obstruction, rapidly progressive glomerulonephritis)
    - Participants who received sustained low-efficiency dialysis (SLED)

Intervention

In the STARRT-AKI trial study, participants were randomized to either the accelerated strategy group (RRT initiated within 12 hours of randomization) or the standard strategy group. For this secondary analysis, the study population was divided into the following groups:

- *Group 1:* CRRT initiated according to the trial's protocol.
- *Group 2:* IHD initiated as RRT modality based on the STARRT-AKI protocol.

Outcome Measures

- *Primary outcome:* Composite outcome of mortality or RRT dependence at 90 days postrandomization.
- *Secondary outcomes:*
    - Components of the primary outcome (mortality or RRT dependence)
    - Ventilator-free days, vasoactive-free days, and ICU-free days at 28 days
    - ICU and hospital LOS
    - Hospital-free days at 90 days

RESULTS

Primary Outcome

The primary outcome, which was a composite of death or RRT dependence at 90 days, showed a difference between the CRRT and IHD groups. Specifically, 51.8% of patients in the CRRT group experienced the composite outcome compared to 54.3% in the IHD group. The unadjusted OR was 0.90 (95% CI: 0.75–1.09). After adjusting for baseline characteristics using overlap weighting, the OR was 0.81 (95% CI: 0.66–0.99), indicating a lower risk of the composite outcome in patients who received CRRT compared to those who received IHD.

Secondary Outcomes

For all-cause mortality at 90 days, 47.3% of patients in the CRRT group and 46% in the IHD group died. The adjusted OR after overlap weighting was 0.90 (95% CI: 0.74–1.11), suggesting no significant difference in mortality between the two groups. However, RRT dependence among survivors at 90 days was lower in the CRRT group (8.4%) compared to the IHD group (15.2%), with an adjusted OR of 0.61 (95% CI: 0.39–0.94), favoring CRRT.

Intensive Care Unit and Hospital Metrics

Continuous RRT was associated with more ICU-free days at 28 days and more hospital-free days at 90 days compared to IHD. However, there were no significant differences in ICU and hospital LOS between the two groups, indicating that the choice of RRT modality did not affect the duration of hospitalization or ICU stay.

Subgroup and Sensitivity Analyses

Subgroup analyses showed no statistically significant interactions across the prespecified subgroups, indicating that the findings were consistent regardless of different patient characteristics or clinical conditions. Sensitivity analyses, including various weighting methods and restricting the cohort to specific patient groups, confirmed the robustness of the primary outcome, supporting the conclusion that CRRT is associated with a lower risk of death or RRT dependence at 90 days compared to IHD.

AUTHORS' CONCLUSION

The authors emphasize that the initial use of CRRT, compared to IHD, significantly reduces the risk of death or RRT dependence at 90 days, primarily by decreasing RRT dependence. They see this as an important advancement in understanding the connection between RRT modality and kidney recovery. The authors suggest that their findings should inform clinical practice and encourage further research through randomized trials to explore the long-term outcomes and cost-effectiveness of CRRT.

STRENGTHS

- *Large sample size:* The study is one of the largest comparisons of CRRT and IHD, allowing detection of significant differences in outcomes.
- *Diverse population:* The STARRT-AKI trial included participants from 15 countries, enhancing the generalizability of the findings.
- *Rigorous data collection:* Data on potential confounders were meticulously collected within the framework of a randomized trial.
- *Advanced statistical methods:* The use of overlap weighting and sensitivity analyses reduced bias and improved the robustness of the findings.

LIMITATIONS

- *Observational nature:* As a secondary analysis, the study is subject to limitations inherent in observational research, including potential residual confounding.
- *Baseline differences:* Despite adjustments, differences in baseline kidney function may have influenced the results.
- *Lack of intradialytic hypotension protocols:* The absence of specific protocols for managing hypotension during IHD sessions may have biased results against IHD.
- *Limited follow-up:* The study focused on outcomes at 90 days, not capturing potential longer-term kidney recovery or mortality effects.
- *Potential for indication bias:* Unmeasured factors related to health system organization could have influenced the choice of RRT modality.

REVIEWERS' VIEWPOINTS

Clinical practice guidelines over 10 years ago suggested that CRRT and IHD are complementary treatments for critically ill patients with AKI. CRRT was recommended for patients with hemodynamic instability and those at increased risk of intracranial hypertension. However, recent meta-analyses and prior randomized trials have not consistently shown the superiority of CRRT over IHD in terms of mortality or kidney recovery. Many trials had methodological limitations, leading to uncertainty in clinical practice regarding the optimal choice of RRT modality for critically ill patients with AKI.

This study provides valuable insights into the comparative effectiveness of CRRT and IHD in critically ill patients with severe AKI, particularly highlighting the potential benefits of CRRT in reducing RRT dependence. However, the observational nature of the analysis and the inherent limitations of secondary data interpretation should be acknowledged. The findings of this study suggest that CRRT may be a more effective initial RRT modality for critically ill patients with severe AKI, particularly in reducing the risk of long-term RRT dependence. Clinicians might consider prioritizing CRRT in patients who are hemodynamically unstable or at higher risk of prolonged kidney injury. Further, the potential cost implications of CRRT should be carefully weighed in clinical decision-making.

TAKE HOME MESSAGE

This study highlights the potential benefits of using CRRT as the initial RRT modality in critically ill patients with severe AKI, particularly in reducing the risk of long-term RRT dependence. While CRRT did not show a significant survival advantage over IHD, its impact on kidney recovery suggests that it may be a preferred option for patients with hemodynamic instability. However, the choice of RRT should be individualized, considering patient-specific factors, resource availability, and the need for further research to confirm these findings.

Phase-3 Trial of Recombinant Human Alkaline Phosphatase for Patients with Sepsis-associated Acute Kidney Injury (REVIVAL)[27]

Pickkers P, Angus DC, Bass K, Bellomo R, van den Berg E, Bernholz J, et al. Phase-3 trial of recombinant human alkaline phosphatase for patients with sepsis-associated acute kidney injury (REVIVAL).

Intensive Care Med. 2024;50:68-78.

BACKGROUND: WHAT IS ALREADY KNOWN?

Ilofotase-alfa [human recombinant alkaline phosphatase (hrAP)] is a proprietary recombinant alkaline phosphatase, constructed from two human isoforms of alkaline phosphatase. It has been shown to have renoprotective effects, thereby projected as a potential novel treatment for patients with sepsis-associated AKI (SA-AKI). The biological rationale behind hrAP is a detoxifying role through dephosphorylation and ameliorating systemic inflammation in sepsis, detoxifying damage-associated molecular patterns (DAMPs) and pathogen-associated molecular patterns (PAMPs) such as lipopolysaccharide (LPS), adenosine triphosphate (ATP), adenosine diphosphate (ADP), and other extracellular substrates that drive acute inflammation, coagulation, and microvascular ischemia found in kidney following sepsis or ischemia-induced damage.[28,29]

CURRENT DILEMMA

A previous phase-2 STOP-AKI study performed in critically ill patients with sepsis without evidence of AKI showed neutral effects for hrAP on the primary efficacy endpoint of improved short-term kidney function (defined as the area under the curve for creatinine clearance over the first 7 days following enrolment), but an improvement in kidney function observed over a 28-day window, along with the occurrence of fewer major adverse kidney events (MAKEs) at 60 and 90 days.[30]

CLINICAL QUESTION

The global phase 3 REVIVAL study assessed the efficacy and safety of ilofotase alfa (human recombinant alkaline phosphatase) for the treatment of patients with SA-AKI.

STUDY TYPE

Phase-3, randomized, double-blind, placebo-controlled, two-arm, parallel-group, sequential, and multicenter trial.

METHODS

The study recruited SA-AKI patients from 107 sites in Europe, North America, Australia, New Zealand, and Japan. The maximum sample size planned was of 1,400 patients in the main trial population providing ~85% power assuming a 35% mortality rate in the placebo group and an 8% absolute treatment effect.

- *Inclusion criteria:*
    - Aged 18 years or older
    - In the ICU or intermediate care unit for clinical reasons
    - *Have sepsis requiring vasopressor therapy, that is:*
        - Suspected or proven bacterial or viral infection
        - On vasopressor therapy (≥0.1 μg/kg/min norepinephrine or equivalent) for sepsis-induced hypotension for at least 1 hour despite adequate fluid resuscitation according to clinical judgment
    - *Have AKI according to at least one of the below KDIGO criteria:*
        - An absolute increase in serum or plasma creatinine (Cr) by ≥0.3 mg/dL (≥26.5 μmol/L) within 48 hours
        - A relative increase in Cr to ≥1.5 times the pre-AKI reference Cr value, which is known or presumed to have occurred within prior 7 days.
        - A decrease in urinary output to <0.5 mL/kg/hour for a minimum of 6 hours following adequate fluid resuscitation.
- If the patient does not have a known history of CKD and there is no pre-AKI reference Cr value available from the past 12 months: a Cr value ≥1.5 times the age/gender/race adjusted normal value, with the increase in Cr presumed to have occurred within prior 7 days.
    - Provision of signed and dated informed consent form in accordance with local regulations.
- *Exclusion criteria:*
    - Known CKD
    - Advanced chronic liver disease defined as a Child–Pugh score of 10–15 (class C).
    - Acute pancreatitis without proven infection
    - Urosepsis related to suspected or proven urinary tract obstruction
    - Main cause of AKI not sepsis
    - Severe burns requiring ICU treatment
    - *Severely immunosuppressed, e.g., due to:*
        - Hematopoietic cell transplantation within past 6 months prior to screening or
        - Acute or chronic graft-versus-host disease
        - Solid organ transplantation
        - Leukopenia not related to sepsis, i.e., preceding sepsis
        - Human immunodeficiency virus (HIV)/acquired immune deficiency syndrome (AIDS) or
        - Receiving chemotherapy within 30 days prior to screening
    - At high risk of being lost to follow-up, e.g., due to known current or recent (within the last 6 months) IV drug abuse or known to be homeless.
    - Limitations to use of mechanical ventilation, RRT or vasopressors, and inotropes
    - Previous administration of recAP
    - Use of a nonmarketed drug within the last month or concurrent or planned

participation in a clinical trial for a nonmarketed drug or device
- Current or planned ECMO or other devices that support hemodynamics
- On RRT, >24 hours before start of trial drug
- Pregnant or nursing women

The "all combined population" includes three cohorts defined as:

1. Patients with SA-AKI with a pre-AKI reference eGFR ≥45 mL/min/1.73 m^2 and no proven or suspected coronavirus disease 2019 (COVID-19) at time of randomization ("main trial population")
2. Patients with a pre-AKI reference eGFR ≥25 and <45 mL/min/1.73 m^2 ("moderate-to-severe CKD population or mCKD") with sepsis and AKI and no proven or suspected COVID-19 at time of randomization
3. Patients with COVID-19-induced sepsis and AKI at time of randomization (COVID-19 population)

The trial randomized only 650 patients out of a planned recruitment of 1,400 patients (46.4%) within 24 hours of the diagnosis of sepsis with AKI to either 3 days of:

- Intravenous ilofotase-alfa (human recombinant alkaline phosphatase) ($n = 330$), or
- Placebo ($n = 319$)

Study medication was administered, within 24 hours if sepsis was present prior to AKI or within 48 hours if AKI was present when sepsis was diagnosed, at 1.6 mg (1,000 U)/kg of patient body weight up to 120 kg, with a fixed dose of 192 mg in patients >120 kg. The study medication was given as a 1-hour infusion once daily for 3 consecutive days.

STUDY ENDPOINTS

- The primary endpoint of the study was 28-day all-cause mortality.
- *Secondary endpoints included majorly:*
  - Long-term MAKEs, which included two definitions: MAKE90A and MAKE90B.
    1. *MAKE90A* was defined as death, >25% decline of eGFR, RRT status at Day 90, any RRT needs through Day 28, and rehospitalization.
    2. *MAKE90B* included death through Day 90, >25% decline of eGFR at Day 28 and Day 90, or RRT at Day 90.
- *Other secondary endpoints included:*
  - Days alive and without the need for organ support through day 28
  - Days alive and free from the ICU through Day 28
  - Time to death through Day 90

RESULTS

- The observed mortality rates in the ilofotase-alfa and placebo groups were 27.9 and 27.9% at 28 days, and 33.9 and 34.8% at 90 days.
- The observed proportion of patients with MAKE90A and MAKE90B were 56.7 and 37.4% in the ilofotase-alfa group versus 64.6 and 42.8% in the placebo group.
- Median (IQR) days alive and free of organ support were 17 (0–24) and 14 (0–24) in the ilofotase-alfa and placebo groups, respectively.
- Number of days alive and discharged from the ICU through Day 28 were 15 (0–22) and 10 (0–22) in the ilofotase-alfa and placebo groups, respectively.
- Adverse events were reported in 67.9 and 75% patients in the ilofotase and placebo group.

AUTHORS' CONCLUSION

Among critically ill patients with SA-AKI, ilofotase-alfa did not improve Day 28 survival.

The REVIVAL study did not reveal any safety concerns but was discontinued for futility based on the primary endpoint of 28-day all-cause mortality after treatment of 650 patients. A prespecified analysis of the key secondary renal endpoint of MAKE90 indicated a significantly ($p = 0.031$) lower rate of subjects experiencing a MAKE90 events in the ilofotase alfa group (56.7%) compared to the placebo group (64.6%). The significant beneficial effect observed on MAKE90 was predominantly driven by the decrease in patients requiring RRT (28.2% ilofotase-alfa vs. 36.4% placebo). In a post-hoc analysis, there was evidence of an interaction between renal function prior to the SA-AKI episode (pre-AKI eGFR) and the incidence of the MAKE90A event ($p = 0.024$), suggesting that the therapeutic efficacy of ilofotase-alfa was more pronounced in patients with a lower pre-AKI eGFR, i.e., more severe preexistent CKD.

STRENGTHS

- Being a multicentric trial, conducted in 107 sites worldwide, REVIVAL study has increased generalizability.
- REVIVAL investigators have focused on improved long-term kidney outcomes as a secondary endpoint. Novel therapies in ICU can be established only through demonstration of measurable effect on short- and long-term organ function.
- RRT dependence is perhaps a more patient-centered and consistent endpoint of a trial focused on long-term kidney outcomes.
- *A strong methodology:* An independent statistician generated a permuted block randomization schedule (block size of 4) for an interactive voice/web response system, which linked sequential patient randomization numbers to treatment codes.
- The group sequential trial design allowed for the results to be reported as the trial was terminated prematurely for futility.

LIMITATIONS

- Being a pharma-driven study, there is a potential bias.
- The trial was terminated prematurely for futility based on the low probability of detecting a difference in the primary efficacy endpoint of 28-day all-cause mortality.
- The proposed effect size with an 8% absolute mortality difference was rather an unrealistic, and too optimistic primary endpoint.
- The observed 28-day mortality rates in both the hrAP and control arms (27.9 and 27.9%) were well below the expected 35% event rate in the control group, negatively impacting the overall power of the planned study.
- With the primary endpoint not met, further statistical testing was considered explorative and further no correction for multiple testing was performed.
- REVIVAL trial included patients who already had AKI when they presented with sepsis in contrast to the STOP-AKI trial and it is plausible that the duration of AKI was longer in these patients, possibly limiting the therapeutic efficacy of ilofotase-alfa.
- The study primarily examined mortality and recruited patients at a later point in their course of critical illness, after evidence of AKI in contrast to the STOP-AKI, which might have led to the cohort less amenable to the biologic activity and risk modification by an early-acting anti-inflammatory intervention. Also, any potential benefit of avoiding the AKI was lost.

- In the REVIVAL, the application of MAKE reflects its lack of standardization with use of two separate definitions, MAKE-A and MAKE-B. MAKE-B definition was prespecified in the trial registration, while the second endpoint (MAKE-A) was first presented in the published protocol and statistical analysis plan. The justification for use of this second endpoint at a late stage in the trial is unclear. The secondary proposed MAKE-A outcome did demonstrate a significant difference in outcome at 28 days, suggesting benefit of hrAP, whereas the findings were neutral for hrAP with the originally planned MAKE-B definition.
- The significance of the observed difference in exposure to RRT in REVIVAL can be questioned, given that there was no difference in days alive and free of RRT up to Day 28.
- REVIVAL was conducted in 107 sites worldwide which increases generalizability but may have also negatively influenced the therapeutic efficacy of the molecule.

REVIEWERS' COMMENTS

Ilofotase-alfa has a significant renoprotective effect in SA-AKI patients with excellent tolerability profile with no survival benefit. The renal effects are most pronounced in patients with preexisting renal impairment. Ilofotase-alfa has a promising potential as a pharmacological recourse in sepsis-associated AKI.

TAKE HOME MESSAGE

REVIVAL trial can be considered as another study showing no survival benefit of another novel drug in sepsis. We await to see if the role of rhAP can be revisited or "revived" in future randomized control studies.

Influence of Therapeutic Plasma Exchange Treatment on Short-term Mortality of Critically Ill Adult Patients with Sepsis-induced Organ Dysfunction: A Systematic Review and Meta-analysis[31]

Kuklin V, Sovershaev M, Bjerner J, Keith P, Scott LK, Thomas OMT, et al. Influence of therapeutic plasma exchange treatment on short-term mortality of critically ill adult patients with sepsis-induced organ dysfunction: a systematic review and meta-analysis.

Crit Care. 2024;28:12.

BACKGROUND: WHAT IS ALREADY KNOWN?

Sepsis, defined by the Third International Consensus, is a severe organ dysfunction caused by an uncontrolled bodily response to infection, involving complex interactions of inflammation, endothelial dysfunction, and abnormal coagulation. Therapeutic plasma exchange (TPE) has been considered as a potential treatment due to its ability to act simultaneously on multiple aspects of the pathway. While some case reports suggest TPE improves outcomes, there is insufficient data to recommend it as standard therapy. There has been limited evidence regarding the impact of plasma exchange in adult patients with sepsis, as most of the existing studies are either case reports, pediatric studies, or observational in nature. However, a meta-analysis of RCTs comparing plasma exchange with standard care in critically ill patients with sepsis or septic shock indicated that plasma exchange might reduce mortality in adults, although no data were reported on ICU or hospital lengths of stay. Additionally, an RCT published in 2002 focused on adults with severe sepsis and septic shock, as defined by the SEPSIS 1.0 criteria, found that, after adjusting for age and infection site, plasma exchange did not significantly reduce mortality ($p = 0.07$). Another RCT on septic shock patients showed that while plasma exchange led to rapid hemodynamic improvement, it did not significantly improve mortality rates or organ function. Given the paucity of evidence in the literature, the American Society for Apheresis currently recommends TPE on a case-by-case basis for sepsis-induced organ dysfunction.[32-38]

CLINICAL QUESTION

Does TPE, when used alongside standard treatment, reduce short-term mortality in critically ill adult patients with sepsis-induced organ dysfunction? This study aims to clarify the potential benefits and risks of TPE specifically in this context, addressing an important gap in the management of sepsis with multiple organ dysfunction.

METHODS

- *Study type:* Systematic review and meta-analysis.
- *Data sources:* Multiple medical and scientific databases were systematically searched to gather relevant studies.
- *Inclusion criteria:* Studies included must have investigated the impact of TPE on sepsis-related mortality and provided sufficient data for analysis.
- *Study selection:* Rigorous selection criteria were applied to identify and include only relevant studies.
- *Population, intervention, comparison, outcomes and study (PICOS) criteria:*
  - *Population:* Critically ill adults with sepsis-induced multiorgan dysfunction.
  - *Intervention:* TPE including both centrifuge and filtration techniques for TPE due to their significant impact on outcomes.
  - *Comparison:* Standard therapy.
  - *Outcomes:* Clinical, laboratory markers, and short-term mortality.
- *Study design:* Randomized controlled trials, observational, and retrospective studies.
- *Data extraction:* Data were extracted independently by multiple reviewers to ensure accuracy, including details on study design, patient characteristics, interventions, and outcomes.
- *Outcome measures:* The primary outcome was short-term mortality, defined as death occurring within 28–30 days of treatment.
- *Data analysis:* Statistical methods were used to pool data from included studies, with sensitivity analyses conducted to explore the impact of study characteristics on outcomes.
- *Quality assessment:* The quality of the included studies was evaluated using standardized tools, with a thorough assessment of the potential for bias to ensure reliability and validity of the findings.

RESULTS

Studies included: 20 studies [5 RCTs and 15 matched cohort studies (MCSs)] met the final criteria for analysis.

- *Meta-analysis:*
  - *Total patients analyzed:* 937 critically ill adults with sepsis-induced organ dysfunction.
    - *TPE group:* 543 received adjunct TPE
    - *Control group:* 394 received standard therapy alone
  - *Meta-analysis specifics:* 11 studies (five RCTs and six MCSs) included, totaling 627 patients.
- *Risk of bias assessment:*
  - *RCTs:* Four rated as good quality with low risk; one had a high risk of bias due to selective reporting.
  - *MCSs:* Four rated as good quality, with some having moderate-to-serious risks of bias due to confounding and participant selection.
  - Blinding was not deemed crucial due to the nature of the TPE procedure.
- *Primary outcomes:*
  - *Median trial size:* 43 patients per trial
  - *Mortality reduction:* RCTs showed lower mortality rates with TPE [RR: 0.62 (95% CI: 0.46, 0.83)].
  - *Subgroup analysis:*
    - *TPE techniques:* Centrifugation showed a significant reduction in short-term mortality [RR: 0.58 (95% CI: 0.45, 0.75)]; filtration technique showed a nonsignificant reduction.
    - *COVID-19 versus non-COVID-19 sepsis:* Non-COVID-19 sepsis showed reduced short-term mortality in both RCTs and MCSs; COVID-19-related sepsis also showed a significant reduction in mortality in MCSs.
- *Secondary outcomes:*
  - *Clinical and laboratory improvements:*
    - *Hemodynamics:* Significant reduction in noradrenaline dose and improvements in arterial blood pressure post-TPE.
    - *Severity scores*: Reduction in APACHE II/III and SOFA scores in multiple studies.
    - *Inflammatory markers*: Reduction in cytokines, lactate dehydrogenase (LDH), ferritin, and other inflammatory markers post-TPE in both RCTs and MCSs.
    - *Protective factors*: Increase in lymphocytes, platelets, and protective factors such as antithrombin-III after TPE.

AUTHORS' VIEWPOINTS

The authors of the study believe that TPE shows potential as an adjunctive treatment for reducing short-term mortality in critically ill patients with sepsis-induced organ dysfunction. While their meta-analysis suggests a significant benefit, particularly with the centrifugation technique and in non-COVID-19 sepsis, they acknowledge the limited quality and quantity of RCTs available. They emphasize the need for more robust, high-quality trials to confirm TPE's efficacy and refine its use in clinical practice.

STRENGTHS

- *Comprehensive data collection:* The study includes a wide range of studies spanning several decades, ensuring a thorough investigation of available evidence.
- *Robust statistical methods:* Advanced statistical techniques, including random effects models, are used to handle heterogeneity and assess the pooled data.
- *Quality assessment:* Rigorous quality assessment tools (Cochrane and ROBINS-I) are employed to evaluate the risk of bias, enhancing the reliability of the conclusions.

- *Diverse study types:* By including both RCTs and MCSs, the study provides a more inclusive assessment of TPE's potential effects.

LIMITATIONS

- *Variability in study designs:* Significant differences in study designs, patient populations, and TPE protocols limit the comparability of results and may introduce variability in outcomes.
- *Heterogeneity:* Variation in TPE techniques, study designs, and patient populations introduces heterogeneity, complicating the comparability of results.
- *Limited sample sizes:* Some of the included studies have small sample sizes, which may limit the statistical power and generalizability of the findings.
- *Risk of bias:* Despite efforts to mitigate bias, some included studies have moderate-to-high risks of bias due to confounding factors and selection processes.
- *Inconsistent outcome reporting:* Variability in how outcomes are defined and reported across studies can complicate the interpretation of the pooled results.
- *Lack of long-term data:* The study focuses primarily on short-term mortality, with limited information on long-term outcomes and potential adverse effects of TPE.

REVIEWERS' VIEWPOINTS

Therapeutic plasma exchange has been proposed as a potential treatment for sepsis with MOF, particularly in cases unresponsive to standard therapies. However, the available data regarding the clinical value of TPE in sepsis are poor. The clinical benefits of TPE are thought to stem from its ability to remove inflammatory mediators and replenish immunoglobulins. Previous studies have shown that TPE can significantly reduce levels of inflammatory biomarkers such as C-reactive protein, α-1 antitrypsin, and cytokines such as tumor necrosis factor-α and interleukin-1β. Additionally, TPE influences the immune system by altering lymphocyte counts, natural killer cell activity, T-suppressor function, and the Th1/Th2 ratio.

This study systematically reviews and analyzes the impact of TPE on short-term mortality in critically ill patients with sepsis-induced organ dysfunction. The authors found that TPE, particularly when performed using centrifugation, is associated with a significant reduction in mortality. This finding aligns with earlier case reports and small-scale studies suggesting TPE's potential benefits. However, the study highlights the limited number of high-quality RCTs and the variability in TPE techniques as significant challenges. Compared to previous meta-analyses, this study provides a more detailed subgroup analysis, including the effect of TPE on COVID-19 versus non-COVID-19 sepsis. While the study advances the understanding of TPE's role in sepsis treatment, the current evidence remains insufficient to recommend it as a routine therapy.

TAKE HOME MESSAGE

Therapeutic plasma exchange may offer a potential benefit in reducing short-term mortality for critically ill patients with sepsis-induced organ dysfunction, particularly when using the centrifugation technique. However, the current evidence is limited by the variability in study designs, techniques, and the small sample sizes of included studies. Despite the promising findings, particularly in non-COVID-19 sepsis, the lack of long-term outcome data and the insufficient number of high-quality RCTs highlight the need for more robust research before TPE can be recommended as a routine treatment in clinical practice.

Initial Renal Replacement Therapy (RRT) Modality Associates with 90-day Postdischarge RRT Dependence in Critically Ill AKI Survivors[39]

Koyner JL, Mackey RH, Echeverri J, Rosenthal NA, Carabuena LA, Bronson-Lowe D, et al. Initial renal replacement therapy (RRT) modality associates with 90-day postdischarge RRT dependence in critically ill AKI survivors.

J Crit Care. 2024;82:154764.

BACKGROUND: WHAT IS ALREADY KNOWN?

Renal replacement therapy in ICUs to support critically ill patients with AKI is most commonly provided as CRRT or standard IHD. CRRT theoretically results in less systemic and thereby intrarenal hypotension and less increase in intracranial pressure, which could be beneficial for long-term renal recovery. But, the current evidence is insufficient to determine whether survival of patients with AKI treated with CRRT differs from those treated with IHD. Several observational studies and few randomized clinical trials (RCTs) and meta-analysis of RCTs suggest better renal recovery for CRRT versus IHD only in special subsets of patients or without reaching statistical significance, which may have been due to small sample size. In a recent secondary analysis of 2,196 patients in the multinational STARRT-AKI trial, patients initiated with CRRT had a 40% lower odds of RRT dependence at 90 days compared to those who initiated with IHD (OR: 0.61; 95% CI: 0.39-0.94).[23]

CLINICAL QUESTION

What is the effect of the RRT modality on RRT dependence at 90-day postdischarge among ICU patients discharged alive after RRT for AKI? With the hypothesis that the slower ultrafiltration and less RRT-induced hypotension with CRRT versus IHD, CRRT would result in less RRT dependence at 90-day postdischarge in critically ill adult AKI survivors, the data-analysis study was conducted to evaluate whether long-term effects on kidney function assessed by ongoing need for RRT, i.e., RRT dependence differ depending on use of CRRT versus IHD.

METHODS

Study type: A retrospective multinational cohort study using US hospital discharge database, and its linked claims database.

All the claims linked to US hospital discharge data [Premier PINC-AI Healthcare Database (PHD)] were analyzed and CRRT was compared with IHD for AKI in adult ICU patients discharged alive from January 1, 2018 to June 30, 2021. The study followed RECORD (REporting of studies Conducted using Observational Routinely collected health Data) guidelines for studies using administrative health data.

- *Inclusion criteria:* Age ≥18 years and with first ICU RRT, either CRRT (performance of urinary filtration, continuous, >18 hours per day) or IHD (performance of urinary filtration, intermittent, <6 hours per day) during the index visit.
- *Exclusion criteria included:*
    - Renal transplant
    - Chronic RRT [end-stage renal disease (ESRD) or >1 RRT event] up to 365 days look back before index hospitalization

- First RRT initiated outside of the ICU
- Use of prolonged intermittent RRT (PIRRT: performance of urinary filtration, intermittent, 6–18 hours per day)
- Occurrence of >1 RRT modality on the first day of initiation, or
- Index admission occurred in hospitals without continuous data submission during the study period (including look back and follow-up)
- The overall survivor cohort excluded patients with discharge status of "expired" or "discharged to hospice."

The primary study cohort was the subset of patients who survived to 90-day postdischarge with linked claims data during days 83–90 postdischarge.

Outcomes: The primary outcome was RRT dependence at 90 days postdischarge, defined as ≥2 days with RRT during last 8 days, i.e., days 83–90 after discharge.

For RRT dependence at hospital discharge, a secondary definition of ≥1 day with RRT in the last 3 days of index hospitalization was also used, for comparison with a prior study.

RESULTS

Of the survivor cohort of 34,804 patients, 3,916 patients had available claims data during days 83–90 postdischarge, but 112 patients [28 CRRT (2.6%) vs. 84 IHD (3.0%), $p = 0.49$] were excluded due to death during days 1–90 postdischarge. The final claims-linked study cohort was 3,804 patients. Of these, 2,740 (72%) were IHD-treated patients and 1,064 (28%) CRRT-treated patients. IHD-treated patients were younger, had more admission to large teaching hospitals, surgery, sepsis, shock, mechanical ventilation, but lower prevalence of comorbidities ($p < 0.05$ for all) in comparison to CRRT-treated patients. Compared to IHD-treated patients, CRRT-treated patients had lower RRT dependence at hospital discharge (26.5 vs. 29.8, $p = 0.04$) and lower RRT dependence at 90 days postdischarge (4.9 vs. 7.4% $p = 0.006$) with weighted adjusted OR (95% CI): 0.68 (0.47–0.97), $p = 0.03$. Results persisted in sensitivity analyses including patients who died during days 1–90 postdischarge ($n = 112$) or excluding patients from hospitals with IHD patients only ($n = 335$), or when excluding patients who switched RRT modalities ($n = 451$). The weighted OR (95% CI) for RRT dependence at 90 days postdischarge for CRRT versus IHD was 0.69 (0.48–0.98), $p = 0.04$, and 0.68 (0.48–0.98) $p = 0.04$ when additionally adjusted for teaching hospital status and LOS.

AUTHORS' CONCLUSION

Adjusted for potential confounders, the odds of RRT dependence at 90-day postdischarge among survivors of RRT for AKI were 30% lower for those treated first with CRRT versus IHD, overall and in several sensitivity analyses. RRT dependence at 90 days postdischarge was still lower for CRRT than IHD-treated patients despite slight imbalance of more severe acute illness among CRRT-treated patients.

STRENGTHS

- A real-world evidence study using a large, geographically diverse, all-payer US hospital discharge database, the Premier PINC-AI Healthcare Database (PHD), and its linked claims database
- Large, multicenter, and nationwide US cohort study with up to 3,804 included patients
- The study used robust and replicable definitions of RRT dependence both at hospital discharge and at 90-day postdischarge follow-up.

- *Robust statistical methods:*
    - The cutting-edge analytic approach, the inverse probability treatment weighting (IPTW) analyses achieved excellent confounder balance between CRRT and IHD-treated patient groups.
    - Robust results across models including sensitivity analyses

LIMITATIONS

- The study cohort with linked claims represents only ~11% of the overall survivor cohort from the PHD.
- There are imitations inherent to observational studies such as inability to prove causality or to adjust for unmeasured or unknown confounders, so there may exist residual indication bias.
- There was no blood pressure data collected in the study, thereby the study did not directly assess the effect of hemodynamic instability on RRT allocation. This could have confounded the results.
- The data does not allow for determination of who ordered and provided CRRT and/or IHD care. This might cause some degree of bias since studies are lacking if provider-based factors impact patient outcomes.

REVIEWERS' CONCLUSION

The results from this nonrandomized study suggest that among ICU survivors of RRT for AKI, CRRT may result in less RRT dependence 90 days after hospital discharge.

TAKE HOME MESSAGE

Continuous renal replacement therapy does not confer a reduction in mortality as compared to IHD but among AKI survivors, there is a higher likelihood of kidney recovery and dialysis independence in CRRT recipients.

The Impact of Higher Protein Dosing on Outcomes in Critically Ill Patients with Acute Kidney Injury: A Post Hoc Analysis of the EFFORT Protein Trial[40]

Stoppe C, Patel JJ, Zarbock A, Lee ZY, Rice TW, Mafrici B, et al. The impact of higher protein dosing on outcomes in critically ill patients with acute kidney injury: a post-hoc analysis of the EFFORT protein trial. ***Crit Care. 2023;27:399.***

BACKGROUND: WHAT IS KNOWN?

The role of protein dosage in critically ill patients is of considerable interest as it is thought to improve clinical outcomes by attenuating protein losses during critical illness and supporting the patients' recovery in later phases. AKI disrupts critical homeostatic processes, including the regulation of acid-base balance, often leading to metabolic acidosis. This condition accelerates proteolysis and protein breakdown while inhibiting amino acid transport between cells. Additionally, the loss of renal function in AKI impairs the body's ability to convert and utilize amino acids effectively. In more severe cases, RRT exacerbates amino acid depletion. Furthermore, the underlying conditions of critical illness—such as sepsis, respiratory failure, and trauma—promote increased protein degradation, resulting in a negative nitrogen balance. This contributes to muscle mass loss, which negatively impacts physical function, recovery, and overall quality of life for survivors.

Theoretically, critically ill patients with AKI may have an increased need for protein compared to those without AKI. Current nutritional guidelines suggest targeting a protein intake of up to 2.0 g/kg of body weight per day (BW/day) for AKI patients who are not receiving RRT, and up to 2.5 g/kg BW/day for those on KRT. However, findings from the recently concluded EFFORT Protein trial, which included mechanically ventilated critically ill patients, indicated that providing a higher protein dose (≥2.2 g/kg/BW/day) did not lead to improved outcomes in terms of time-to-discharge alive (TTDA) or 60-day mortality compared to a usual protein dose (<1.2 g/kg/BW/day).[41]

CLINICAL QUESTION

The clinical question of this study is whether administering a higher protein dose (≥2.2 g/kg BW/day) compared to a usual protein dose (<1.2 g/kg BW/day) improves outcomes in critically ill patients who have developed AKI.

METHODS

Study Design

This post-hoc analysis was based on the EFFORT Protein trial conducted across 85 ICUs in 15 different countries.

Participants

The original trial enrolled adult critically ill patients who were:

- Mechanically ventilated within 96 hours of ICU admission and
- Considered at high nutritional risk. High nutritional risk was defined by specific criteria, including a BMI of ≤25 or ≥35 kg/m^2, moderate-to-severe malnutrition, a clinical frailty scale score of 5 or higher, a SARC-F score of 4 or higher, or a projected duration of mechanical ventilation longer than 4 days.

Patients were excluded if they were:

- Moribund
- Pregnant, or
- If equipoise regarding protein dosing was not present.

For this post-hoc analysis, a subset of patients with AKI, as defined by the KDIGO classification, was included.

Intervention

In the trial, patients were randomly assigned to receive either a high protein dose (≥2.2 g/kg of BW/day) or a usual protein dose (≤1.2 g/kg of BW/day). The protein dosing was initiated as soon as possible after randomization and continued for up to 28 days in the ICU. Energy intake was determined by the clinical care team, with pre-ICU dry weight used to calculate the nutrition targets. For patients with a BMI above 30 kg/m^2, an ideal body weight based on a BMI of 25 kg/m^2 was applied.

Outcomes

The primary outcome for this post-hoc analysis was the TTDA from the hospital, where death was considered a competing risk.

Secondary outcomes included 60-day mortality, the duration and incidence of KRT after randomization, and urea levels measured during the first 12 days after randomization.

Statistical Analysis

For the primary analysis of TTDA, the study used a Cox proportional hazards model that allowed for death as a competing risk and accounted for ICU as a shared frailty (random effect). Since the Fine-Gray model was not available for simultaneous use with the random effect model in SAS software, death after the last event time was censored to approximate the Fine-Gray estimates. For the secondary analysis, relative risks for 60-day mortality were estimated using a mixed log-binomial model with ICU as a random effect, calculated via maximum likelihood estimation.

The study also conducted subgroup analyses to explore the effect of protein dosing on TTDA and 60-day mortality across various subgroups, including AKI stage, KRT use, presence of CKD, blood urea nitrogen to creatinine ratio, age, BMI, and sepsis status. The interaction between protein dosing and these subgroups was tested but not adjusted for multiplicity, as none of the interactions reached statistical significance.

Ethical Considerations

The original EFFORT Protein trial protocol was approved by the Research Ethics Committees of Queen's University in Canada and Vanderbilt University in the USA, with additional local ethical approvals obtained as necessary. Informed consent was either waived or obtained from patient surrogates, depending on the site's requirements.

RESULTS

Patient Characteristics

- A total of 1,329 patients were randomized in the original EFFORT Protein trial.
- For this analysis, 312 patients who developed AKI within the first 7 days of ICU admission were included.
    - *High-protein group:* 163 patients (25.3% developed AKI)
    - *Usual-protein group:* 149 patients (22.7% developed AKI)
- *AKI stages in the cohort:*
    - 38.5% at AKI stage 1
    - 23.7% at AKI stage 2
    - 37.8% at AKI stage 3
- Baseline characteristics, including the proportion of patients with CKD and the number receiving KRT, were similar between groups.

Protein and Energy Delivery

- *High-protein group:* Received an average of 1.5 ± 0.5 g/kg BW/day.
- *Usual-protein group:* Received an average of 0.9 ± 0.3 g/kg BW/day.

Energy Intake

- *High-protein group:* 17.4 ± 6.5 kcal/kg/day
- *Usual-protein group:* 15.6 ± 6.1 kcal/kg/day ($p = 0.01$)

Time-to-discharge alive: High-protein intake was associated with a slower TTDA. HR: 0.5 (95% CI: 0.4–0.8, $p = 0.001$). This negative effect was consistent across all subgroups, including different AKI stages.

Mortality: High-protein intake was linked to higher 60-day mortality [RR: 1.4 (95% CI: 1.1–1.8, $p = 0.02$)]. Mortality increased across all AKI stages, but the effect was less pronounced in patients who received KRT.

Renal replacement therapy: No significant difference in the duration of KRT between groups:

- *High-protein group:* Median of 5 days
- *Usual-protein group:* Median of 6 days ($p = 0.21$)
- *Incidence of new RRT postrandomization:* 20.5% overall, with no significant difference between groups.

Urea levels: Urea levels were higher in the high-protein group.

- *High-protein group:* 19.7 ± 9.8 mmol/L
- *Usual-protein group:* 17.6 ± 9.7 mmol/L ($p = 0.04$)

- However, this difference did not reach statistical significance after adjusting for multiple comparisons.

AUTHORS' VIEWPOINTS

The authors of this study believe that the current nutritional guidelines recommending high-protein intake for critically ill patients with AKI need to be reconsidered. Their viewpoint is based on the findings that higher protein dosing (≥2.2 g/kg/day) was associated with slower recovery, as indicated by a delayed TTDA, and increased 60-day mortality across all AKI stages. They express particular concern that these negative outcomes were most significant in AKI patients who did not receive RRT.

The authors also suggest that although RRT appeared to mitigate the harmful effects of high-protein dosing, the interaction was not statistically significant. This raises important questions about whether critically ill patients, particularly those with AKI, can effectively utilize high-protein intake. They emphasize that despite theoretical and experimental considerations, the real-world clinical scenario suggests that excessive protein intake may increase metabolic stress rather than provide benefit in these patients.

STRENGTHS

- *Large sample size:* The study used data from the largest RCT to date on protein dosing in critically ill patients, providing robust data to support its conclusions.
- *Diverse population:* The study was conducted across 85 ICUs in 15 countries, representing a wide range of practice settings and enhancing the generalizability of the findings.
- *Subgroup analysis:* The study performed detailed subgroup analyses, allowing for an in-depth exploration of how different stages of AKI and KRT use affected the relationship between protein dosing and clinical outcomes.
- *Real-world relevance:* The pragmatic design of the trial reflects real-world clinical practice, making the findings more applicable to everyday medical care.
- *Focus on AKI patients:* This study is one of the few that specifically looks at the effect of protein dosing in patients with AKI, a particularly vulnerable group, and highlights important considerations for nutritional support in this population.

LIMITATIONS

- *Post-hoc analysis:* Since the analysis was performed post-hoc, it is exploratory in nature, which means the results should be interpreted as hypothesis-generating rather than definitive.
- *Lack of adjustment for multiple comparisons:* In the subgroup analyses, *p*-values were not adjusted for multiplicity, increasing the risk of type I errors (false positives).
- *Unaccounted variability in KRT use:* The study did not evaluate the modality of KRT, which could influence the protein requirements and clinical outcomes of patients, introducing variability in the results.
- *Potential for confounding:* As AKI was primarily diagnosed after randomization, it remains unclear whether higher protein dosing contributed to the development of AKI or worsened outcomes after AKI had already developed.
- *Inability to establish causality:* Being a post-hoc analysis, the study is limited in its ability to establish causality, and the findings should be considered in the context of generating hypotheses for future research.

REVIEWERS' VIEWPOINTS

- This study addresses an important gap in the understanding of protein dosing in critically ill patients with AKI. While existing nutritional guidelines advocate for higher protein intake in such patients, evidence supporting these recommendations has been limited and often of low quality. By analyzing data from the largest trial to date on protein dosing in critically ill patients, the study offers valuable insights into the potential risks associated with high-protein intake, particularly in those not receiving RRT.
- As a post-hoc analysis, the study's conclusions should be approached with caution. While the findings are compelling, they remain exploratory, and prospective, adequately powered trials would be necessary to confirm these results and refine protein dosing guidelines for AKI patients.
- Although the study performed detailed subgroup analyses, the lack of adjustments for multiple comparisons raises concerns about the potential for false positives. It would have been beneficial if the authors had accounted for multiplicity to provide more robust conclusions.
- The study raises an important question regarding whether high protein intake exacerbates AKI or worsens outcomes in patients with existing AKI. However, it lacks clarity on causality due to its observational nature, making it difficult to determine whether the negative outcomes are directly attributable to high-protein intake or other confounding factors.
- The study's pragmatic design enhances its relevance to clinical practice. However, the variability in KRT practices across sites could introduce biases, and it would be helpful to see standardized approaches to KRT in future studies to better isolate the effects of protein intake.

TAKE HOME MESSAGE

The current nutritional guidelines for critically ill AKI patients recommending higher protein doses may need to be reconsidered. This is a significant finding and underscores the need for a more individualized approach to nutrition support in these patients.

REFERENCES

1. Dong V, Robinson AM, Dionne JC, Cardoso FS, Rewa OG, Karvellas CJ. Continuous renal replacement therapy and survival in acute liver failure: a systematic review and meta-analysis. J Crit Care. 2024;81:154513.
2. Cardoso FS, Gottfried M, Tujios S, Olson JC, Karvellas CJ, US Acute Liver Failure Study Group. Continuous renal replacement therapy is associated with reduced serum ammonia levels and mortality in acute liver failure. Hepatology. 2018;67(2):711-20.
3. Warrillow S, Fisher C, Tibballs H, Bailey M, McArthur C, Lawson-Smith P, et al. Continuous renal replacement therapy and its impact on hyperammonaemia in acute liver failure. Crit Care Resusc. 2020;22(2):158-65.
4. Fisher C, Baldwin I, Fealy N, Naorungroj T, Bellomo R. Ammonia clearance with different continuous renal replacement therapy techniques in patients with liver failure. Blood Purif. 2022;51(10):840-6.
5. Bianchi Bosisio NSM, Romero-González G, De Silvestri A, Husain-Syad F, Ferrari F. Doppler-based evaluation of intrarenal venous flow as a new tool to predict acute kidney injury: A systematic review and meta-analysis. Nefrol (Engl Ed). 2023;43(Suppl 2):57-66.
6. Firth JD, Raine AE, Ledingham JG. Raised venous pressure: a direct cause of renal sodium retention in oedema? Lancet. 1988;1(8593):1033-5.
7. Geri G, Ferrer L, Tran N, Celi LA, Jamme M, Lee J, et al. Cardio-pulmonary-renal interactions in ICU patients. Role of

mechanical ventilation, venous congestion and perfusion deficit on worsening of renal function: Insights from the MIMIC-III database. J Crit Care. 2021;64:100-7.

8. Tang WHW, Kitai T. Intrarenal venous flow: A window into the congestive kidney failure phenotype of heart failure? JACC Heart Fail. 2016;4(8):683-6.
9. Wiersema R, Kaufmann T, van der Veen HN, de Haas RJ, Franssen CFM, Koeze J, et al. Diagnostic accuracy of arterial and venous renal Doppler assessment for acute kidney injury in critically ill patients: A prospective study. J Crit Care. 2020;59:57-62.
10. Li T, Wu B, Li L, Bian A, Ni J, Liu K, et al. Automated electronic alert for the care and outcomes of adults with acute kidney injury: A randomized clinical trial. JAMA Netw Open. 2024;7(1):e2351710.
11. Colpaert K, Hoste EA, Steurbaut K, Benoit D, Van Hoecke S, De Turck F, et al. Impact of real-time electronic alerting of acute kidney injury on therapeutic intervention and progression of RIFLE class. Crit Care Med. 2012;40(4):1164-70.
12. Park S, Baek SH, Ahn S, Lee KH, Hwang H, Ryu J, et al. Impact of electronic acute kidney injury (AKI) alerts with automated nephrologist consultation on detection and severity of AKI: A quality improvement study. Am J Kidney Dis. 2018;71(1):9-19.
13. Wu MJ, Huang SC, Chen CH, Cheng CY, Tsai SF. An early warning system for the differential diagnosis of in-hospital acute kidney injury for better patient outcome: Study of a quality improvement initiative. Int J Environ Res Public Health. 2022;19(6):3704.
14. Wilson FP, Shashaty M, Testani J, Aqeel I, Borovskiy Y, Ellenberg SS, et al. Automated, electronic alerts for acute kidney injury: a single-blind, parallel-group, randomised controlled trial. Lancet. 2015;385(9981):1966-74.
15. Landoni G, Monaco F, Ti LK, Baiardo Redaelli M, Bradic N, Comis M, et al. A randomized trial of intravenous amino acids for kidney protection. N Engl J Med. 2024;391(8):687-98.
16. Brown JR, Baker RA, Shore-Lesserson L, Fox AA, Mongero LB, Lobdell KW, et al. The society of thoracic surgeons/society of cardiovascular anesthesiologists/American society for extracorporeal technology clinical practice guidelines for the prevention of adult cardiac surgery-associated acute kidney injury. Anesth Analg. 2023;136(1):176-84.
17. Zhu R, Allingstrup MJ, Perner A, Doig GS; Nephro-Protective Trial Investigators Group. The effect of IV amino acid supplementation on mortality in ICU patients may be dependent on kidney function: post hoc subgroup analyses of a multicenter randomized trial. Crit Care Med. 2018;46:1293-301.
18. Pu H, Doig GS, Heighes PT, Allingstrup MJ, Wang A, Brereton J, et al. Intravenous amino acid therapy for kidney protection in cardiac surgery patients: A pilot randomized controlled trial. J Thorac Cardiovasc Surg. 2019;157(6):2356-66.
19. Kunz JV, Hansmann H, Fähndrich M, Pigorsch M, Bethke N, Peters H, et al. Standard vs. carbone dioxide adapted kidney replacement therapy in hypercapnic ARDS patients: a randomized controlled pilot trial (BigBIC). Crit Care. 2024;28(1):198.
20. Panitchote A, Mehkri O, Hastings A, Hanane T, Demirjian S, Torbic H, et al. Factors associated with acute kidney injury in acute respiratory distress syndrome. Ann Intensive Care. 2019;9(1):74.
21. Gupta S, Coca SG, Chan L, Melamed ML, Brenner SK, Hayek SS, et al. AKI treated with renal replacement therapy in critically ill patients with COVID-19. J Am Soc Nephrol. 2021;32(1):161-76.
22. Wald R, Gaudry S, da Costa BR, Adhikari NKJ, Bellomo R, Du B, et al. Initiation of continuous renal replacement therapy versus intermittent hemodialysis in critically ill patients with severe acute kidney injury: a secondary analysis of STARRT-AKI trial. Intensive Care Med. 2023;49(11):1305-16.
23. STARRT-AKI Investigators; Canadian Critical Care Trials Group; Australian and New Zealand Intensive Care Society Clinical Trials Group; United Kingdom Critical Care Research Group; Canadian Nephrology Trials Network; Irish Critical Care Trials

Group, et al. Timing of initiation of renal-replacement therapy in acute kidney injury. N Engl J Med. 2020;383(3):240-51.

24. Ostermann M, Bellomo R, Burdmann EA, Doi K, Endre ZH, Goldstein SL, et al. Controversies in acute kidney injury: conclusions from a Kidney Disease: Improving Global Outcomes (KDIGO) Conference. Kidney Int. 2020;98(2):294-309.
25. Ye Z, Wang Y, Ge L, Guyatt GH, Collister D, Alhazzani W, et al. Comparing renal replacement therapy modalities in critically ill patients with acute kidney injury: A systematic review and network meta-analysis. Crit Care Explor. 2021;3(5):e0399.
26. Uehlinger DE, Jakob SM, Ferrari P, Eichelberger M, Huynh-Do U, Marti HP, et al. Comparison of continuous and intermittent renal replacement therapy for acute renal failure. Nephrol Dial Transplant. 2005;20(8):1630-7.
27. Pickkers P, Angus DC, Bass K, Bellomo R, van den Berg E, Bernholz J, et al. Phase-3 trial of recombinant human alkaline phosphatase for patients with sepsis-associated acute kidney injury (REVIVAL). Intensive Care Med. 2024;50(1):68-78.
28. Pickkers P, Angus DC, Arend J, Bellomo R, van den Berg E, Bernholz J, et al. Study protocol of a randomised, double-blind, placebo-controlled, two-arm parallel-group, multi-centre phase 3 pivotal trial to investigate the efficacy and safety of recombinant human alkaline phosphatase for treatment of patients with sepsis-associated acute kidney injury. BMJ Open. 2023;13(4):e065613.
29. Kellum JA, Chawla LS, Keener C, Singbartl K, Palevsky PM, Pike FL, et al. The effects of alternative resuscitation strategies on acute kidney injury in patients with septic shock. Am J Respir Crit Care Med. 2016;193(3):281-7.
30. Su F, Brands R, Wang Z, Verdant C, Bruhn A, Cai Y, et al. Beneficial effects of alkaline phosphatase in septic shock. Crit Care Med. 2006;34(8):2182-7.
31. Kuklin V, Sovershaev M, Bjerner J, Keith P, Scott LK, Thomas OMT, et al. Influence of therapeutic plasma exchange treatment on short-term mortality of critically ill adult patients with sepsis-induced organ dysfunction: a systematic review and meta-analysis. Crit Care. 2024;28(1):12.
32. Snow TAC, Littlewood S, Corredor C, Singer M, Arulkumaran N. Effect of extracorporeal blood purification on mortality in sepsis: A meta-analysis and trial sequential analysis. Blood Purif. 2021;50(4-5):462-72.
33. Connelly-Smith L, Alquist CR, Aqui NA, Hofmann JC, Klingel R, Onwuemene OA, et al. Guidelines on the use of therapeutic apheresis in clinical practice: evidence-based approach from the writing committee of the American Society for apheresis: The ninth Special Issue. J Clin Apher. 2023;38(2):77-278.
34. Weng J, Chen M, Fang D, Liu D, Guo R, Yang S. Therapeutic plasma exchange protects patients with sepsis-associated disseminated intravascular coagulation by improving endothelial function. Clin Appl Thromb Hemost. 2021;27:10760296211053312.
35. Bagshaw SM, Darmon M, Ostermann M, Finkelstein FO, Wald R, Tolwani AJ, et al. Current state of the art for renal replacement therapy in critically ill patients with acute kidney injury. Intensive Care Med. 2017;43(6):841-54.
36. Schefold JC, von Haehling S, Pschowski R, Bender T, Berkmann C, Briegel S, et al. The effect of continuous versus intermittent renal replacement therapy on the outcome of critically ill patients with acute renal failure (CONVINT): a prospective randomized controlled trial. Crit Care. 2014;18(1):R11.
37. Bell M, Granath F, Schön S, Ekbom A. Martling Continuous renal replacement therapy is associated with less chronic renal failure than intermittent haemodialysis after acute renal failure. Intensive Care Med. 2007;33:773-80.
38. Bonnassieux M, Duclos A, Schneider AG, Schmidt A, Bénard S, Cancalon C. Renal replacement therapy modality in the ICU and renal recovery at hospital discharge. Crit Care Med. 2018;46(2):e102-e110.

39. Koyner JL, Mackey RH, Echeverri J, Rosenthal NA, Carabuena LA, Bronson-Lowe D, et al. Initial renal replacement therapy (RRT) modality associates with 90-day postdischarge RRT dependence in critically ill AKI survivors. J Crit Care. 2024;82:154764.
40. Stoppe C, Patel JJ, Zarbock A, Lee ZY, Rice TW, Mafrici B, et al. The impact of higher protein dosing on outcomes in critically ill patients with acute kidney injury: a post hoc analysis of the EFFORT protein trial. Crit Care. (London, England). 2023;27(1):399.
41. Heyland DK, Patel J, Compher C, Rice TW, Bear DE, Lee ZY, et al. The effect of higher protein dosing in critically ill patients with high nutritional risk (EFFORT Protein): an international, multicentre, pragmatic, registry-based randomised trial. Lancet (London, England). 2023;401(10376): 568–76.

SECTION 6

Antimicrobials

Section Editor: *Sumesh Arora*

Continuous vs. Intermittent β-Lactam Antibiotic Infusions in Critically Ill Patients with Sepsis: The BLING III Randomized Clinical Trial

Dulhunty JM, Brett SJ, De Waele JJ, Rajbhandari D, Billot L, Cotta MO, et al.; BLING III Study Investigators. Continuous vs Intermittent β-Lactam Antibiotic Infusions in Critically Ill Patients With Sepsis: The BLING III Randomized Clinical Trial.

JAMA. 2024;332(8):629-37.

CLINICAL QUESTION OR PROBLEM

Beta-lactam rings containing antibiotics (penicillins, cephalosporins, monobactams, carbapenems, etc.) exhibit time-dependent killing. Time-dependent killing refers to the observation that the prolonged exposure to drugs above minimum inhibitory concentration (MIC) is the most important factor in the clearance of microorganisms. The duration of exposure is typically measured as the duration of time spent above MIC between the dosing interval is referred to as time above MIC (t >MIC). To prolong t >MIC, for drugs with a short half-life, the drug either must be administered frequently or as a continuous infusion. Continuous infusion has long been proposed to improve the efficacy of the beta-lactam antibiotics. However, there is no conclusive evidence that continuous infusion of beta-lactam antibiotics results in improved microbiological cure or patient-centered outcomes.

The Beta-Lactam Infusion Group (BLING) III trial was done to answer the question if there is a difference in mortality between continuous and intermittent infusions of β-lactam antibiotics in critically ill patients with sepsis.[1]

WHAT IS ALREADY KNOWN?

We know that the beta-lactam antibiotics exhibit time-dependent killing of bacteria. We do not know if this results in improved microbiological cures or improved patient-centered outcomes such as mortality. Piperacillin-tazobactam or meropenem were the antibiotics chosen for this study.

STUDY DESIGN

The salient features of the BLING III trial are outlined in **Table 1**.

TABLE 1: Study design BLING III trial.

Setting	Multicenter, International, in 104 ICUs
Countries	Australia, Belgium, France, Malaysia, New Zealand, Sweden, and the UK
Blinding	Open label
Randomization	Yes. 1:1 in intervention and control arm, using minimization algorithm and stratification by study site
Informed consent	Yes. Written consent or documented verbal consent during the COVID-19 pandemic
Sample size calculation	Assuming 27.5 baseline mortality, 7,000 patients were required for 90% power to detect a 3.5% difference in all-cause 90-day mortality with an α of 0.05. Sample size calculation allowed for a 5% loss to follow-up
Primary outcome	Intention to treat analysis

POPULATION STUDIED INCLUDING DEMOGRAPHICS

Adult patients admitted to the intensive care unit (ICU) who satisfied the following criteria:

- A documented site or a strong suspicion of infection
- Treatment with piperacillin-tazobactam or meropenem within the previous 24 hours
- Development of at least one organ dysfunction in the previous 24 hours

INTERVENTION(S) STUDIED

Intervention Arm

Continuous infusion of piperacillin-tazobactam or meropenem.

Control Arm

Intermittent infusion of piperacillin-tazobactam or meropenem.

COMPARATOR USED

Intermittent infusion of piperacillin-tazobactam or meropenem, as outlined above.

OUTCOMES EVALUATED

Primary Outcome

The primary outcome was all-cause mortality at 90 days from randomization.

Secondary Outcomes

The secondary outcomes were:

- Clinical cure, defined as cessation of the antimicrobial therapy within 14 days without the need for recommencement within 48 hours for the same episode of infection.
- New acquisition, colonization, or infection with a multi-resistant organism or *Clostridium difficile*
- All-cause ICU mortality
- All-cause hospital mortality

SUBGROUP ANALYSIS

Predefined subgroup for analysis included:

- Presence or absence of pulmonary infection
- Type of beta-lactam used
- Age >65 years
- Sex
- APACHE >25

STATISTICAL ANALYSIS

The primary analysis consisted of logistic regression of the primary outcome (survival or death at day 90) with the treatment allocation (continuous infusion vs intermittent dosing). All tests were two sided, with a nominal significance level at 5%.

STATISTICAL NOTE

Logistic Regression is an analysis technique used when the dependent outcome variable is binary. In this case, the dependent variable is mortality at day 90 is: Yes or no. The independent variable in logistic regression may be continuous or categorical. In this case, the independent variable is categorical—continuous infusion or variable infusion. The regression analysis provides "log odds". Log odds are difficult to interpret. The output is therefore provided as an odds ratio. The function that converts the log odds to probability is called the Logistic function. The Logistic regression in this case, therefore, provides the probability of the dependent outcome (death) as a function of an independent categorical variable (continuous infusion vs. intermittent infusion).[2]

RESULTS

A total of 7,202 patients were randomized, of whom 7,031 were included in the primary analysis, and 6,950 in the safety analysis. In 59% of the patients, the lungs were the primary site of infection. At baseline, the two groups were similar. The me dian duration of therapy in the continuous infusion group was 5.8 days and in the intermittent infusion group was 5.7 days.

Primary Outcomes

At 90 days from randomization, 24.9% of patients in the continuous infusion group had died, compared to 26.8% of patients in the intermittent infusion group.

The absolute difference in mortality between the two groups was −1.9% (95% CI: −4.9% to 1.1%). The confidence interval in this difference crosses zero. This means that the difference between the two groups is not statistically significant.

The odds ratio of death in the continuous infusion group was 0.91 (95% CI: 0.89–1.01); with a p value of 0.08. The confidence interval of the odds ratio crosses 1. This means that the difference between the two groups is not statistically significant.

Secondary Outcomes

Clinical cure at day 14, one of the secondary outcomes was better in the continuous infusion group. 55.7% of patients in the continuous infusion group achieved clinical cure, compared to 50% in the intermittent infusion group [absolute difference 5.7% (95% CI: 2.4–9.1), OR 1.26 (1.15–1.38), $p < 0.001$].

There was no difference between the groups for any of the other secondary outcome measures. These include ICU mortality and hospital mortality.

There was one serious adverse event, encephalopathy, in the continuous infusion group, which was potentially related to meropenem.

AUTHORS' VIEWPOINT

The primary outcome of mortality at 90 days from the randomization showed a 1.9% drop in the continuous infusion group, but it did not reach statistical significance. The authors are of the opinion that this still represents a clinically significant decrease in mortality with a number needed to treat 50, to prevent one death. The authors also point out that the clinical cure rate is significantly better in the continuous infusion group.

STRENGTH OF THE STUDY

This is a well-conducted study. It follows a significant body of work by the same investigators in their previous feasibility and phase II study.[3,4] The primary outcome is a categorical patient-centered variable (death at 90 days) which is not subject to adjudication bias.

DRAWBACKS OF THE STUDY

This is an open-label study. The authors comment that the blinding was not possible. Most of the participating countries are high-income countries, so the results of the study may not be transferrable to lower-income countries. The impact of additional antibiotics or the results of antimicrobial susceptibility on the outcome has not been studied in this study.

REVIEWERS' VIEWPOINT

The authors should be congratulated on doing a robust and pragmatic study, with a patient-centered primary outcome which is not susceptible to bias.

In the discussion, the authors appear to suggest that despite the result not reaching statistical significance, continuous infusion is clinically beneficial for the patient. The authors quote a similar decrease in mortality in the recently concluded MERCY trial that compared continuous with intermittent infusion of meropenem.[5] The reference is misleading in the way that the results of the MERCY trial did not reach statistical significance either.

It is worth pointing out that the hospital mortality and ICU mortality in continuous infusion and intermittent infusion were no different.

Achieving a clinical cure is an important secondary outcome. The definition of clinical cure (discontinuation of the antibiotics within 14 days, and not restarting for the same clinical problem within 48 hours) is, however, in my opinion, subject to bias in an open-label study. That clinical cure rate is higher with continuous infusion and should be interpreted with caution.

Continuous infusion of antibiotics generally requires a dedicated lumen for infusion. In critically ill patients, dedicating one lumen to the antibiotic may increase the need for inserting additional intravenous cannulas. This may increase the risk of secondary infection and the workload on the healthcare staff. This aspect of treatment with continuous infusion has not been reported.

IMPACT ON CURRENT PRACTICE AND TAKE-HOME MESSAGE

While there are theoretical benefits to using a continuous infusion of beta-lactam antibiotics as a continuous infusion, based on the results of this study, continuous infusion of beta-lactam antibiotics cannot be routinely recommended.

Antimicrobial Prophylaxis with Ampicillin-sulbactam Compared with Cefazolin for Esophagectomy: Nationwide Inpatient Database Study in Japan

Hirano Y, Konishi T, Kaneko H, Itoh H, Matsuda S, Kawakubo H, et al. Antimicrobial Prophylaxis With Ampicillin-sulbactam Compared With Cefazolin for Esophagectomy: Nationwide Inpatient Database Study in Japan.

Ann Surg*. *2024;279:640-7.

CLINICAL QUESTION OR PROBLEM

A retrospective registry study to evaluate the difference in short-term postoperative complications after esophagectomy for esophageal cancer between the use of cefazolin and ampicillin-sulbactam for postoperative prophylaxis. Short-term complications include surgical site infections, anastomotic leak, or postoperative respiratory failure.

WHAT IS ALREADY KNOWN?

Esophageal cancer is the 8th most common cancer worldwide.[6] Locally advanced tumors are best treated with a multimodal approach, which includes esophagectomy with adjuvant or neoadjuvant chemoradiotherapy or immunotherapy.[7] Esophagectomy is a complex surgical procedure with a high risk of postoperative complications. An anastomotic leak is defined as a full-thickness gastrointestinal defect involving the esophagus, anastomosis, staple line, or conduit, irrespective of the presentation or method of identification.[8] Pulmonary complications are frequent after Ivor Lewis Oesophagectomy (ILO) and may occur in >50% of patients.[9] Antimicrobial prophylaxis is recommended for clean contaminated gastrointestinal procedures. Procedure-specific antimicrobial prophylaxis may reduce the risk of postoperative complications after procedures such as pancreaticoduodenectomy,[10] colorectal surgery,[11] and pulmonary resection.[12] There are no studies on procedure-specific antimicrobial prophylaxis following esophagectomy. Some guidelines recommend the use of cefazolin without any evidence of specific benefit after esophagectomy.[13]

STUDY DESIGN

The salient features of this study are outlined in **Table 2**.

POPULATION STUDIED INCLUDING DEMOGRAPHICS

Adult patients who received cefazolin or ampicillin-sulbactam on the day of surgery and on postoperative day 1 after esophagectomy for esophageal cancer, from July 2010 to March 2019. The use of

TABLE 2: Study design.

Setting	Retrospective, multicenter, national registry (Diagnosis, Procedure Combination database) study. Submission of data to the repository is mandatory for all university hospitals in Japan
Countries	Japan
Blinding	Not applicable
Randomization	Not applicable
Informed consent	Waived
Ethics approval	Yes, the institute review board of the University of Tokyo
Sample size calculation	Not applicable

these antibiotics on the day of surgery was deemed as antibiotic prophylaxis for surgery. Transhiatal esophagectomies, which form only a minority of cases in Japan, were not included in this study.

The exclusion criteria were as follows:

- Age <18 years
- Missing data on body mass index
- Preoperative antibiotics
- Concomitant laryngeal surgery for cancer
- Intestinal reconstruction
- Reoperation on day 1 postoperative
- Discharge on day 2 after surgery

INTERVENTION(S) STUDIED

The following two groups were compared:

1. Use of cefazolin on the day of esophagectomy for esophageal cancer and continued at least on postoperative day 1.
2. Use of ampicillin-sulbactam on the day of esophagectomy for esophageal cancer and continued at least on postoperative day 1.

OUTCOMES EVALUATED

The primary outcomes were as follows:

- Surgical site infection
- Anastomotic leak
- Respiratory failure (The authors did not distinguish between pneumonia and respiratory failure due to atelectasis, or other reasons, as they could be exceedingly difficult to distinguish from each other. Respiratory failure was defined as the need for mechanical ventilation lasting more than 2 days after surgery.)

Secondary outcomes:

- Severe respiratory failure lasting >7 days after surgery
- *Clostridium difficile* colitis
- Noninfectious complications
- 30-day mortality
- Postoperative length of stay
- Total hospitalization cost

STATISTICAL ANALYSIS

Overlap propensity score weighting analysis was used to compare the cefazolin group to the ampicillin-sulbactam group. The overlap weighting analysis adjusts for measured potential confounding variables without excluding participants from the original sample.

STATISTICAL NOTE: PROPENSITY SCORE ANALYSIS

The propensity score analysis is a well-established and commonly used technique to evaluate the effect of a treatment or intervention in observational studies. Unlike prospective randomized controlled studies, it is often not possible to have a control group in observational studies like those evaluating rare diseases or review of registries (e.g., this study). Propensity score matching is a statistical method for reducing bias and estimating treatment effect when it is not possible to randomly assign patients to one or the other group. A simple but excellent multimedia demonstration of propensity score analysis is available on the web page by Mercuri et al.[14]

Sensitivity analyses were done using the 1:1 propensity score matching.

RESULTS

During the study period, there were 27,299 patients who were screened. 9,527 were excluded because they had one or more exclusion criteria, most commonly because the antibiotics were not given the next day ($n = 4{,}586$). 17,772 patients from 732 hospitals were analyzed. Cefazolin was administered to 90.5% of patients ($n = 16{,}077$), while ampicillin-sulbactam to 9.5% ($n = 1{,}695$).

Ampicillin-sulbactam was more likely to be used in patients with three-field lymph node dissection (as opposed to two-field lymph node dissection), longer duration of anesthesia, epidural anesthesia, prophylactic corticosteroid administration, or transfusion on the day of surgery.

Primary Outcomes

After overlap weighting, the risk of the primary outcomes was lower in the ampicillin-sulbactam group. The numbers are as follows:

- *Surgical site infection*: 10.6% versus 18.9%; odds ratio: 0.51; 95% CI: 0.43–0.60
- *Anastomotic leak*: 9.2% versus 16.5%; odds ratio: 0.51; 95% CI: 0.43–0.61
- *Respiratory failure*: 12.6 versus 17.8%; odds ratio: 0.66; 95% CI: 0.57–0.77

Secondary Outcomes

The ampicillin-sulbactam group also demonstrated lower hospital length of stay and lower hospitalization cost. The risk of *Clostridium difficile* colitis, infectious complications, and mortality did not differ in the two groups.

AUTHORS' VIEWPOINT

The use of ampicillin-sulbactam, compared to cefazolin, in patients undergoing esophagectomy for esophageal cancer is associated with a lower incidence of surgical site infection, anastomotic leak, and respiratory failure. This is the first study that has related the choice of antibiotics for surgical prophylaxis to these outcome measures. Multiple antibiotics have been used in different settings, but in the absence of evidence, the choice of antibiotics is left to the treating teams.

Recent evidence suggests that the esophageal microbiome consists of various streptococcus species and anaerobes, including *Veillonella*, *Prevotella*, and *Fusobacterium*.[15] Cefazolin acts against the streptococci but not against the anaerobes. There is, therefore, biological plausibility that the use of antibiotics that cover anaerobes will reduce the risk of surgical site infections.

STRENGTH OF THE STUDY

This is a very large study that covered over 10 years of data from all university hospitals across Japan and many nonteaching hospitals. The quality of the data had been validated in the past in published literature. The exclusion criteria were strict, and despite removing the patients who fulfilled the exclusion criteria, there were over 7,000 patients. The statistical analysis is rigorous. There is biological plausibility for the observed results, and they are in keeping with emerging evidence for site-specific prophylaxis for several other surgeries such as pancreaticoduodenectomy, colorectal surgery, etc.[9-11]

DRAWBACKS OF THE STUDY

This is a retrospective study and therefore suffers from the drawbacks of retrospective studies. However, in this case, the statistical analysis is robust, and the authors have gone the extra mile in their propensity analysis. It generates a useful hypothesis and sets the stage for a future prospective study. Minimally invasive surgery is coming up in a big way, and it is possible that the results of this study may not hold up with the new approach. The optimum duration of antimicrobial prophylaxis remains unclear. Patients who undergo intestinal reconstruction instead of a gastric pull-up should benefit from an individualized approach, but they were not included in this study.

REVIEWERS' VIEWPOINT

This is an excellent retrospective study. It has been well conducted. The statistical analysis is rigorous. There is biological plausibility in the results. The current practice of using cefazolin in most units is based on culture and dogma, and this study challenges the usual practice. It sets the stage for future studies. In the meantime, the results of this study should be discussed by the intensive care, infectious diseases, and surgical team in individual hospitals and potentially site-specific antibiotic prophylaxis considered for esophagectomy.

IMPACT ON CURRENT PRACTICE AND TAKE-HOME MESSAGE

Emerging evidence suggests that we are at the dawn of site-specific antibiotic prophylaxis. We need to review our current practice in light of emerging practices and consider the use of antibiotics that cover the esophageal microbiome. Local sensitivity patterns should be considered.

Ceftriaxone to Prevent Early Ventilator-Associated Pneumonia in Patients with Acute Brain Injury: A Multicentre, Randomised, Double-Blind, Placebo-Controlled, Assessor-Masked Superiority Trial

Dahyot-Fizelier C, Lasocki S, Kerforne T, Perrigault PF, Geeraerts T, Asehnoune K, et al.; PROPHY-VAP Study Group and the ATLANREA Study Group. Ceftriaxone to prevent early ventilator-associated pneumonia in patients with acute brain injury: a multicentre, randomised, double-blind, placebo-controlled, assessor-masked superiority trial.

Lancet Respir Med. 2024;12:375-85.

CLINICAL QUESTION OR PROBLEM

The ProphyVAP study evaluated the effectiveness of a single dose of 2 g of intravenous ceftriaxone, administered within 12 hours of endotracheal intubation, on the occurrence of early VAP in comatose patients with acute brain injury. Early ventilator-associated pneumonia (VAP), between days 2 and 7 of endotracheal intubation, was confirmed by masked assessors.[16]

WHAT IS ALREADY KNOWN?

Ventilated patients with acute brain injury are at high risk of developing VAP, with a reported incidence of 20–71% in patients with traumatic brain injury[17] and 28–76% in patients with stroke.[18] The development of VAP is a risk factor for mortality, prolonged intensive care unit (ICU) and hospital length of stay, and poor neurological outcomes.[19] Small studies have evaluated the role of prophylactic antibiotics in preventing VAP, either a single dose or as a short course.[20] A short course of antibiotics in patients managed with 32–34° targeted temperature after cardiac arrest has been shown to reduce the incidence of VAP.

STUDY DESIGN

The salient features of the ProphyVAP trial are outlined in **Table 3**.

POPULATION STUDIED INCLUDING DEMOGRAPHICS

Comatose (GCS ≤12) adult patients (>18 years), who needed endotracheal intubation and were predicted to require mechanical ventilation for >48 hours after traumatic brain injury or stroke or subarachnoid hemorrhage were eligible.

TABLE 3: Study design ProphyVAP study.	
Setting	Multicenter, 8 French ICUs
Countries	France
Blinding	Yes. Drugs prepared by nonparticipants. Opaque vials. Ventilator-associated pneumonia (VAP) confirmation by blinded assessors
Randomization	Yes. 1:1 in intervention vs. placebo. Stratified to center and severity of unconsciousness [Glasgow Coma Scale (GCS) <8]
Informed consent	Yes. Modified intention to treat analysis: If the participant refused consent, their data was not used
Sample size calculation	Assuming VAP risk of 30%, the intervention aimed at reducing the risk to half, with 90% power and a two-sided type-I error of 0.05
Primary outcome analysis	Modified intention to treat analysis (Those who did not consent or refused the use of their data were excluded)

Participants were excluded if they satisfied any of the following criteria.

- Coma due to tumor
- Ongoing antibiotic therapy
- High risk of death within 48 hours
- Previous hospitalization in the last 1 month
- Need for prophylactic antibiotics (e.g., after surgery)
- Endotracheal tube with subglottic suction drainage
- Nasotracheal intubation

INTERVENTION(S) STUDIED

Intervention Arm

A single dose of ceftriaxone, 2 g, intravenously, within 12 hours of endotracheal intubation. Prepared from a especially made vial compounded for the study purposes by a nurse, not from the ICU where the patient was being managed.

Control Arm

A single dose of saline, prepared from a especially made vial compounded for the study purposes by a nurse, not from the ICU where the patient was being managed.

COMPARATOR USED

Saline, as outlined above, a VAP prevention bundle which included interventions such as head end elevation, heated humidifier use, proton pump inhibitor use, oral hygiene, etc., was used in all patients.

OUTCOMES EVALUATED

Primary Outcome

Early VAP, between days 2 and 7. A standardized approach to diagnosis, as determined by the American Thoracic Society criteria, was used.[21] After the diagnosis of VAP was made by the treating team, a central adjudication committee, composed of two senior intensive care specialists, reviewed the data. This committee was blinded to the allocation. This committee made the final diagnosis of VAP.

Secondary Outcomes

The secondary outcomes studied were as follows:

- Late VAP, >7 days after intubation
- VAP any time until day 28
- Ventilator-free days on day 28
- Antibiotics-free days on day 60
- Neurological outcome
- ICU-free days and hospital-free days on day 28

STATISTICAL ANALYSIS

A sample size of 354 patients was decided assuming a VAP risk of 30%, the intervention aimed at reducing the risk to half, with 90% power and a two-sided type-I error of 0.05. Chi-square or Fischer exact test was used for categorical data and the Mann-Whitney U test for numerical data. This is an ambitious effect size.

STATISTICAL NOTE

Why do we use the term "ventilator-free days" (VFD), instead of "days on ventilator"?

It would be more appropriate to call VFD as "alive and ventilator-free days". VFD is a composite measure, that accounts for the patient being alive and free of mechanical ventilation. For the calculation of VFD, one point is given for each day that the patient is free of ventilation and alive.

For example, ventilator-free days are to be calculated at day 28 in the following two scenarios:

1. Patient intubated and then extubated after 2 days. Alive at day 28. VFD = 26.
2. Patient intubated, died on day 2, while intubated. VFD = 0.

Calculation of VFD may be confusing if the patient receives noninvasive ventilation, intermittent ventilation through a tracheostomy, or dies a few days after extubation. The definition of VFD is often imprecise in clinical trials and must be checked carefully when reviewing the results.

RESULTS

345 patients were randomized, but 319 were included in the final analysis due to exclusion for various reasons (withdrawal of consent, refusal of family to give consent or use data, patients under legal protection, etc.). The patient characteristics were balanced in the two groups. Of the 319 included in the final analysis, 162 received ceftriaxone, and 169 received placebo.

160 cases of VAP were reported in 139 patients by the investigators. These were referred to the adjudication committee. The adjudication committee judged that of these 93 episodes were VAP, in 90 patients. So, 90 patients out of 319 (28%) had at least one episode of VAP. Early VAP represented 82% of all episodes.

Primary Outcome

Early VAP occurred in 14% of the patients in the ceftriaxone group, and 32% of patients in the control group. The hazard ratio for the development of VAP in the ceftriaxone group was 0.60 (95% CI: 0.38–0.95), $p = 0.30$.

Secondary Outcomes

A few selected secondary outcomes are listed in **Table 4**.

AUTHORS' VIEWPOINT

For patients with acute brain injury, who need endotracheal intubation, a single dose of ceftriaxone within 12 hours of intubation reduced the risk of early VAP (2–7 days), VAP within 28 days, exposure to antibiotics, and the duration of mechanical ventilation. The authors sought to reduce the risk of VAP by 50%. This is an ambitious effect size, and the authors have been successful in demonstrating that. Patients with acute brain injury are at high risk of VAP. Pneumonia itself may worsen the outcome of brain injury. The results are in keeping with some of the recent trials, like the ANTHARTIC trial, in which the use of augmentin reduced the risk of VAP after cardiac arrest.[22] The authors are careful to point out that the impact of this approach on antimicrobial resistance and on the microbiome remains to be studied.

TABLE 4: Selected secondary outcomes.

Outcome	*Ceftriaxone group*	*Control group*	*Hazard ratio (HR) or p value*
Ventilator-associated pneumonia (VAP) any time until day 28: 20% vs. 36%; HR 0.62 (0.42–0.98)	20%	36%	HR 0.62
Ventilator-free days at day 28	9 (IQR: 0–22)	5 (IQR: 0–18)	$p = 0.023$
Antibiotics-free days at day 60	21 (IQR: 13–28)	15 (8–21)	$p < 0.0001$
Mortality day 28	15%	25%	HR 0.62 (0.39–0.97)
Mortality at 60 days	20%	30%	0.074

STRENGTH OF THE STUDY

This is a well-conducted study. It is multi-centered, randomized, blinded, and has a precise statistical plan.

DRAWBACKS OF THE STUDY

If the impact of the use of ceftriaxone on the development of resistance and on the microbiome were studied, it would have strengthened the safety profile of the intervention.

REVIEWERS' VIEWPOINT

This is a well-conducted study. In recent years, efforts to prevent VAP have centered around the use of selective decontamination of the digestive tract or selective oral decontamination. While some studies have shown a reduction in VAP, almost all those studies have fallen short of a comprehensive evaluation of the impact of the intervention on the development of resistance or microbiome.

IMPACT ON CURRENT PRACTICE AND TAKE-HOME MESSAGE

There is no doubt that further studies are required to confirm the findings of this study and to confirm the impact of the single dose of ceftriaxone on the development of antibiotic resistance and on the composition of the gut microbiome. Until more evidence is available, should we use the study intervention? It is hard to argue against giving ceftriaxone to prevent intubation in patients with acute brain injury getting intubated. Should we expand it to other groups of patients, who are perhaps not at such a high risk of aspiration? That decision will need to be individualized.

Postoperative Prophylactic Antibiotic Therapy after Pancreaticoduodenectomy in Bile Duct-Stented Patients Reduces Postoperative Major Complications

Steffani M, Jäger C, Hüser N, Friess H, Hartmann D, Demir IE, et al. Postoperative prophylactic antibiotic therapy after pancreaticoduodenectomy in bile duct-stented patients reduces postoperative major complications.

Surgery. 2024;176:1162-8.

CLINICAL QUESTION OR PROBLEM

Patients presenting for pancreaticoduodenectomy (PD), or Whipple's procedure, often have biliary obstruction in the preoperative period. Prior to surgery, they often require relief of biliary obstruction and placement of a biliary stent. This study evaluated the impact of postoperative antibiotic prophylaxis (with piperacillin-tazobactam, imipenem, or other antibiotics) on postoperative complications after PD.[23]

WHAT IS ALREADY KNOWN?

Patients with tumors of the pancreatic head or the bile duct (e.g., cholangiocarcinoma) commonly present with biliary obstruction and jaundice. They often require preoperative biliary decompression and stent placement.[24] Infections (wound, intra-abdominal, or elsewhere) are among the most common serious complications. Preoperative biliary stent placement may improve morbidity and mortality after PD.[25] Biliary stent placement is also an increasingly recognized risk factor for the development of postoperative infection.[26]

The placement of a biliary stent alters the normal biliary microbiome from bacteria such as *E. coli* to other bacteria (e.g., *Enterococcus faecium, Enterococcus faecalis, Enterobacter cloacae,* and *Klebsiella*).[27] The presence of contaminated bile at the time of surgery is associated with an increased risk of wound infection. There are, however, no standardized guidelines for perioperative antibiotic prophylaxis after PD.

STUDY DESIGN

The salient features of the trial are outlined in **Table 5**.

POPULATION STUDIED INCLUDING DEMOGRAPHICS

In this retrospective study, patients who underwent PD between 2007 and 2015 at Klinikum Rechts der Isar of the Technical University of Munich, who underwent preoperative bile duct stenting, and had intraoperative bile culture were included in the study. Intraoperatively, the patients received ampicillin-sulbactam in the first few years of the study and piperacillin-tazobactam in the latter years. An intraoperative bile

TABLE 5: Study design.

Setting	Single center, Klinikum Rechts der Isar of the Technical University of Munich
Countries	Germany
Design	Retrospective and observational
Blinding	Not applicable
Randomization	Not applicable
Informed consent	Yes. No details in the study on how it was obtained
Sample size calculation	15-year study period without sample size calculation
Ethics approval	Yes

sample was taken. Postoperative antibiotic therapy was tailored to bile culture results.

INTERVENTION(S) STUDIED

Intervention Arm

Since there were no guidelines available for postoperative prophylactic antibiotics, the choice was made by the surgeons based on intraoperative findings, and preoperative clinical and laboratory status. The other group received broad spectrum antibiotics (mostly piperacillin-tazobactam). This group was called the antibiotic prophylaxis group.

Control Arm (Nonantibiotic Prophylaxis Group)

Some patients received prophylaxis according to the WHO guidelines for surgery. This group of patients was called the nonantibiotic prophylaxis group. The authors have not reported which antibiotic (e.g., first-generation cephalosporin) was used in these patients.

OUTCOMES EVALUATED

Primary Outcomes

There was no primary outcome for this retrospective study. The following outcomes were evaluated:

- Death within 30 days of surgery
- Postoperative complications, major or minor as evaluated by the Clavien-Dindo classification.[28] Class 0–II was classified as minor complications, and III–V as major complications.
- Postoperative wound infections
- Postoperative pancreatic fistula

STATISTICAL ANALYSIS

Categorical data was analyzed using the chi-square test or Fischer exact test. Continuous variables were evaluated using the Kruskal-Wallis test or Mann-Whitney U test. The odds ratio and the confidence intervals were calculated using logistic regression.

STATISTICAL NOTE

Retrospective observational studies suffer from several drawbacks, and therefore, even when their conclusions appear to be convincing, generally need to be confirmed with prospective studies. While they may demonstrate association, a cause-effect relationship can generally not be ascertained from retrospective data. This, however, does not mean that retrospective studies have no role. They are vital in the study of rare diseases. Retrospective data generates a hypothesis, which serves as the basis for prospective studies.

Some common drawbacks of retrospective studies are:

- Since the information is obtained from medical records, there is often missed data.
- Lack of control over sampling
- Selection bias
- Recall bias

RESULTS

370 fulfilled the criteria for inclusion. 291 patients were included in the antibiotic prophylaxis group, and 79 patients were in the nonantibiotic prophylaxis group. While the number of patients in the two groups is quite different, the characteristics of the patients in the two groups were evenly matched. Most patients had carcinoma of the pancreas or biliary duct.

OUTCOMES

There was no primary outcome in this retrospective study. The overall number of complications in the two groups was similar. However, more major complications (Clavien-Dindo class III–V) occurred in the nonantibiotic prophylaxis group.

These included:

- Longer ICU stay in nonantibiotic prophylaxis group (15.2% vs. 7.6%; $p = 0.037$)
- More reoperations in the nonantibiotic prophylaxis group (16.5 vs. 8.6%; $p = 0.034$)
- More pneumonia nonantibiotic prophylaxis group (3.8 vs. 0.7%; $p = 0.034$)

There was no significant difference in the number of surgical site infections, deep abdominal infections, sepsis, urinary tract infection, cholangitis, or pancreatic fistula.

Logistic regression demonstrated that antibiotic prophylaxis was associated with significantly fewer postoperative major complications [OR: 0.547 (95% CI: 0.327–0.915); $p = 0.02$].

Positive bile culture was noted in 87% of patients in the nonantibiotic prophylaxis group and 94% in the antibiotic prophylaxis group. The most common organisms isolated included *E. faecium*, *E. faecalis*, *E. cloacae*, and *Klebsiella*.

AUTHORS' VIEWPOINT

The authors concluded that antibiotic prophylaxis is associated with reduced risk of major complications.

STRENGTH OF THE STUDY

This study, while it has the shortcomings of a retrospective study, adds to a growing body of evidence that:

- Patients who undergo biliary stenting prior to PD have a higher risk of biliary infection.
- The antibiotic prophylaxis used for surgery to other parts of the body (e.g., neurosurgery, orthopedic surgery, etc.), typically with first-generation cephalosporins to primarily prevent Gram-positive infections is not adequate for patients undergoing major gastrointestinal surgery with complex reconstruction.

DRAWBACKS OF THE STUDY

This is a retrospective study and suffers from the limitations of such studies as outlined in the statistical note above. It should also be noted that the number of patients in the two groups is quite different. Also, the authors do not report the nature of antibiotics in the nonantibiotic prophylaxis group, which did receive some antibiotics.

REVIEWERS' VIEWPOINT

There is no doubt that this study suffers from several drawbacks, as noted above, and any conclusions drawn to change practice solely based on this study alone would be imprudent. There are still no guidelines from any infectious disease society or surgical society on the choice of prophylactic antibiotics for patients undergoing PD.

We know that the risk of biliary colonization with pathogenic bacteria is common after biliary stenting.[27] Just like appropriate antimicrobials are required for surgery on an infected organ (say, septic arthritis or a liver abscess), similarly, appropriate antibiotic therapy is required when the risk of biliary contamination is high, e.g., after biliary stenting.

A review of this study provided me an opportunity to study in detail the nuances of antimicrobial use after PD.[24] I am now more cautious of the knowledge that a patient admitted to my intensive care unit (ICU) after Whipple's procedure had a biliary stent, the results of their preoperative biliary culture, whether intraoperative biliary culture was taken, and whether pus was present at the time of dissection of the biliary duct. This knowledge allows me to use broad-spectrum antibiotics in appropriate patients.

IMPACT ON CURRENT PRACTICE AND TAKE-HOME MESSAGE

As intensive care physicians looking after patients admitted to our ICU after Whipple's procedure, we should pay close attention to preoperative biliary interventions, preoperative and intraoperative bile culture, and where a high risk of infection is likely, use appropriate broad-spectrum antibiotics.

REFERENCES

1. Dulhunty JM, Brett SJ, De Waele JJ, Rajbhandari D, Billot L, Cotta MO, et al. Continuous vs Intermittent beta-lactam Antibiotic Infusions in Critically Ill Patients With Sepsis: The BLING III Randomized Clinical Trial. JAMA. 2024;332(8):629-37.
2. IBM. Interpreting logistic regression: IBM. [online] Available from https://www.ibm.com/topics/logistic-regression [Last accessed January, 2025].
3. Dulhunty JM, Roberts JA, Davis JS, Webb SA, Bellomo R, Gomersall C, et al. Continuous infusion of beta-lactam antibiotics in severe sepsis: a multicenter double-blind, randomized controlled trial. Clin Infect Dis. 2013;56(2):236-44.
4. Dulhunty JM, Roberts JA, Davis JS, Webb SA, Bellomo R, Gomersall C, et al. A Multicenter Randomized Trial of Continuous versus Intermittent β-Lactam Infusion in Severe Sepsis. Am J Respir Crit Care Med. 2015;192(11):1298-305.
5. Monti G, Bradic N, Marzaroli M, Konkayev A, Fominskiy E, Kotani Y, et al. Continuous vs Intermittent Meropenem Administration in Critically Ill Patients With Sepsis: The MERCY Randomized Clinical Trial. JAMA. 2023;330(2):141-51.
6. Napier KJ, Scheerer M, Misra S. Esophageal cancer: A Review of epidemiology, pathogenesis, staging workup and treatment modalities. World J Gastrointest Oncol. 2014;6(5):112-20.
7. Morgan MA, Lewis WG, Casbard A, Roberts SA, Adams R, Clark GW, et al. Stage-for-stage comparison of definitive chemoradiotherapy, surgery alone and neoadjuvant chemotherapy for oesophageal carcinoma. Br J Surg. 2009;96(11):1300-7.
8. Low DE, Alderson D, Cecconello I, Chang AC, Darling GE, D'Journo XB, et al. International Consensus on Standardization of Data Collection for Complications Associated With Esophagectomy: Esophagectomy Complications Consensus Group (ECCG). Ann Surg. 2015;262(2):286-94.
9. Hulscher JB, van Sandick JW, de Boer AG, Wijnhoven BP, Tijssen JG, Fockens P, et al. Extended transthoracic resection compared with limited transhiatal resection for adenocarcinoma of the esophagus. N Engl J Med. 2002;347(21):1662-9.
10. D'Angelica MI, Ellis RJ, Liu JB, Brajcich BC, Gönen M, Thompson VM, et al. Piperacillin-Tazobactam Compared With Cefoxitin as Antimicrobial Prophylaxis for Pancreatoduodenectomy: A Randomized Clinical Trial. JAMA. 2023;329(18):1579-88.
11. Castagneto-Gissey L, Russo MF, Casella-Mariolo J, Serao A, Marcellinaro R, D'Andrea V, et al. The Role of Antibiotic Prophylaxis in Anastomotic Leak Prevention during Elective Colorectal Surgery: Systematic Review and Meta-Analysis of Randomized Controlled Trials. Antibiotics (Basel). 2023;12(2).
12. Schussler O, Dermine H, Alifano M, Casetta A, Coignard S, Roche N, et al. Should we change antibiotic prophylaxis for lung surgery? Postoperative pneumonia is the critical issue. Ann Thorac Surg. 2008;86(6):1727-33.
13. Ohge H, Mayumi T, Haji S, Kitagawa Y, Kobayashi M, Mizuguchi T, et al. The Japan Society for Surgical Infection: guidelines for the prevention, detection, and management of gastroenterological surgical site infection, 2018. Surg Today. 2021;51(1):1-31.
14. Eugenio Mercuri FM, Osorio AN, et al. (2022). Propensity score matching methodology: why and how it is used. Video Journal of Biomedicine. [online] Available from https://www.biomedicine.video/animated-videos/propensity-score-matching-methodology-why-and-how-it-is-used [Last accessed January, 2025].
15. Di Pilato V, Freschi G, Ringressi MN, Pallecchi L, Rossolini GM, Bechi P. The esophageal microbiota in health and disease. Ann N Y Acad Sci. 2016;1381(1):21-33.
16. Dahyot-Fizelier C, Lasocki S, Kerforne T, Perrigault PF, Geeraerts T, Asehnoune K,

et al. Ceftriaxone to prevent early ventilator-associated pneumonia in patients with acute brain injury: a multicentre, randomised, double-blind, placebo-controlled, assessor-masked superiority trial. Lancet Respir Med. 2024;12(5):375-85.

17. Robba C, Rebora P, Banzato E, Wiegers EJA, Stocchetti N, Menon DK, et al. Incidence, Risk Factors, and Effects on Outcome of Ventilator-Associated Pneumonia in Patients With Traumatic Brain Injury: Analysis of a Large, Multicenter, Prospective, Observational Longitudinal Study. Chest. 2020;158(6):2292-303.
18. Yuan MZ, Li F, Tian X, Wang W, Jia M, Wang XF, et al. Risk factors for lung infection in stroke patients: a meta-analysis of observational studies. Expert Rev Anti Infect Ther. 2015;13(10):1289-98.
19. Rincón-Ferrari MD, Flores-Cordero JM, Leal-Noval SR, Murillo-Cabezas F, Cayuelas A, Muñoz-Sánchez MA, et al. Impact of ventilator-associated pneumonia in patients with severe head injury. J Trauma. 2004;57(6):1234-40.
20. Vallés J, Peredo R, Burgueño MJ, Rodrigues de Freitas AP, Millán S, Espasa M, et al. Efficacy of single-dose antibiotic against early-onset pneumonia in comatose patients who are ventilated. Chest. 2013;143(5):1219-25.
21. Society AT, America IDSo. Guidelines for the management of adults with hospital-acquired, ventilator-associated, and healthcare-associated pneumonia. Am J Respir Crit Care Med. 2005;171(4):388-416.
22. François B, Cariou A, Clere-Jehl R, Dequin PF, Renon-Carron F, Daix T, et al. Prevention of Early Ventilator-Associated Pneumonia after Cardiac Arrest. N Engl J Med. 2019;381(19):1831-42.
23. Steffani M, Jäger C, Hüser N, Friess H, Hartmann D, Demir IE, et al. Postoperative prophylactic antibiotic therapy after pancreaticoduodenectomy in bile duct-stented patients reduces postoperative major complications. Surgery. 2024;176(4):1162-1168.
24. van der Gaag NA, Kloek JJ, de Castro SM, Busch OR, van Gulik TM, Gouma DJ. Preoperative biliary drainage in patients with obstructive jaundice: history and current status. J Gastrointest Surg. 2009;13(4):814-20.
25. Klinkenbijl JH, Jeekel J, Schmitz PI, Rombout PA, Nix GA, Bruining HA, et al. Carcinoma of the pancreas and periampullary region: palliation versus cure. Br J Surg. 1993;80(12):1575-8.
26. DeOliveira ML, Winter JM, Schafer M, Cunningham SC, Cameron JL, Yeo CJ, et al. Assessment of complications after pancreatic surgery: A novel grading system applied to 633 patients undergoing pancreaticoduodenectomy. Ann Surg. 2006;244(6):931-7; discussion 7-9.
27. Goel N, Nadler A, Reddy S, Hoffman JP, Pitt HA. Biliary microbiome in pancreatic cancer: alterations with neoadjuvant therapy. HPB (Oxford). 2019;21(12):1753-60.
28. Dindo D, Demartines N, Clavien PA. Classification of surgical complications: a new proposal with evaluation in a cohort of 6336 patients and results of a survey. Ann Surg. 2004;240(2):205-13.

SECTION

7

Sepsis

Section Editor: *Manoj Y Singh*

Continuous vs Intermittent β-Lactam Antibiotic Infusions in Critically Ill Patients With Sepsis: The BLING III Randomized Clinical Trial[1]

Dulhunty JM, Brett SJ, De Waele JJ, Rajbhandari D, Billot L, Cotta MO, et al. Continuous vs Intermittent β-Lactam Antibiotic Infusions in Critically Ill Patients With Sepsis: The BLING III Randomized Clinical Trial. ***JAMA. 2024;332:629-37.***

CLINICAL QUESTION OR PROBLEM

Does the administration of beta-lactam antibiotics via a continuous infusion versus intermittent infusion in patients admitted to the intensive care unit (ICU) with presumed reduce 90-day mortality?

WHAT IS ALREADY KNOWN?

Pharmacodynamically, beta-lactam have time-dependent bactericidal activity. It makes obvious sense that the efficacy of these antibiotics is much better when administered as a continuous infusion. But the level above the minimum inhibitory concentration (MIC) for longer duration can also be achieved by frequent intermittent dosing of the antibiotics. Given sepsis is a hyperdynamic state, it can potentially increase drug clearance as the cardiac output is augmented. In addition, the capillary leak can also increase the overall volume of distribution.

Two previous studies have not shown any mortality benefit with continuous infusion. The MERCY trial [multicenter, randomized controlled trial (RCT) with 607 patients] showed a nonsignificant 2% reduction in overall 28-day mortality but no difference at 90-day all-cause mortality.[2] BLING II trial (multicenter, RCT, 432 patients) had failed to demonstrate ICU-free days at 18 and 20 days.[3]

STUDY DESIGN

- Multicenter, open-label RCT (randomization using web-based system with 1:1 ratio)
- *Power calculation*: Based on BLING II, a sample size of 7,000 to achieve 90% power to detect a 3.5% difference in all-cause mortality at 90 days including a 5% loss to follow-up based on baseline mortality of 27.5%
- Clinical cure was defined as completion of beta-lactam antibiotic by day 14 without

recommencement of antibiotics within 48 hours of cessation for the same infective episode.
- 104 ICUs across 7 countries (Australia, New Zealand, Belgium, France, Sweden, and Malaysia)

POPULATION STUDIED INCLUDING DEMOGRAPHICS

- *Inclusion:*
  - Adults with age >18 years
  - Strong suspicion or documented site of infection
  - Patients admitted to ICU and expected to remain in ICU for at least another 24 hours
  - A beta-lactam antibiotic commenced in the last 24 hours.
- *Exclusion:*
  - Receipt of piperacillin-tazobactam or meropenem for >24 hours during the current infectious episode
  - Patient known or suspected to be pregnant
  - Known allergy to piperacillin-tazobactam, meropenem, or penicillin
  - Requiring renal replacement therapy (RRT) (acute or chronic)
  - Previously enrolled in BLING III
  - Palliative treatment only, limits to care, death is imminent, or death is likely within 90 days due to underlying process
- A total of 7,202 patients were included in the study.
  - Average age was 59.3 years, 65% male
  - Very well-matched groups in both arms in terms of APCHE II scores, vasopressor or inotrope requirements, source of admission, and site of infection.

INTERVENTION(S) STUDIED

- Continuous infusion of beta-lactam antibiotic (for clinician-prescribed duration OR until ICU discharge)
- Infusion over 24 hours began with a bolus of intermittent dose as a load.
- Median duration was 5.8 days.

COMPARATOR USED

- Intermittent infusion of beta-lactam mover 30 minutes
- Median duration was 5.7 days.

OUTCOMES EVALUATED

- *Primary outcomes:*
  - *No significant difference in all-cause mortality at day 90*: 24.9% (continuous) versus 26.8% (intermittent)
  - *Adjusted absolute risk reduction (ARR):* −2.2% (95% CI: −5.5 to 1.1) OR 0.89 (95% CI: 0.79–0.99), $p = 0.04$
  - *Number needed to treat (NNT):* 52
- *Secondary outcomes comparing continuous versus intermittent infusion:*
  - Clinical cure: 55.7% versus 50.0%: ARR 5.7% (95% CI: 2.4–9.1); $p < 0.$
- No significant difference in:
  - New acquisition/colonization/infection with multidrug-resistant organism (MRO) or *Clostridioides difficile*: 7.2 versus 7.5%; ARR: −0.3%; $p = 0.65$
  - All-cause ICU mortality: 17.1 versus 18.4% ARR: −1.3%; $p = 0.35$
  - All-cause hospital mortality: 23.3 versus 25%; ARR −1.8%; $p = 0.27$
  - Days alive and free of ICU, hospital, mechanical ventilation, or RRT by day 90
- *Adverse events*: No significant difference in the two groups

STRENGTH OF THE STUDY

- Multicenter study design, with well-balanced baseline characteristics after randomization.
- Doses and duration of antibiotics were similar in the two groups.
- Minimal loss of follow-up

DRAWBACKS OF THE STUDY

- Unblinded
- The study definition of cure is not universal and 48 hours may not be long enough to state if a cure is achieved.
- Difficult to rule out systemic inflammatory response syndrome (SIRS).
- Nearly one-third of patients had protocol violations in each arm with delays in the administration of antibiotics.

AUTHORS' VIEWPOINT

The use of continuous infusion of beta-lactam antibiotics did not meet statistical significance in 90-day all-cause mortality but was associated with a better cure rate of infection. One may use a continuous infusion treating multi-resistant organisms.

IMPACT ON CURRENT PRACTICE AND TAKE-HOME MESSAGE

While there is no evidence to harm with the use of continuous infusion of beta-lactams, one can consider its use especially if an access is available to reduce staff load and decrease the frequency of access to a venous cannula or central line.

Lower vs. Higher Fluid Volumes in Adult Patients with Sepsis. An updated Systematic Review with Meta-Analysis and Trial Sequential Analysis[4]

Sivapalan P, Ellekjaer KL, Jessen MK, Meyhoff TS, Cronhjort M, Hjortrup PB, et al. Lower vs Higher Fluid Volumes in Adult Patients With Sepsis: An Updated Systematic Review With Meta-Analysis and Trial Sequential Analysis.

Chest*. *2023;164:892-912.

CLINICAL QUESTION OR PROBLEM

Does the administration of lower versus higher fluid volumes improve various patient-centered outcomes in adult patients with sepsis?

WHAT IS ALREADY KNOWN?

Fluid resuscitation forms an essential component when resuscitating a patient with suspected or confirmed sepsis. Since the ground-breaking EGDT trial by Rivers et al., there has been a paradigm shift in how we approach after initial fluid resuscitation. Fluid administration must be monitored to avoid positive fluid balance and fluid overload, which has been associated with multiple adverse outcomes including increased mortality, prolonged mechanical ventilation, and worsening of acute kidney injury (AKI). Recently two major trials Conservative versus Liberal Approach to Fluid Therapy of Septic Shock in Intensive Care (CLASSIC)[5] and the Crystalloid Liberal or Vasopressors Early Resuscitation in Sepsis (CLOVERS) trials[6] were designed to address whether a restrictive versus a liberal approach in fluid management would improve outcomes in patients with sepsis. In both trials, no difference was detected in the primary outcome of 90-day mortality. Nevertheless, there are several reasons why liberal fluid strategy should be avoided.[7] In a CLOVERS trial, restrictive fluid was not associated with worse mortality. Fluid responsiveness does not equate to the fact that a patient needs fluids. Moreover, fluid responders in AMDROMEDA-SHOCK study[8] demonstrated that fluid responsiveness was lost within 8 hours after fluid bolus therapy.

STUDY DESIGN

Systematic review with meta-analysis and trial sequential analysis of randomized clinical trials assesses lower versus higher intravenous (IV) fluid volumes in adult patients with sepsis.

POPULATION STUDIED INCLUDING DEMOGRAPHICS

Adult patients with sepsis (as defined in the original trials) independent of hospital setting.

TYPES OF STUDIES

- *Included:* All RCTs comparing different strategies intended to obtain a separation in IV fluid volumes in hospitalized adults with sepsis. No restrictions regarding language, publication source, or status were placed. RCTs with a preplanned strategy for separation of IV fluid volumes or balances regardless of whether a separation was obtained.
- *Excluded:* Quasi-randomized trials because of selection bias and crossover trials because of the nature of the design. Trials comparing different types of fluids and trials of resuscitation of severe blood loss and burns.

OUTCOME MEASURED

- *Primary:* The coprimary outcomes were all-cause mortality, serious adverse events (SAEs), and health-related quality of life.
- *Secondary:* Duration of mechanical ventilation, ventilator-free days, duration of vasopressor or inotropes, vasopressor-free days, use of RRT, duration of RRT, RRT-free days, and incidence of AKI.

SEARCH METHODS

All major databases include Cochrane Library, MEDLINE, Embase, Science Citation Index Expanded, Conference Proceedings Citation Index, and BIOSIS previews and Epistemologies.

INTERVENTION(S) STUDIED

Lower versus higher IV fluid volumes in adult patients with sepsis.

RESULTS

- A total of 13 trials were included in the meta-analysis of which 10 included patients from ICU and 3 from emergency department (ED) settings. 6 were single center and 7 were multicenter trials.
- *Primary outcomes:* The meta-analysis of all-cause mortality in eight trials with low risk of bias showed a relative risk of 0.99 (97% CI: 0.89–1.10). Six trials with predefined definitions of SAEs showed a relative risk of 0.95 (97% CI: 0.83–1.07; low certainty evidence). Health-related quality of life was not reported.
- *Secondary outcomes:*
  - 7 trials reported duration of mechanical ventilation and a meta-analysis of 4 trials with low risk of bias showed no statistically significant difference in the two study groups.
  - 10 trials reported ventilator-free days of which 5 were included in the

meta-analysis as had low risk of bias and showed no difference between in two study groups.

- 7 trials reported circulatory support and duration of vasopressors and 6 were included in the meta-analysis and showed no difference in the two study groups. Vasopressor-free days were not statistically different.
- 9 trials reported the use of RRT while 3 reported the incidence of AKI. Of the studies included in the meta-analysis showed no difference in outcomes.

DRAWBACKS OF THE STUDY

- The separation of fluid volumes between the groups was unsuccessful in five trials, which may have contributed to the finding of no difference in the outcomes.
- The definitions of sepsis and septic shock were not consistent across the trials, which may influence mortality because this varies according to the definitions used.
- The heterogeneity in the patient population and interventions may have been present because seven trials included patients in the ICU, three trials included patients from the ED, and three trials included patients from both settings.
- Some fluid trials used more complex protocols including a bundle of interventions. We allowed all types of IV fluid, and one trial used hydroxyethyl starch with well-known harms in patients with sepsis.
- Definitions of SAEs vary across trials and SAEs are likely underreported.

AUTHORS' VIEWPOINT

- In this systematic review of adult patients with sepsis, lower IV fluid volumes probably result in little to no difference in all-cause mortality compared with higher IV fluid volume.
- This meta-analysis suggests that lower IV fluid volumes result in little to no difference in SAEs; however, we need more robust RCTs to study these in more detail.

IMPACT ON CURRENT PRACTICE AND TAKE-HOME MESSAGE

Among adult patients with sepsis, lower IV fluid volumes probably result in little to no difference in all-cause mortality and SAEs when compared with higher fluid volumes, but the interpretation is limited by imprecision in effect estimates, which does not exclude potential benefit or harm.

Cefepime vs. Piperacillin-Tazobactam in Adults Hospitalized with Acute Infection. The ACORN Randomized Clinical Trial[9]

Qian ET, Casey JD, Wright A, Wang L, Shotwell MS, Siemann JK, et al.; Vanderbilt Center for Learning Healthcare and the Pragmatic Critical Care Research Group. Cefepime vs Piperacillin-Tazobactam in Adults Hospitalized With Acute Infection: The ACORN Randomized Clinical Trial.

JAMA. 2023;330:1557-67.

CLINICAL QUESTION OR PROBLEM

Does the administration of cefepime or piperacillin-tazobactam (pip-taz) result in an increased incidence of AKI or death by day 14 in acutely ill adults in the ED and ICU?

WHAT IS ALREADY KNOWN?

Sepsis is one of the leading causes of admission to critical care environments, especially ICU. Given the undifferentiated nature, many guidelines recommend antipseudomonal antibiotics. Antibiotic usage does come with adverse effects (namely nephrotoxicity by pip-taz and neurotoxicity by cefepime), especially in patients with altered pharmacokinetics secondary to organ dysfunction. Limited studies have evaluated these risks.

STUDY DESIGN

- A pragmatic, single-center, open-label, parallel-group RCT (randomization without stratification in a 1:1 ratio).
- Data was collected on electronic medical record (EMR) and clinicians were asked to document the reason for starting or stopping unassigned antibiotics for 7 days following randomization.

POPULATION STUDIED INCLUDING DEMOGRAPHICS

- *Inclusion*:
    - Adults with age >18 years in ED or medical ICU
    - <12 hours from presentation and a treating clinician starting an antipseudomonal cephalosporin or penicillin
- *Exclusion*:
    - Known allergy to antipseudomonal antibiotics
    - Not needing an antipseudomonal antibiotic or have received the same in the last 7 days

RESULTS

- A total of 2,634 patients were included in the study.
    - 1,277 to cefepime and 1,357 to pip-taz
    - Very well-matched groups in both arms in terms of age, hours from presentation to enrolment, suspected sites of infections, sepsis, SOFA scores, vasopressor or mechanical ventilation requirements, chronic kidney disease (CKD), and AKI at enrollment.

INTERVENTION STUDIED

- Cefepime was administered 2 g over 5 minutes every 8 hours compared to 3.375 g of pip-taz over 30 minutes for administered followed by every 8 hours over 4 hours.
- No other antipseudomonal antibiotics allowed
- Duration of therapy and addition of other antibiotics (e.g., vancomycin) at clinician's discretion

- Dedicated clinical pharmacists in both ED and ICU

OUTCOMES EVALUATED

- *Primary outcomes*: Comparing cefepime versus pip-taz
    - AKI (any stage) or death by day 14, OR 0.95 (95% CI 0.80–1.13)
    - *Death:* 7.6 versus 6.0%, ARR 1.6%, (95% CI -0.5 to 3.6)
- *Secondary outcomes comparing cefepime versus pip-taz*:
    - *Major adverse kidney events (MAKE) at day 14:* 10.2 versus 8.8%, ARR 1.4%; 95% CI: -1.0 to 3.8
    - *Delirium or coma incidence*: 20.8 versus 17.3%
        - *ARR:* 3.4%, (95% CI: 0.3–6.6)
        - *NNT:* 28
- No difference in vasopressor-free days, ventilator-free days, ICU free-days, and hospital-free days by day 28.

STRENGTH OF THE STUDY

- Large study addressing an important and frequently used intervention with limited good-quality evidence
- Strong internal validity
- Leveraging the EMR to recruit and conducting multiple sensitivity analyses for both the primary and secondary outcomes enhances robustness.

DRAWBACKS OF THE STUDY

- Single center, unblinded study
- Approximately 20% of patients received an alternate antibiotic within the first 14 days; however, exposure was similar in both groups.
- Median duration of antibiotic exposure was short and only ~50% of the population was retrospectively deemed to meet sepsis III criteria by study investigators.
- This may bias toward the null but is reflective of the undifferentiated nature of ED presentations which made up a large proportion of randomizations.
- Relatively low rates of critically unwell patients.

AUTHORS' VIEWPOINT

Most of us usually use pip-taz in our clinical practice and is associated with lower adverse outcomes compared to cefepime.

IMPACT ON CURRENT PRACTICE AND TAKE-HOME MESSAGE

There is no need to change our practice and when considering the use of cefepime it is important to keep in mind its potential risk of neurotoxicity, especially in the critically ill with altered pharmacokinetics or blood-brain barrier disruption.

REFERENCES

1. Dulhunty JM, Brett SJ, De Waele JJ, Rajbhandari D, Billot L, Cotta MO, et al. Continuous vs Intermittent beta-Lactam Antibiotic Infusions in Critically Ill Patients With Sepsis: The BLING III Randomized Clinical Trial. JAMA. 2024;332(8):629-37.
2. Monti G, Bradic N, Marzaroli M, Konkayev A, Fominskiy E, Kotani Y, et al. Continuous vs Intermittent Meropenem Administration in Critically Ill Patients With Sepsis: The MERCY Randomized Clinical Trial. JAMA. 2023;330(2):141-51.
3. Udy AA, Dulhunty JM, Roberts JA, Davis JS, Webb SAR, Bellomo R, et al. Association between augmented renal clearance and clinical outcomes in patients receiving beta-lactam antibiotic therapy by continuous or intermittent infusion: a nested cohort study of the BLING-II randomised, placebo-controlled, clinical trial. Int J Antimicrob Agents. 2017;49(5):624-30.
4. Sivapalan P, Ellekjaer KL, Jessen MK, Meyhoff TS, Cronhjort M, Hjortrup PB, et al. Lower vs

Higher Fluid Volumes in Adult Patients With Sepsis: An Updated Systematic Review With Meta-Analysis and Trial Sequential Analysis. Chest. 2023;164(4):892-912.

5. Meyhoff TS, Hjortrup PB, Wetterslev J, Sivapalan P, Laake JH, Cronhjort M, et al. Restriction of Intravenous Fluid in ICU Patients with Septic Shock. N Engl J Med. 2022;386(26):2459-70.
6. National Heart, Lung, and Blood Institute Prevention and Early Treatment of Acute Lung Injury Clinical Trials Network; Shapiro NI, Douglas IS, Brower RG, et al. Early Restrictive or Liberal Fluid Management for Sepsis-Induced Hypotension. N Engl J Med. 2023;388(6):499-510.
7. Taniguchi TM, Taniguchi LU. Fluid management in sepsis: 5 reasons why less fluid might be more rational. Crit Care Sci. 2024;36:e20240111en.
8. Kattan E, Ospina-Tascon GA, Teboul JL, Castro R, Cecconi M, Ferri G, et al. Systematic assessment of fluid responsiveness during early septic shock resuscitation: secondary analysis of the ANDROMEDA-SHOCK trial. Crit Care. 2020;24(1):23.
9. Qian ET, Casey JD, Wright A, Wang L, Shotwell MS, Siemann JK, et al. Cefepime vs Piperacillin-Tazobactam in Adults Hospitalized With Acute Infection: The ACORN Randomized Clinical Trial. JAMA. 2023;330(16):1557-67.

SECTION

8

Hematology

Section Editor: Gunjan Chanchalani

Early and Empirical High-Dose Cryoprecipitate for Hemorrhage after Traumatic Injury: The CRYOSTAT-2 Randomized Clinical Trial[1]

Davenport R, Curry N, Fox EE, Thomas H, Lucas J, Evans A, et al. Early and Empirical High-Dose Cryoprecipitate for Hemorrhage after Traumatic Injury: The CRYOSTAT-2 Randomized Clinical Trial.

JAMA. 2023;330:1882-91.

BACKGROUND

Hemorrhage is the most common preventable cause of early death in patients with trauma which is further exacerbated by coagulation factor consumption including acute fibrinogen deficiency. It has been shown that one-third of patients with trauma have fibrinogen concentration <2 g/L on admission and in up to three-fourths of the patients with trauma-induced coagulopathy.

CRYOSTAT[2] pilot randomized controlled trial found that early transfusion of cryoprecipitate was feasible with a mean time of 60 minutes in a major hemorrhage protocol and raised fibrinogens levels.

CLINICAL QUESTION

Does transfusion of early and empirical high-dose cryoprecipitate in addition to standard care improve survival in bleeding patients with trauma who require activation of a major hemorrhage protocol?

STUDY DESIGN

- Multicenter—26 UK and US major trauma centers
- International
- Randomized clinical trial, 1:1 assigned
- Open label
- Intention-to-treat

POPULATION

- Injured adult patients >16 years of age
- Requiring activation of hospital's major hemorrhage protocol with evidence of active hemorrhage, systolic blood pressure <90 mm Hg at any time and receiving at least one unit of blood component transfusion.
- Patients in the whom 3 hours had elapsed from the time of injury or those having

injuries incompatible with life were excluded from the study.

INTERVENTION

Cryoprecipitate group—three pools of cryoprecipitate (6 g fibrinogen equivalent) administered in addition to standard care within 90 minutes of randomization and 3 hours of injury.

CONTROL

Standard care—reviewed for guideline adherence for local major hemorrhage protocol.

OUTCOMES

- *Primary outcomes:* All-cause 28-day mortality in the intention-to-treat population was 26.1% in the standard care group versus 25.3% in the cryoprecipitate group.
- No difference in transfusion requirements and safety events—thrombosis.

SUBGROUP ANALYSIS

- The penetrating injury group had worser 28-day mortality in cryoprecipitate group [16.2 vs. 10%, odds ratio (OR): 1.74].
- The blunt injury group had 28-day mortality of 30.4% in cryoprecipitate group versus 34.8% in standard care group [OR: 0.82 (0.62–1.09)].

STUDY STRENGTHS

- Relatively balanced study and control group at baseline
- Allocation concealment.

STUDY WEAKNESSES

- Unblinded
- Fibrinogen levels were not measured.
- Less than one-fourth of the patients enrolled in the study required massive transfusion.
- Crossover between groups—15% of the patients in the cryoprecipitate group did not receive the transfusion as either their bleeding was controlled or they had died. While 32% in the control group received cryoprecipitate.

REVIEWER COMMENTS

PAMPer trial[3] had shown that prehospital administration of thawed plasma in patients at risk of hemorrhage shock was safe and resulted in lower 30-day mortality as compared to standard care resuscitation. Further randomized blinded studies are needed to confirm the role of early administration cryoprecipitate in prehospital trauma settings.

Administration of blood products in bleeding trauma patients needing massive transfusion should be guided by rotational thromboelastometry (ROTEM).

Andexanet for Factor Xa Inhibitor–Associated Acute Intracerebral Hemorrhage[4]

Connolly SJ, Sharma M, Cohen AT, Demchuk AM, Członkowska A, Lindgren AG, et al. Andexanet for Factor Xa Inhibitor–Associated Acute Intracerebral Hemorrhage.

N Engl J Med. 2024;390(19):1745-55.

BACKGROUND

Use of factor Xa inhibitors for anticoagulation has increased over the past years, with possibility of intracerebral hemorrhage as one of the consequences of their use. Andexanet alfa is a modified recombinant inactive form of factor Xa, which on administration binds the factor Xa inhibitor molecules, rapidly reducing their activity and restoring thrombin production.

ANNEXA-4 study[5] was a single arm, multicenter, prospective cohort study of the use of Andexanet alfa in patients with acute major bleeding at any site, that showed clinical hemostasis in almost 80% of the patients, with 18% having a thrombotic episode on 30-day follow-up.

CLINICAL QUESTION

Does the administration of Andexanet alfa in patients who have recently taken factor Xa inhibitors with an intracerebral hemorrhage result in better hemostatic efficacy?

STUDY DESIGN

- Multicenter, international—131 sites in 23 countries
- Open label
- Blinded outcome assessment
- Randomized 1:1.

POPULATION

- Patients with intracerebral hemorrhage (amendment in protocol excluded subdural or subarachnoid hemorrhage)—hematoma volume 0.5–60 mL with maximum National Institutes of Health Stroke Scale (NIHSS) score of 35.
- Should be on factor Xa inhibitor, with most recent dose taken within 15 hours before randomization.
- The time from onset of symptoms to baseline imaging scan of 12 hours or less (Amended protocol reduced this time to 6 hours or less)
- Patience with Glasgow Coma Scale (GCS) score of <7 at the time of consent were excluded
- Also, patients who were planned for surgery within 12 hours of enrolment were excluded.
- Patients with thrombotic event within 2 weeks before enrolment were excluded.

INTERVENTION

- Received Andexanet alfa bolus dose over 15–30 minutes followed by a continuous infusion over next 2 hours.
- The dose of the drug (58 patients received high-dose, and 200 patients received low-dose) was in accordance with the label approved by the Food and Drug Administration.

CONTROL

Usual care or could include administration of prothrombin complex concentrate (PCC). 85.5% of control group received PCC.

OUTCOMES

- 530 patients assigned—263 patients in Andexanet group and 267 in control group
- Prespecified interim analysis included 452 patients.

Primary Outcomes

- *Hemostatic efficacy*: Hemostatic efficacy was achieved in 150 of 224 patients (67.0%) receiving Andexanet and in 121 of 228 (53.1%) receiving usual care [adjusted difference: 13.4 percentage points; 95% confidence interval (CI): 4.6–22.2; p = 0.003].
- Hemostatic efficacy was defined as achieved if all the following criteria were met—a change in hematoma volume of 20% or less (excellent efficacy) or 35% or less (good efficacy) within 12 hours after baseline, an worsening in NIHSS score of <7 points at 12 hours, and no rescue therapy is used such as Andexanet alfa, PCC, or surgery to decompress the hematoma within 3–12 hours after randomization.
- This efficacy was mainly driven by limitation in hematoma volume expansion of <35%—165 of 215 patients (76.7%) receiving Andexanet and in 137 of 212 (64.6%) receiving usual care (adjusted difference: 12.1 percentage points; 95% CI: 3.6–20.5).
- Results from the other two components did not differ between the two groups.

Secondary Outcomes

- Hematoma volume expansion of >12.5%—24 of 216 patients (11.1%) receiving Andexanet and in 36 of 214 (16.8%) receiving usual care (adjusted difference: 5.6 percentage points; 95% CI: 12.0–0.8).
- Results from the other two components did not differ between the two groups.
- The median reduction from baseline to the 1-to-2-hour nadir in antifactor Xa activity was 94.5% with Andexanet and 26.9% with usual care ($p < 0.001$).

SAFETY ENDPOINT

- Safety was analyzed in all 530 enrolled patients.
- Thrombotic events occurred more often in Andexanet group [27 of 263 patients (10.3%)] than in usual care group [15 of 267 (5.6%)] (difference: 4.6 percentage points; 95% CI: 0.1–9.2; p = 0.048); With increased incidence of ischemic stroke in Andexanet group [17 patients (6.5%) vs. 4 patients (1.5%), respectively].

POST-HOC ANALYSIS

There were no appreciable differences between the groups in the score on the modified Rankin Scale or in death within 30 days.

STUDY STRENGTHS

- International RCT—131 sites in 23 countries
- Relatively balanced study and control group, except in location of hemorrhage
- Robust safety analysis.

STUDY WEAKNESSES

- Unblinded
- Funded
- Primary outcome was hematoma volume change which may or may not be clinically important. Major go to call amendments were done which included inclusion criteria and primary and secondary endpoints.
- Excluded patients with GCS <7, that is patients with large intracerebral bleeds.

REVIEWER COMMENTS

The trial showed a rapid improvement in factor Xa activity in the Andexanet group with better control of hematoma expansion; however, the increased thrombotic events, especially ischemic stroke is a concern. Though the groups were relatively balanced, only 85.5% received PCC in the usual care group. Also, patients with large intracerebral bleeds were excluded. Long-term follow-up with analysis of functional outcomes was lacking.

A meta-analysis and systematic review of 22 studies, both retrospective and controlled did not find any statistically significant advantage of the use of Andexanet alfa over four-factor PCC for anticoagulation reversal of direct oral anticoagulants (DOACs), in terms of mortality and instead found an increased risk of thromboembolic events associated with use of Andexanet alfa.[6]

With the results of ANNEXA-1 trial, it is difficult to recommend the use of Andexanet alfa in patients on factor Xa inhibitors with intracerebral hemorrhage.

Liberal or Restrictive Transfusion Strategy in Patients with Traumatic Brain Injury[7]

Turgeon AF, Fergusson DA, Clayton L, Patton MP, Neveu X, Walsh TS, et al. Liberal or Restrictive Transfusion Strategy in Patients with Traumatic Brain Injury.

N Engl J Med. 2024;391:722-35.

BACKGROUND

TRICC trial,[8] published in 1999, suggested a restrictive transfusion strategy in patients with traumatic brain injury as against the previous target of 9–10 g/dL. Subgroup of less acutely ill (APACHE II <20) and age <55 years had a significantly lower mortality with restrictive blood transfusion.

Studies comparing transfusion strategies in traumatic brain injury with long-term neurological function as the outcome had not been conducted.

CLINICAL QUESTION

Whether a liberal transfusion strategy (transfusion if Hb <10 g/dL) as compared with a restrictive strategy (transfusion if Hb <7 g/dL) in critically ill adult patients with traumatic brain injury, would lead to better functional outcomes as assessed by the score on the Glasgow Outcome Scale-Extended (GOS-E) at 6 months.

STUDY DESIGN

- Pragmatic
- 1:1 randomization
- Intention-to-treat analysis
- Open label
- Blinded outcome assessment
- 34 centers in Canada, UK, France, and Brazil.

POPULATION

- Critically ill adults with moderate-to-severe traumatic brain injury.
- Age >18 years—mean age 48.7 years.
- Acute, moderate, or severe traumatic brain injury—the mean injury severity score was 30.

INTERVENTION

Liberal group—transfusion if hemoglobin (Hb) <10 g/dL or lower.

CONTROL

Restrictive group—transfusion if Hb <7 g/dL or lower.

OUTCOMES

Primary Outcomes

- GOS-E at 6 months was <4 (unfavorable) in 68.4% in the liberal-strategy group and 73.5% in the restrictive-strategy group
- Adjusted absolute difference, restrictive strategy versus liberal strategy, 5.4 percentage points; (95% CI: –2.9 to 13.7).
- Findings were consistent across subgroups and also with the worst, intermediate, and best predicted prognoses.

Secondary Outcomes

- *Mortality:* No significant difference in mortality in intensive care unit (ICU) (17.1 vs. 15.3%), mortality in hospital (23 vs. 21.5%), mortality at 6 months (26.8 vs. 26.3%).
- No significant difference in functional independence measure or other measures of functional outcome

Tertiary Outcomes

Median number of red cell units transfused was 3 (2–5) in the liberal group, 98.9% of patients received at least 1 unit of packed cells, mean Hb 10.8 g/dL.

Median number of red cell units transfused was 0 (0–1) in the restrictive group, 38.4% of patients received at least 1 unit of packed cells, mean Hb 8.8 g/dL.

SAFETY ENDPOINT

- Six patients in the liberal group had a mild reaction to transfusion, 1 in the restrictive group.
- Venous thromboembolism (VTE) was the same in each group.
- Acute respiratory distress syndrome (ARDS) was 3.3% in liberal group and 0.8% in restrictive group.

STUDY STRENGTHS

- Pragmatic, intention-to-treat analysis
- Multicenter study

STUDY WEAKNESSES

- Open label
- The groups were not balanced at baseline. More patients in the restrictive group had GCS motor score of 1, and no pupillary reactivity.

REVIEWER COMMENTS

Maintenance of brain perfusion and oxygenation is crucial in patients with moderate-to-severe traumatic brain injury to improve outcomes. Early resuscitation should focus on maintaining cerebral perfusion by restoring the circulatory blood volume and maintaining adequate blood pressure. Improving the oxygen carrying capacity of the blood by maintaining a liberal hemoglobin level may play a role in the same.

Although transfusion of leukodepleted red blood cells (RBCs) may be relatively safe in the current era, it does possess significant risks. A personalized approach with monitoring of brain oxygenation is important in planning the hemoglobin target and meticulous use of RBCs.

The 2020 Seattle International Severe Traumatic Brain Injury Consensus Conference (SIBICC)[9] algorithm focuses on improving cerebral oxygenation based on brain tissue oxygen ($PbtO_2$) monitoring. When $PbtO_2$ levels fall below 20 mm Hg, they specifically suggest considering transfusion of packed RBCs if Hb levels drop below 9 g/dL.

A secondary analysis of CENTER-TBI trial[10] found that in critically ill traumatic brain injury patients, increasing hemoglobin level was independently associated with decrease in unfavorable neurological outcomes as well as mortality.

The results of recently published large multicenter randomized trial, the TRAIN study,[11] have demonstrated lower unfavorable neurological outcomes at 180 days with liberal blood transfusion (Hb transfusion threshold of 9 g/dL) in acute brain injury patients.

Further research is needed in optimizing transfusion protocols in order to enhance long-term functional outcomes in patients with traumatic brain injury, with use of more noninvasive monitoring techniques. Also, clinicians must consider underlying cardiac comorbidities when making decisions about appropriate transfusion thresholds.

Review of studies on use of Tranexamic Acid over the last year

Tranexamic acid is an antifibrinolytic agent that inhibits plasminogen activation and thus stabilizes clot formation. The drug has been widely used in various bleeding conditions.

Tranexamic acid is included in the essential medicines list of World Health Organization (WHO). Last 1 year saw the publication of various studies and articles on Tranexamic acid in various bleeding conditions.

The consensus of Brazilian association of hematology, hemotherapy, and cellular therapy on patient blood management[12] recommended the use of tranexamic acid to reduce blood loss and transfusion use in cardiac and noncardiac surgeries with expected blood loss >500 mL, without causing serious adverse effects.

Intravenous tranexamic acid has been used in cardiac surgery to reduce the risk of bleeding and need for transfusion for many years. The DEPOSITION randomized control trial[13] included 3,242 patients compared the use of intravenous or topical tranexamic acid in patients undergoing cardiac surgery with cardiopulmonary bypass. An 8.3% of absolute increase in transfusion was seen in patients with topical administration of tranexamic acid without reducing the seizure incidents.

The PATCH-Trauma trial[14] (Prehospital Tranexamic Acid for severe trauma) by the ANZICS trial group was a pragmatic double-blinded placebo control trial in which adult patients with major trauma and having a high risk of coagulopathy received Tranexamic acid within 3 hours of injury or placebo. The trial found no significant difference in the primary outcome of survival with a favorable functional outcome at 6 months. However, mortality was slightly reduced in the tranexamic acid group at 24 hours (9.7 vs. 14.1%) and 28 days (17.3 vs. 21.8%), similar to the findings of CRASH-2 trial.[15]

A meta-analysis of 11 randomized control trials found that early administration of tranexamic acid within 3 hours, significantly decrease the likelihood of intracranial hemorrhage expansion in patients with traumatic brain injury.[16]

The TICH-NOAC[17] was a double-blind, randomized, placebo-controlled trial assessed the efficacy and safety of tranexamic acid in patients on nonvitamin K antagonist oral anticoagulants (NOACs) with intracerebral hemorrhage. Though the trial was discontinued prematurely due to exhausted funding, no evidence was found to support the use of tranexamic acid to prevent hematoma expansion in this group of patients. But there were no major safety concerns either.

The STOP-MSU[18] was an investigator-led, double-blind, multicenter, randomized, phase 2 trial in patients with acute spontaneous intracerebral hemorrhage. In this, tranexamic acid was administered within 2 hours of symptom onset compared to dose-matched placebo. No difference in hematoma expansion, functional outcome, or safety was found in the two groups.

The post hoc subgroup analysis of ULTRA trial[19] published in 2021, showed that the use of tranexamic acid in good grade aneurysmal subarachnoid hemorrhage (aSAH) had worse clinical outcomes and no difference in clinical outcomes in poor grade aSAH. Another subgroup analysis assessing the time of administration of tranexamic acid in aneurysmal SAH found no difference in the functional outcome.[20]

A randomized controlled trial of the use of tranexamic acid in cirrhotic patients with upper gastrointestinal bleed[21] found significantly reduced failure to control bleeding by day 5 and reduced failure to prevent rebleeding up to 6 weeks in patients with advanced liver cirrhosis (Child-Turcotte-Pugh class B or C).

REVIEWER COMMENTS

There is competing evidence regarding the benefit and harm in the use of tranexamic acid in various bleeding situations. There is no available clinical trial which can mitigate this knowledge gap and it is yet to prove the safety and efficacy of the use of tranexamic acid in patients with spontaneous or traumatic intracerebral hemorrhage.

Tranexamic acid continues to show promise in reducing risk of rebleeding, in major surgeries but has not yet demonstrated a significant improvement in clinical outcomes.

With the current available evidence, early use of tranexamic acid in bleeding patients within 3 hours, especially orthopedic surgery and cardiac surgery or polytrauma, may be considered.

Further studies are needed to define its role in critical care hematology, and also to identify the treatment window of administration.

Guidelines and Position Statements Published on Critical Care Hematology through the Year

A clinical guideline on reversal of DOACs in patients with life-threatening bleeding was published and the consensus was reached via the Delphi process.[22] They recommended reversal of DOAC without awaiting laboratory results in patients undergoing urgent surgery or having intracerebral hemorrhage. Either direct reversal agents (idarucizumab for dabigatran/Andexanet alfa for direct factor Xa inhibitors) or nonspecific hemostatic agents

(PCC/activated PCC) should be started for most urgent and emergency procedures and bleeding.

The International Society on Thrombosis and Hemostasis (ISTH) guidelines for use of antithrombotics in COVID-19 patients have been updated[23] after the publication of more evidence since 2022. The updated guidelines do not recommend the use of intermediate dose or therapeutic dose of low-molecular weight heparin (LMWH) or unfractionated heparin (UFH) or addition of antiplatelet, over the prophylactic dose of LMWH or UFH in critically ill hospitalized patients for COVID-19.

The consensus of Brazilian association on preoperative management of patients anemia recommends early detection, identifying underlying causes, nutritional support, iron replacement, erythropoietin therapy, preoperative optimization, and collaborative care.[24]

The British Society of Haematology guidelines recommend against routine testing of coagulation profile in patient undergoing procedures with low risk of bleeding.[25] In patients undergoing a procedure that has a high risk of bleeding, liver disease, malnutrition, prolonged antibiotic use, and a risk of coagulopathy. They recommend platelet transfusion in patients with platelet count <30 × 10^9/L, requiring a tunneled central venous catheter.

REFERENCES

1. Davenport R, Curry N, Fox EE, Thomas H, Lucas J, Evans A, et al. Early and Empirical High-Dose Cryoprecipitate for Hemorrhage after Traumatic Injury: The CRYOSTAT-2 Randomized Clinical Trial. JAMA. 2023; 330(19):1882-91.
2. Curry N, Rourke C, Davenport R, Beer S, Pankhurst L, Deary A, et al. Early cryoprecipitate for major haemorrhage in trauma: a randomised controlled feasibility trial. Br J Anaesth. 2015;115(1):76-83.
3. Sperry JL, Guyette FX, Brown JB, Yazer MH, Triulzi DJ, Early-Young BJ, et al. Prehospital Plasma during Air Medical Transport in Trauma Patients at Risk for Hemorrhagic Shock. N Engl J Med. 2018;379(4):315-26.
4. Connolly SJ, Sharma M, Cohen AT, Demchuk AM, Członkowska A, Lindgren AG, et al. Andexanet for Factor Xa Inhibitor-Associated Acute Intracerebral Hemorrhage. N Engl J Med. 2024;390(19):1745-55.
5. Connolly SJ, Milling TJ Jr, Eikelboom JW, Gibson CM, Curnutte JT, Gold A, et al. Andexanet Alfa for Acute Major Bleeding Associated with Factor Xa Inhibitors. N Engl J Med. 2016;375(12):1131-41.
6. Orso D, Fonda F, Brussa A, Comisso I, Auci E, Sartori M, et al. Andexanet alpha versus four-factor prothrombin complex concentrate in DOACs anticoagulation reversal: an updated systematic review and meta-analysis. Crit Care. 2024;28(1):221.
7. Turgeon AF, Fergusson DA, Clayton L, Patton MP, Neveu X, Walsh TS, et al. Liberal or Restrictive Transfusion Strategy in Patients with Traumatic Brain Injury. N Engl J Med. 2024;391(8):722-35.
8. Hébert PC, Wells G, Blajchman MA, Marshall J, Martin C, Pagliarello G, et al. A multicenter, randomized, controlled clinical trial of transfusion requirements in critical care. Transfusion Requirements in Critical Care Investigators, Canadian Critical Care Trials Group. N Engl J Med. 1999;340(6):409-17.
9. Chesnut R, Aguilera S, Buki A, Bulger E, Citerio G, Cooper DJ, et al. A management algorithm for adult patients with both brain oxygen and intracranial pressure monitoring: the Seattle International Severe Traumatic Brain Injury Consensus Conference (SIBICC). Intensive Care Med. 2020;46(5):919-29.
10. Guglielmi A, Graziano F, Bogossian EG, Turgeon AF, Taccone FS, Citerio G, et al. Haemoglobin values, transfusion practices, and long-term outcomes in critically ill patients with traumatic brain injury: a secondary analysis of CENTER-TBI. Crit Care. 2024;28(1):199.

11. Taccone FS, Rynkowski Bittencourt C, Møller K, Lormans P, Quintana-Díaz M, Caricato A, et al. Restrictive vs Liberal Transfusion Strategy in Patients With Acute Brain Injury: The TRAIN Randomized Clinical Trial. JAMA. 2024;332(19):1623-33.
12. Montano-Pedroso JC, Perini FV, Donizetti E, Oliveira LC, Rodrigues RDR, Rizzo SRCP, et al. Consensus of the Brazilian association of hematology, hemotherapy and cellular therapy on patient blood management: Antifibrinolytics. Hematol Transfus Cell Ther. 2024;46 Suppl 1(Suppl 1):S40-S47.
13. Lamy A, Sirota DA, Jacques F, Poostizadeh A, Noiseux N, Efremov S, et al. Topical Versus Intravenous Tranexamic Acid in Patients Undergoing Cardiac Surgery: The DEPOSITION Randomized Controlled Trial. Circulation. 2024;150(17):1315-23.
14. PATCH-Trauma Investigators and the ANZICS Clinical Trials Group; Gruen RL, Mitra B, Bernard SA, McArthur CJ, Burns B, et al. Prehospital Tranexamic Acid for Severe Trauma. N Engl J Med. 2023;389(2):127-36.
15. CRASH-2 trial collaborators; Shakur H, Roberts I, Bautista R, Caballero J, Coats T, et al. Effects of tranexamic acid on death, vascular occlusive events, and blood transfusion in trauma patients with significant haemorrhage (CRASH-2): a randomised, placebo-controlled trial. Lancet. 2010;376(9734):23-32.
16. Zhang M, Liu T. Efficacy and safety of tranexamic acid in acute traumatic brain injury: A meta-analysis of randomized controlled trials. Am J Emerg Med. 2024;80:35-43.
17. Polymeris AA, Karwacki GM, Siepen BM, Schaedelin S, Tsakiris DA, Stippich C, et al. Tranexamic Acid for Intracerebral Hemorrhage in Patients on Non-Vitamin K Antagonist Oral Anticoagulants (TICH-NOAC): A Multicenter, Randomized, Placebo-Controlled, Phase 2 Trial. Stroke. 2023;54(9):2223-34.
18. Yassi N, Zhao H, Churilov L, Wu TY, Ma H, Nguyen HT, et al. Tranexamic acid versus placebo in individuals with intracerebral haemorrhage treated within 2 hours of symptom onset (STOP-MSU): an international, double-blind, randomised, phase 2 trial. Lancet Neurol. 2024;23(6): 577-87.
19. Tjerkstra MA, Post R, Germans MR, Vergouwen MDI, Jellema K, Koot RW, et al. Ultra-Early and Short-Term Tranexamic Acid Treatment in Patients with Good- and Poor-Grade Aneurysmal Subarachnoid Hemorrhage. Neurology. 2024;102(12): e209169.
20. Germans MR, Tjerkstra MA, Post R, Brenner A, Vergouwen MD, Rinkel GJ, et al. Impact of time to start of tranexamic acid treatment on rebleed risk and outcome in aneurysmal subarachnoid hemorrhage. Eur Stroke J. 2024;9(3):658-66.
21. Kumar M, Venishetty S, Jindal A, Bihari C, Maiwall R, Vijayaraghavan R, et al. Tranexamic acid in upper gastrointestinal bleed in patients with cirrhosis: A randomized controlled trial. Hepatology. 2024; 80(2):376-88.
22. Grottke O, Afshari A, Ahmed A, Arnaoutoglou E, Bolliger D, Fenger-Eriksen C, et al. Clinical guideline on reversal of direct oral anticoagulants in patients with life threatening bleeding. Eur J Anaesthesiol. 2024;41(5):327-50.
23. Schulman S, Arnold DM, Bradbury CA, Broxmeyer L, Connors JM, Falanga A, et al. 2023 ISTH update of the 2022 ISTH guidelines for antithrombotic treatment in COVID-19. J Thromb Haemost. 2024;22(6):1779-97.
24. Benites BD, Leite F, Soriano S, da Silva RL, Alves SOC, Rizzo SRCP, et al. Consensus of the Brazilian association of hematology, hemotherapy and cellular therapy on patient blood management: Preoperative Phase - Preoperative management of the patient's anemia. Hematol Transfus Cell Ther. 2024;46 Suppl 1(Suppl 1):S17-S23.
25. Lester W, Bent C, Alikhan R, Roberts L, Gordon-Walker T, Trenfield S, et al. A British Society for Haematology guideline on the assessment and management of bleeding risk prior to invasive procedures. Br J Haematol. 2024;204(5):1697-13.

SECTION

9

Ethics, Organization, and Outcomes in Intensive Care Unit

Section Editor: *Prashant Nasa*

Associate Editor: *Deven Juneja*

ETHICS

Setting Up a Just and Fair ICU Triage Process during a Pandemic: A Systematic Review

Chakraborty R, Achour N. Setting Up a Just and Fair ICU Triage Process during a Pandemic: A Systematic Review.

Healthcare. 2024;12(2):146.

CLINICAL QUESTION OR PROBLEM

This review evaluates the guidelines on pandemic planning in the Indian subcontinent in the context of COVID-19 management, with a focus on ethical principles for intensive care unit (ICU) triaging.

WHAT IS ALREADY KNOWN?

Triage is a complex and dynamic decision-making process with ethical challenges in prioritizing access to care, involving admission and treatment. Equitable access to available healthcare facilities and resources, especially during disasters such as COVID-19, is an ongoing debate. Despite pandemic preparedness, the triage for admission to ICUs was made when overwhelmed with critical cases and resources. A closer examination of the ICU triaging principles revealed a considerable variation among countries that produced ICU guidelines for triage during mass casualties with a wide range of concepts, including saving the most lives through medical prognosis, adopting age, life expectancy, and quality of life (QoL).

STUDY DESIGN

A systematic review of qualitative research.

POPULATION STUDIED INCLUDING DEMOGRAPHICS

National and regional pandemic guidelines and policies, including ministry or department of health websites of India, Nepal, Bangladesh, Sri Lanka, and Pakistan.

INTERVENTION(S) STUDIED

Not applicable

COMPARATOR USED

Not applicable

OUTCOMES EVALUATED

Ethical principles guiding patient prioritization.

AUTHORS' VIEWPOINT

Broad themes were identified: (1) Need of ethics for ICU triaging during pandemics, (2) disagreements on the (ethical) framework, (3) ICU triage protocols are to be transparent, (4) ICU triaging needs an equitable approach with consideration of underlying health inequities, and (5) need of regional mapping of capacities and better modeling. None of the reviewed guidelines was comprehensive to match all the themes. Moreover, there was a lack of mention of the term "fairness", in these guidelines, and the only discussion was focused on protection, despite an extensive diversity in religious, cultural, and political beliefs, as well as socioeconomic inequities. The Nepalese guidelines were relatively better than others in matching the themes.

STRENGTH OF THE STUDY

Focus only on the South Asia guidelines and include the recent guidelines.

DRAWBACKS OF THE STUDY

After analyzing different ethical guidelines, this study emphasizes that there is a need for a just and fair framework, mainly a social justice-based framework, in ICU triage in the subcontinent to address the existing health inequities.

In the crisis hours of a pandemic, an open and transparent ethical ICU triage can help avert many irrational strategies impacting the service delivery and can also save many unwanted and premature deaths. Inequalities in society are unavoidable. However, if they are thoughtfully incorporated into the pandemic planning, many real-time disasters can be averted. And for this, more research, with a vision of social justice, is needed in this domain.

LIMITATIONS

The review included secondary literature and gray literature. The study failed to extract information related to the implementation of these guidelines.

REVIEWERS' VIEWPOINT

The lack of inclusion of important ethical principles like a just and fair framework in these guidelines is concerning. This could have considerable implications for our population with widespread existing health and socioeconomic inequities.

IMPACT ON CURRENT PRACTICE AND TAKE-HOME MESSAGE

Current guidelines on pandemic preparedness and ICU triaging were drafted during the pandemic. A review based on an audit of their implementation's ethical implications using a comprehensive ethical framework is needed.

Perspectives of ICU Patients on Deferred Consent in the Context of Post-ICU Quality of Life: A Substudy of a Randomized Clinical Trial

van der Wal LI, Grim CCA, Del Prado MR, van Westerloo DJ, Schultz MJ, Helmerhorst HJF, et al.; ICONIC Investigators. Perspectives of ICU Patients on Deferred Consent in the Context of Post-ICU Quality of Life: A Substudy of a Randomized Clinical Trial.

Crit Care Med. 2024;52:694-703.

CLINICAL QUESTION OR PROBLEM

To evaluate the opinion of former ICU patients on their participation in a clinical trial with deferred consent and influence of the QoL following hospital discharge on their reflections. The hypothesis was that patients with impaired QoL after hospital or ICU discharge are less likely to accept deferred consent.

WHAT IS ALREADY KNOWN?

Deferred consent means when consent cannot be sought from patients and/or legal representatives before commencing (trial) treatment due to insufficient time, with the condition that consent must be sought by a legal representative as soon as circumstances allow it. Despite its increased use in clinical trials in the ICU, there is a concern that the acceptance of deferred consent is likely to be higher in patients with favorable outcomes compared to those with unfavorable outcomes.

STUDY DESIGN

Cross-sectional questionnaire. This is a substudy of the Conservative versus Liberal Oxygenation Targets in Intensive Care Unit Patients (ICONIC) trial, a multicentric, randomized parallel-group trial.

POPULATION STUDIED INCLUDING DEMOGRAPHICS

The original trial was conducted in eight ICUs in the Netherlands and one ICU in Italy, including 664 patients between November 2018 and November 2021. 362 (55%) of 664 included patients in the original trial were by deferred consent, and only Dutch-speaking patients, who were alive 6 months after the original study, were included in the current study. 197 patients completed the questionnaire. Noteworthy, an additional 125 patients initially enrolled with deferred consent were subsequently excluded, because of declined consent by the legal representative of the patient.

INTERVENTION(S) STUDIED

Patient perspectives and experiences on the deferred consent procedure.

COMPARATOR USED

Low and high QoL after discharge using EQ-5D-5L questionnaire.

OUTCOMES EVALUATED

Recollection, perception, and experience of the patients on the deferred consent.

AUTHORS' VIEWPOINT

Despite obtaining deferred consent, nearly 65% of participating patients needed to be made aware of their participation in the ICONIC study. However, most patients were positive regarding using deferred consent, and most individuals preferred legal representatives to provide it. Patients with higher QoL had more acceptance for deferred consent than those with low QoL.

STRENGTH OF THE STUDY

The trial integrated a variable through QoL assessment into evaluating patients' opinions. The study had a high inclusion rate compared to previous studies in this area. Finally, the trial was pragmatic, including patients with a real-life experience of deferred consent in the ICONIC trial, rather than previous studies in which hypothetical scenarios were used among participants.

DRAWBACKS OF THE STUDY

Only half of the eligible patients were enrolled, and nonresponders may have different opinions. The duration of 6 months between the original study and the questionnaire may be considered relatively long as the opinions of participants may have changed over time. Finally, the study was performed in a high-income country, and the generalization of findings beyond this specific cultural population and the context of a low-risk study is questionable.

REVIEWERS' VIEWPOINT

Deferred consent is an ethical method to obtain consent for a clinical trial, especially in ICU settings where delay in randomization may affect the outcome. However, such trials should also be performed in resource-limited settings to understand the cultural differences and ethical implications of deferred consent.

IMPACT ON CURRENT PRACTICE AND TAKE-HOME MESSAGE

Deferred consent is a feasible ethical method for randomizing and enrolling critically ill patients in clinical trials where informed consent is challenging, provided the intervention is low-risk and appropriate monitoring and regulatory oversight are available.

End-of-life Care in the Intensive Care Unit and Ethics of Withholding/Withdrawal of Life-sustaining Treatments

Cortegiani A, Ippolito M, Mercadante S. End-of-life Care in the Intensive Care Unit and Ethics of Withholding/Withdrawal of Life-sustaining Treatments.

Anesthesiol Clin. 2024;42:407-19.

CLINICAL QUESTION OR PROBLEM

To identify major end-of-life issues in ICU and the general principles, practice, and ethics of limitation of life-sustaining treatments in the form of withholding and withdrawal of care.

WHAT IS ALREADY KNOWN?

End-of-life issues are an integral component of ICU care. As per general estimates, on average, one-fifth of patients admitted to ICUs receive futile therapy. In a cross-sectional survey, 66–89% of ICU nurses provided futile treatment during their careers. Despite several studies discussing the approach to the care of the dying patient, there are no reliable estimates of the magnitude of end-of-life care in the ICU. Moreover, ICU competencies in end-of-life care, life-sustaining care, and intensive treatment must be defined in the context of its limitations and cultural and legal differences.

STUDY DESIGN

A narrative review of the key elements of end-of-life care in the ICU and the ethics of withholding/withdrawal life-sustaining treatments.

POPULATION STUDIED INCLUDING DEMOGRAPHICS

Critically ill patients

INTERVENTION(S) STUDIED

Not applicable

COMPARATOR USED

Not applicable

OUTCOMES EVALUATED

Not applicable

AUTHORS' VIEWPOINT

End-of-life decisions can be stressful for patients, families, and clinicians. Withholding and withdrawal of life-sustaining treatment contribute to 12% of deaths globally in ICUs and 80% of deaths in the ICUs of Western countries. Hence, the end-of-life care decision follows the evaluation of the appropriateness of support, shared decision-making and care goals with patients and families, and consensus among the ICU team. Their application is highly variable according to geographic location and ethical, spiritual, moral, and religious factors as long as provider experience. End-of-life decisions must incorporate palliative care and communication, optimizing comfort for patients and families, and facilitating eventual bereavement.

STRENGTH OF THE STUDY

Not applicable

DRAWBACKS OF THE STUDY

Not applicable

REVIEWERS' VIEWPOINT

The transition from full-code treatments to "no escalation" and comfort care, together with withdrawing and withholding life-sustaining treatments, has emerged as a universal need for care in the ICU. However, end-of-life decisions must consider cultural, religious, and geographic location differences. Specific competencies, training, and experience are needed to implement such procedures, offering physicians an opportunity to go beyond the impotence generated by unavoidable death and to focus on patients' dignity and wishes. They should be seen as a "limitation" of not proportioned support. Incorporating palliative care into the process may support patients and their families.

IMPACT ON CURRENT PRACTICE AND TAKE-HOME MESSAGE

This is an updated review of global practices regarding end-of-life decisions, considering the impact of such decisions on patient- and family-centered care and the influence of diversity of culture, religion, and geography on end-of-life care practices. The review dwelled on the challenges and potential solutions for effective end-of-life care, with a focus on physician competencies in these areas.

Family Centeredness of Care: A Cross-sectional Study in Intensive Care Units Part of the European Society of Intensive Care Medicine

Azoulay É, Kentish-Barnes N, Boulanger C, Mistraletti G, van Mol M, Heras-La Calle G, et al. Family centeredness of care: a cross-sectional study in intensive care units part of the European society of intensive care medicine.

Ann Intensive Care. 2024;14:77.

CLINICAL QUESTION OR PROBLEM

To identify the variations in family-centered care practices in ICUs worldwide.

WHAT IS ALREADY KNOWN?

Family-centered care understands values and addresses the needs of the family as a stakeholder involved in healthcare delivery. Family-centered care has been shown to improve health outcomes, especially patient and family satisfaction, care experience, staff satisfaction, and ICU resource utilization.

STUDY DESIGN

Cross-sectional study involving members/nonmembers registered on the mailing list of the ESICM.

POPULATION STUDIED INCLUDING DEMOGRAPHICS

A physician or a nurse documented the local practices of each participating ICU, with a focus on key components of family-centered care.

INTERVENTION(S) STUDIED

Healthcare professionals were asked to complete a questionnaire between August and December 2022, with areas covered were family-centered care, work environment, ethical climate, and burnout among healthcare professionals.

COMPARATOR USED

Not applicable

OUTCOMES EVALUATED

Variations in the ICU visitation policies, team-family interactions, and practices on the end-of-life care in the participating ICUs.

AUTHORS' VIEWPOINT

The survey response rate was 53%, with 24% of invited ICUs completing the survey, with 62% located in Europe and 9% in Asia. Participants ranked family-centered care highly important [median 7/10 on visual analogue scale (VAS)]. Mean visiting hours were 6 (2–22) h/day, with 54% of ICUs allowing night visitation and 29% allowing family members to sleep in the ICU. Waiting rooms for visitors were available in 86% of ICUs, and receptionists were available in 34% of ICUs. <18% of ICUs had a nurse facilitator, and social workers were available in 58% of ICUs.

STRENGTH OF THE STUDY

Including ICUs from diverse global regions provides a snapshot and understanding of challenges in family-centered care in ICUs worldwide. Despite considerable differences in cultural and system in ICUs worldwide, the importance of family-centered care is recognized universally and hugely by healthcare professionals.

DRAWBACKS OF THE STUDY

The cross-sectional nature of the study relies on self-reported data from healthcare professionals only with a low participation rate.

REVIEWERS' VIEWPOINT

There is a need to integrate family-centered care into ICU culture and work environment. Healthcare systems should strive for a more comprehensive and compassionate approach by addressing organizational impediments to the well-being of healthcare personnel and recognizing the link to ethical decision-making. As the healthcare landscape shifts toward patient-centered approaches, incorporating family-centered care emerges as an essential component for providing holistic and sympathetic treatment in ICUs.

IMPACT ON CURRENT PRACTICE AND TAKE-HOME MESSAGE

There is a considerable gap in the support provided to family of ICU patients with a direct impact on their satisfaction and experience. The key elements that need to be addressed are visitation policies, team-family communications, and end-of-life discussions. Family-centered care means family members are actively involved in the care of patients and impacts communication strategies.

ORGANIZATION

Associations of the Staffing Structure of Intensive Care Units and High Care Units on In-Hospital Mortality among Patients with Sepsis: A Cross-sectional Study of Japanese Nationwide Claims Data

Umegaki T, Nishimoto K, Kamibayashi T. Associations of the staffing structure of intensive care units and high care units on in-hospital mortality among patients with sepsis: a cross-sectional study of Japanese nationwide claims data.

***BMJ Open.* 2024;14:e085763.**

CLINICAL QUESTION OR PROBLEM

This study evaluates the association between organizational structure in the ICU or high care unit (HCU) and hospital mortality among patients with sepsis in acute care hospitals in Japan.

WHAT IS ALREADY KNOWN?

Optimal treatment of sepsis depends on the availability of early and effective healthcare provisions with optimum resources. In Japan, HCUs share similar organization and functions to high-dependency units of other countries, designed for less critically ill patients. However, many Japanese hospitals that lack ICUs or, due to the unavailability of an ICU bed, treat critically ill patients in HCUs. Moreover, ICUs are graded as Level 1, which meets the criteria needed for nurse-to-patient ratio (minimum ratio of 1:2) and experienced medical staff (≥5 years) and evaluate the needs of patients for appropriate needs, and Level 2, which does not meet the criteria. Higher insurance reimbursement is paid to Level 1 ICUs than Level 2 ICUs.

STUDY DESIGN

Cross-sectional study of adult patients with sepsis between April 1, 2018 and March 31, 2019.

POPULATION STUDIED INCLUDING DEMOGRAPHICS

A physician or a nurse documented the local practices of each participating ICU, focusing on key components of family-centered care.

INTERVENTION(S) STUDIED

Not applicable

COMPARATOR USED

Not applicable

OUTCOMES EVALUATED

In-hospital mortality, ICU/HCU stay (days), and overall hospital stay (days).

AUTHORS' VIEWPOINT

Before matching, the patients in HCU had the highest survival rate. However, after adjusting for the covariates, compared with the Level 1 ICUs, the in-hospital mortality was higher for Level 2 ICUs, 1.12 (95% CI: 1.04–1.21), and HCUs, 1.17 (95% CI: 1.08–1.26). The outcome was worse in patients with blood-borne infections and immunological disorders.

STRENGTH OF THE STUDY

Country-wide collection of data with clear demarcation of organization staffing.

DRAWBACKS OF THE STUDY

Severity assessment of patients using sequential organ failure assessment (SOFA) was unavailable, and differentiation of community and hospital-acquired sepsis was not performed. There was no information on hospital and ICU size, absolute staffing numbers, and physician-patient ratio.

REVIEWERS' VIEWPOINT

Lower in-hospital mortality among patients with sepsis was associated with ICUs that fulfill more stringent staffing criteria. Differences in organizational structure may be associated with outcomes in sepsis patients.

IMPACT ON CURRENT PRACTICE AND TAKE-HOME MESSAGE

There is a considerable gap in the organizational structure in different ICUs and the care provided by them. It is important to evaluate objective measures such as nurse-patient or physician-patient ratios and the experience of the healthcare staff in relation to outcomes in Indian ICUs. This will help in quality improvement and healthcare delivery and will promote adequate staffing as recommended by regulators.

OUTCOMES

Prevalence of Frailty and Association with Patient Centered Outcomes: A Prospective Registry-Embedded Cohort Study from India

Tirupakuzhi Vijayaraghavan BK, Rashan A, Ranganathan L, Venkataraman R, Tripathy S, Jayakumar D, et al.; IRIS collaborative. Prevalence of frailty and association with patient centered outcomes: A prospective registry-embedded cohort study from India.

J Crit Care. 2024;80:154509.

CLINICAL QUESTION OR PROBLEM

To study the prevalence, risk factors of frailty on admission to ICU among critically ill patients in India and the impact of frailty on patient-centered outcomes

WHAT IS ALREADY KNOWN?

Previous studies demonstrated an association between preadmission frailty and mortality and poor health-related QoL. However, most studies were from high-income countries, and there is limited data from lower-middle-income countries (LMICs).

STUDY DESIGN

Prospective Indian Registry of IntenSive care (IRIS) based cohort study across 7 ICUs (from four hospitals) from June 11, 2021 to December 26, 2021.

POPULATION STUDIED INCLUDING DEMOGRAPHICS

Adult (≥18 years) critically ill patients admitted for the first time during the current hospitalization, and with an anticipated ICU stay of ≥48 hours.

INTERVENTION(S) STUDIED

Clinical Frailty Scale (CFS) is a 9-point scoring system for a multidimensional estimate of a patient's baseline frailty status. A CFS score of at least 5 is defined as low frailty.

COMPARATOR USED

Not applicable

OUTCOMES EVALUATED

The primary outcome was ICU mortality. The secondary outcomes were in-hospital mortality, AKI, and measures of organ support (resources utilization) need for invasive or noninvasive ventilation, vasopressors, receipt of RRT, length of ICU, and hospital stay. All outcomes were censored on day 28.

AUTHORS' VIEWPOINT

Frailty is common among critically ill patients in India, with 20% of ICU admissions having CFS above 5 in this cohort and is associated with worse clinical outcomes. The Charlson comorbidity index and malnourishment at admission were independent risk factors.

STRENGTH OF THE STUDY

The largest study on frailty from India was conducted in ICUs of a mix of public and private hospitals.

DRAWBACKS OF THE STUDY

Lack of follow-up for longer-term outcomes beyond hospital discharge and use of CFS only for the frailty assessment.

REVIEWERS' VIEWPOINT

A well-conducted prospective study to understand the impact of frailty on the prognosis and need of ICU resources from the Indian context.

IMPACT ON CURRENT PRACTICE AND TAKE-HOME MESSAGE

Clinical Frailty Scale at admission is a good tool to help predict patients admitted to the ICU with worse outcomes in patients with higher frailty scores. Future research must focus on strategies for improving outcomes, resource utilization, and long-term outcomes after discharge for frail ICU patients.

SECTION 10

Sonography/Imaging

Section Editor: *Shrikanth Srinivasan*

Associate Editors: *Velmurugan Selvam, Magesh Parthiban*

Passive Leg Raising Test Using the Carotid Flow Velocity–Time Integral to Predict Fluid Responsiveness

Cheong I, Otero Castro V, Sosa FA, Tort Oribe B, Frúchtenicht MF, Tamagnone FM, et al. Passive leg raising test using the carotid flow velocity-time integral to predict fluid responsiveness.

J Ultrasound. 2024;27:97-104.

CLINICAL QUESTION

Can changes in carotid flow velocity–time integral (CF VTI) measured during a passive leg raising (PLR) test accurately predict fluid responsiveness (FR) in critically ill patients?

WHAT IS ALREADY KNOWN?

Fluid resuscitation aims to improve cardiac output and organ perfusion in critically ill patients. However, only about 50% of patients respond positively to fluid administration, and excessive fluids can increase mortality risks. Therefore, predicting FR is crucial. Traditional static indicators, such as central venous pressure, have shown poor accuracy in predicting FR, as they do not reliably correlate with intravascular volume or cardiac output. The PLR test is a reversible, noninvasive method that can simulate the effects of a fluid bolus by shifting blood to the central circulation, allowing clinicians to assess a patient's FR. When used with real-time stroke volume measurements via transthoracic echocardiography (TTE), PLR is considered a reliable predictor. TTE, which measures stroke volume changes via left ventricular outflow tract (LVOT) VTI, is often difficult to perform in critically ill patients due to positioning limitations and interference from ventilation. Carotid artery flow, measured by Doppler ultrasound, has been explored as a surrogate for stroke volume. However, technical limitations, especially the alignment of the Doppler angle, have posed challenges, leading to inconsistent results in predicting FR.

STUDY DESIGN

This study is a performance diagnostic accuracy study designed to evaluate the effectiveness of using CF VTI changes during the PLR test to predict FR in critically ill patients. The research was conducted between February and April 2022 across two intensive care units (ICUs) in Argentina, aiming to provide a simpler and potentially more accessible alternative to traditional echocardiographic assessments for FR in challenging ICU settings.

POPULATION STUDIED INCLUDING DEMOGRAPHICS

The study included 50 patients out of 62 eligible patients from two ICUs in Argentina. Patients who presented signs of hypoperfusion (e.g., low mean arterial pressure, elevated heart rate, low urine output, or high lactate levels) were identified as potential candidates for fluid resuscitation. The median age was 68, with 64% male participants. Common reasons for ICU admission were surgery, sepsis, septic shock, and pneumonia.

INTERVENTION AND COMPARATOR

The study protocol involved a sequence of measurements under varying patient positions and conditions:

- *Baseline measurements:* Patients were initially positioned in a semirecumbent posture with the head of the bed elevated to 45°. Baseline measurements of CF VTI, LVOT VTI, blood pressure, heart rate, and other vital parameters were recorded.
- *PLR test:* Patients were repositioned by laying them flat with both legs elevated to 45° to perform the PLR test, which mimics a transient increase in preload. After 1 minute in this position, CF VTI and other hemodynamic parameters were recorded again. This maneuver temporarily increases venous return and allows clinicians to observe changes in flow and volume that can indicate whether the patient would respond to a true fluid bolus.
- *Fluid challenge:* After returning to the semirecumbent position, each patient received a 500 mL bolus of Ringer's Lactate over a 15-minute period. Postbolus measurements of LVOT VTI and other hemodynamic parameters were then collected. An increase of at least 15% in LVOT VTI after the fluid bolus categorized a patient as a fluid responder. This outcome was used as the gold standard for FR and was compared to the changes observed in CF VTI during the PLR test.

RESULTS

The study's main finding was that an increase of at least 11% in the CF VTI during the PLR test was predictive of FR. Fluid responders were defined as those showing a 15% or greater increase in LVOT VTI following a 500 mL fluid bolus. Of the 50 patients, 22 (44%) were classified as fluid responders based on this criterion. The area under the receiver operating characteristic (ROC) curve for CF VTI change during PLR was 0.869, indicating a high level of diagnostic accuracy. The 11% increase threshold in CF VTI during PLR provided a sensitivity of 77.3% and specificity of 78.6%. The positive predictive value (PPV) was 73.9%, and the negative predictive value (NPV) was 81.5%. For CF VTI, responders showed a median increase of 18.1% during PLR, while nonresponders had a median increase of only 5%, with a significant p value ($p < 0.0001$) indicating a meaningful difference between the two groups.

STRENGTH OF THE STUDY

- *Innovative approach:* This study introduces a novel technique that could potentially replace echocardiography in predicting FR, which is relevant in challenging ICU conditions.
- *Clear protocol:* The study's methodology is transparent, with detailed descriptions that allow for replicability.

- *Statistical validation:* The use of ROC analysis and other statistical methods adds robustness to the findings, lending credibility to the CF VTI cutoff threshold for predicting FR.

DRAWBACKS OF THE STUDY

- *Small sample size:* With only 50 patients, the study may not be broadly generalizable.
- *Single-center limitation:* Conducted within two ICUs in the same region, the results may lack external validity in other healthcare settings.
- *Technical limitations:* The reliance on accurate Doppler angle alignment introduces the potential for variability in CF VTI measurements, particularly for practitioners with less ultrasound experience.

REVIEWERS' VIEWPOINT

The study introduces an innovative approach by examining CF VTI changes during PLR as a potential alternative measure for FR, which could be especially beneficial in ICU settings where echocardiography may be difficult to implement. The suggested CF VTI cutoff of an 11% increase during PLR allows for a quick bedside evaluation that may enhance timely fluid management decisions, particularly in resource-constrained environments.

However, accurately distinguishing between responders and nonresponders in FR assessment requires an optimal fluid challenge technique. In this study, a 500 mL bolus over 15 minutes was used, a method that could be suboptimal, as it may increase the risk of fluid overload in nonresponders and potentially lead to false-positive results. Recent studies have shown that rapid alternative methods, including the PLR, a mini-fluid challenge (100 mL over 1 minute), and the end-expiratory occlusion test, have superior predictive accuracy and are more suitable for assessing FR compared to a 500 mL bolus administered over 15 minutes. These techniques minimize the risks associated with excessive fluid administration and provide quicker results, which could significantly improve clinical decision-making in the ICU.

The study is further limited by its small sample size and single-center design, which restrict the generalizability of its findings. Future multicenter studies with larger and more diverse populations, as well as comparisons to these rapid FR assessment techniques, would strengthen the evidence for CF VTI changes during PLR as a reliable and practical FR measure. Including long-term outcomes in future studies would also help clarify the broader clinical impact of this approach in critical care settings.

IMPACT ON CURRENT PRACTICE AND TAKE-HOME MESSAGE

The study suggests that CF VTI during PLR could be a practical, noninvasive tool to predict FR in critically ill patients, offering a potentially simpler alternative to echocardiography in situations where its use is limited. The take-home message is that CF VTI during PLR may improve bedside assessment of FR, though further research is needed to confirm these results across broader populations.

Utility of Ultrasound in the Diagnostic Work-up of Suspected Pulmonary Embolism: An Open-Label Multicentre Randomized Controlled Trial (the PRIME Study)

Falster C, Mørkenborg MD, Thrane M, Clausen J, Arvig M, Brockhattingen K, et al. Utility of ultrasound in the diagnostic work-up of suspected pulmonary embolism: an open-label multicentre randomized controlled trial (the PRIME study).

Lancet Reg Health Eur. 2024;42:100941.

CLINICAL QUESTION OR PROBLEM

Could an integrated ultrasonography of lung, cardiac, and lower extremity veins reduce the need for diagnostic imaging in patients with suspected pulmonary embolism (PE)?

WHAT IS ALREADY KNOWN?

- Diagnosing PE is often challenging due to its nonspecific clinical presentation and the lack of a reliable screening tool to reduce unnecessary diagnostic imaging referrals.
- Current guidelines recommend stratifying patients with suspected PE into risk categories based on clinical decision rules, such as the Wells or Revised Geneva score. For patients with low risk, a subsequent D-dimer test within the normal reference range can help rule out PE.
- Studies such as ADJUST-PE and PEGeD have shown that adjustable D-dimer cut-off levels, based on age or pretest probability, can reduce unnecessary imaging referrals while maintaining an acceptable failure rate.
- However, the utility of D-dimer remains questionable, particularly as age and comorbidities increase, leading to a significant drop in specificity (down to 10%).
- While ultrasonography has good specificity, its role is limited by lower sensitivity. An integrated, tailored ultrasonographic approach could potentially enhance both sensitivity and specificity in selecting patients who truly require imaging.
- Preliminary descriptive studies support this, reporting a 50% reduction in imaging referrals. This study is the first randomized controlled trial (RCT) to investigate the pragmatic utility of such an approach.

STUDY DESIGN

This trial was a randomized, open-label, multicenter study in which patients were randomized in a 1:1 ratio to either multiorgan ultrasound investigation (intervention) or referral for CT pulmonary angiography or lung scintigraphy (control). Randomization was conducted using a web-based system with permuted blocks of random numbers to ensure equal patient distribution across study arms at all participating centers. Both the investigator and the participating patient were aware of the group allocation, and outcome assessors and data analysts were also not blinded to the randomization results. Ethical approval was obtained from the regional scientific committee and the institutional review boards of all participating sites, with informed consent obtained from all participants before enrollment. A sample size of 120 patients was required to achieve 90% power with a significance level of 0.05 to detect a 15% absolute reduction in imaging referrals; a total of 150 patients were enrolled to account for a 25% attrition and loss to follow-up.

SETTING

- *Patients were recruited from six Danish hospitals:* One tertiary hospital and five secondary hospitals.
- Study period—June 18th, 2021 to February 1st, 2023.

POPULATION STUDIED INCLUDING DEMOGRAPHICS

- *Inclusion:*
  - All patients aged 18 years or more admitted in an emergency with a suspicion of PE
  - Wells score 0–6 and an elevated age-adjusted D-dimer or Wells score >6
- *Exclusion:*
  - Hemodynamically unstable (systolic blood pressure <90 mm Hg for at least two consecutive measurements)
  - Pregnant patients
  - Diagnosed with a PE within 6 months or had permanent mental disability
  - Ultrasound done prior to enrollment

BASELINE CHARACTERISTICS

A total of 218 patients were screened for eligibility out of which 68 patients were excluded. Final analysis was done for the remaining 150 patients who were randomized to either an ultrasound group (intervention) ($n = 73$) or usual diagnostic imaging ($n = 77$). No patient was excluded after randomization or was lost to follow-up. Demographics and other baseline characteristics were similar between the groups (control group vs. FOCUS group)

- *Age:* 71 (57.5–79) years versus 66 (56–77) years
- *Gender:* Females 52.1% versus 49.4%
- *BMI:* 26.3 (23.1–29.3) versus 27.7 (24.7–30.8)
- Comorbidities including hypertension, coronary artery disease, diabetes mellitus, etc., were similar between the groups.
- Most common symptoms at presentation were dyspnea (79.3%) and chest pain (44.7%) which were similar in both the groups.
- *Well's score:* 3 (1.5–4.5) versus 3 (1.5–6)
- *D-dimer:* 1.7 (1.2–4.6) versus 2.1 (1.1–5.6) (mg/L)

Control Group

Patients in the control group underwent CT pulmonary angiography or lung scintigraphy per national and local guidelines.

Intervention Ultrasound Group Protocol

Patients randomized to the ultrasound group had a multiorgan ultrasound of the heart, lungs, and lower extremity veins performed by a certified investigator according to Danish Society for Emergency Medicine guidelines.

- *Cardiac ultrasound:* Focused on detecting right ventricular strain (e.g., D-sign and McConnell's sign), reduced left ventricular function, chamber enlargement, pericardial effusion, and valve pathology
- *Lung ultrasound:* The lung ultrasound assessed 14 predefined zones for pleural line visualization, lung consolidations, lung sliding, B-lines, and pleural effusion.
- *Lower extremity venous ultrasound:* Assessed the femoral and popliteal veins for compressibility to detect deep vein thrombosis (DVT), with a linear or curved probe as needed.
- *Categorization based on ultrasound findings:* Patients were categorized based on ultrasound findings into categories such as confirmed PE, PE dismissed, or indeterminate.
- *PE confirmed:* If PE was confirmed by ultrasound, the risk was assessed

using the simplified PE severity index, cardiac troponin levels, and right ventricular dysfunction. Patients with intermediate-low to intermediate-high risk patients were admitted and referred for CT pulmonary angiography or lung scintigraphy for final diagnosis confirmation. Outpatient treatment for low-risk patients with anticoagulation and were monitored without further diagnostic imaging. Therefore, only patients with a deep venous thrombus or at least two subpleural infarctions could forgo further diagnostic imaging, as the presence of right ventricular strain indicates at least an intermediate-low risk.

- *PE indeterminate:* If PE could not be definitively ruled out or confirmed, the patient was referred for CT pulmonary angiography or lung scintigraphy.
- *PE dismissed:* If PE was ruled out by ultrasound (no PE findings or alternative diagnosis confirmed), the patient was either discharged or referred for further investigation if necessary. Discharged patients were advised to contact a healthcare provider if symptoms worsened or did not improve within 2 weeks.
- Three months later, two independent reviewers examined electronic patient records to assess secondary outcomes. All diagnostic work-up related to venous thromboembolism was managed by the Danish healthcare system and recorded in patient files. Discrepancies were resolved through consensus or a third assessor's review.

OUTCOMES EVALUATED

Control group versus USG group:

- In all 73 patients in the intervention group, a complete multiorgan ultrasound was feasible and ruled out PE in 30 of them. With 20 cases dismissed based on the absence of right ventricular strain, subpleural consolidations, and deep venous thrombus and the remaining 10 patients, ultrasound identified an alternative diagnosis.
- PE was confirmed in 11 patients, mainly by detecting a proximal deep venous thrombus, with subsequent CT pulmonary angiography or lung scintigraphy confirming PE in 8.
- An additional 32 patients were referred for diagnostic imaging when ultrasound could not definitively confirm or rule out PE, of whom 12 were diagnosed with PE.
- Of the 77 patients in the control group, 75 underwent CT or lung scintigraphy.

Primary Outcome

The ultrasound group had 40 out of 73 patients referred for further imaging, leading to a 45.2% reduction in imaging referrals ($p < 0.001$).

Secondary Outcomes

- At enrollment, 31.5% of ultrasound group patients and 33.8% of controls had PE.
- In the ultrasound group, 4.0% of patients without anticoagulation were diagnosed with PE during follow-up, all of whom had had PE initially dismissed by ultrasound.
- No PE was diagnosed in the control group during follow-up.
- Adverse events were more common in the ultrasound group (43.8%) compared to the control group (22.6%), though no bleeding complications occurred in the ultrasound group.
- Referral to emergency care occurred in 35.6% of ultrasound patients and 24.7% of controls.
- Mortality during follow-up was higher in the ultrasound group (12.3%) compared

to the control group (7.8%), but no deaths were due to missed PE.

- Cancer diagnoses during follow-up were similar in both groups (6.8% in ultrasound and 7.8% in control).
- A reduction in imaging referrals could save approximately €156.60 per patient, with no additional costs for ultrasound.

AUTHORS' VIEWPOINT

Integrating multiorgan ultrasound in the diagnostic work-up for suspected PE could reduce the need for further imaging. However, the failure rate is concerning, and future studies must be adequately powered to assess safety. Additionally, refining the protocol—perhaps by limiting it to low-probability patients or incorporating D-dimer—could improve the negative predictive value and reduce the risk of misdiagnosis.

STRENGTH OF THE STUDY

- Multicentric RCT
- Low rate of protocol violations
- Trial protocol and statistical analysis plans were published prior.
- Ultrasonography was performed by investigators certified in all three modalities by the Danish Society for Emergency Medicine.
- Pragmatic trial

DRAWBACKS OF THE STUDY

- The study protocol did not incorporate D-dimer levels in decision-making, relying solely on pretest probability and ultrasound findings. Given that D-dimer correlates with PE likelihood, future studies should consider integrating it as a safety threshold.
- The authors acknowledge moderate inter-rater variability in interpreting ultrasound findings, which could affect the reliability of the approach. Proper training and competency assessments are crucial to ensure consistency across different physicians.
- Recruitment across six hospitals was slower than in similar studies, which may introduce selection bias.
- Not all eligible patients may have been considered for inclusion, as only a small number of physicians were trained in the required ultrasound modalities.
- While the patient population in this study had clinical characteristics similar to those in a large-scale PE study, the findings may not be universally applicable, especially given variability in physician expertise and the specific protocol used.

REVIEWERS' VIEWPOINT

The findings of this study suggest that integrating multiorgan ultrasound into the diagnostic work-up for suspected PE could be a promising approach, particularly in reducing reliance on further imaging such as CT pulmonary angiography or lung scintigraphy. The significant reduction in imaging referrals by 45.2% demonstrates the potential for ultrasound to streamline the diagnostic process, leading to both cost savings and improved patient flow in emergency settings. Additionally, ultrasound in this study provided alternative diagnoses in 13.7% of cases, a positive finding showing that ultrasound can sometimes identify other conditions, thus avoiding unnecessary treatments or investigations. However, despite these promising results, the study also highlights serious concerns, particularly the high failure rate of 4.0% in the ultrasound group after 3 months, which exceeds the acceptable threshold of around 2.0% as per international guidelines. This failure rate raises significant concerns about the safety and accuracy of relying solely on ultrasound to rule out PE. Furthermore, inter-rater variability in ultrasound interpretation could lead to inconsistent results depending on the physician performing the examination.

IMPACT ON CURRENT PRACTICE AND TAKE-HOME MESSAGE

- Integrating ultrasound into the diagnostic pathway for suspected PE could reduce the need for further diagnostic imaging by nearly 50%, helping to lower healthcare costs and reduce patient exposure to radiation.
- This trial shows a higher-than-acceptable failure rate (4.0%) in ruling out PE with ultrasound alone, highlighting the need for future studies with larger sample sizes and adequate power to more definitively assess the safety of this approach.
- The current protocol, which does not integrate D-dimer levels, may not be optimal. Including D-dimer levels, particularly when elevated, could help refine decision-making and improve the diagnostic accuracy of ultrasound, thereby reducing the risk of misdiagnosis.
- Given the moderate inter-rater variability in ultrasound interpretation, ensuring that physicians are properly trained and assessed for competency in all ultrasound modalities is crucial. Standardized training and competency requirements would improve consistency and reliability in clinical practice.
- The findings emphasize the need for further well-powered studies to validate this approach, especially focusing on low-probability PE patients to increase the negative predictive value of ultrasound in this context.

SECTION

11

Nutrition/Metabolic

Section Editor: *Ketan Kargirwar*

Associate Editor: *Sanket Hansora*

Association of Glutamine and Glutamate Metabolism with Mortality among Patients at Nutritional Risk – A Secondary Analysis of the Randomized Clinical Trial EFFORT

Wunderle C, von Arx D, Mueller SC, Bernasconi L, Neyer P, Tribolet P, et al. Association of glutamine and glutamate metabolism with mortality among patients at nutritional risk – A secondary analysis of the randomized clinical trial EFFORT.

Nutrients. 2024;16:222.

CLINICAL QUESTION OR PROBLEM

This article investigates the association between glutamine (GLN) and glutamate metabolism and clinical outcomes such as short-term and long-term mortality. It also explores the relationship between glutamine/glutamate levels and:

- Malnutrition parameters
- Effectiveness of nutritional support

The main aim is to evaluate the prognostic impact of GLN metabolism through a secondary analysis of the EFFORT (Effect of Early Nutritional Support on Frailty, Functional Outcome, and the Recovery of Malnourished Medical Inpatient Trials).

This analysis aims to provide insights into how GLN metabolism can influence recovery, malnutrition outcomes, and mortality, contributing to better nutritional strategies for malnourished medical inpatients.

WHAT IS ALREADY KNOWN?

- *Importance of nutrition in critical illness*:
    - Critically ill patients often face catabolic stress, leading to malnutrition and poor clinical outcomes.
    - Optimal nutrition support has been shown to improve outcomes in these patients.
- *Role of glutamine and glutamate*:
    - Glutamine (GLN) is a crucial immune nutrient, whose plasma levels significantly drop during critical illnesses.
    - This decline in GLN may reduce the host's resistance to infections, resulting in poorer outcomes.
    - Glutamine and its metabolite glutamate serve as primary energy substrates for immune cells, supporting immune function and energy metabolism.

- *Evidence on GLN supplementation:*
  - *Animal studies have demonstrated that GLN supplementation can:*
    - Reduce bacterial translocation
    - Improve survival rates
  - In clinical settings, GLN supplementation has shown benefits in cancer patients, critically ill patients, and those with burn injuries.
- *Clinical trials and guidelines:*
  - The 2019 ESPEN guidelines recommended GLN supplementation for critically ill patients.
  - However, the RE-ENERGIZE trial (a large RCT with 1,209 patients) found no significant effect of GLN supplementation on time to hospital discharge.
  - *Other RCTs have reported that enteral GLN supplementation can:*
    - Decrease infection rates
    - Reduce hospital length of stay (LOS)
    - Lower mortality rates
- *Gap in knowledge:*
  - Most research on GLN supplementation focuses on critically ill patients in intensive care units (ICUs).
  - Little is known about GLN metabolism in patients with severe, but not critical illnesses.

STUDY DESIGN AND POPULATIONS

Study Type

- This research is a secondary analysis of the EFFORT trial.
- The EFFORT trial is a pragmatic, investigator-initiated, open-label, non-commercial, multicenter, and randomized controlled trial.

Setting

Conducted across eight Swiss hospitals, comprising both secondary and tertiary care centers.

Patient Screening

- *Screening tool:* Nutritional Risk Screening 2002 (NRS 2002), a validated tool for identifying patients at risk of malnutrition.
- *Total screened:* 5,015 patients
- *Excluded:* 1,878 patients
- Eligible for inclusion: 3,137 patients

Randomization

- *Refusals:* 1,049 patients declined participation
- *Final randomized cohort:* 2,088 patients

Enrollment Period

Patients were enrolled between April 1st, 2014 and February 28th, 2018.

Inclusion Criteria

- *Age:* Patients aged 18 years or older.
- *Nutritional risk:* An NRS 2002 score of 3 or greater, indicating a risk of malnutrition.
- *Hospital stay:* Expected length of hospital stay of at least 5 days.
- *Consent:* Patients who provided valid consent within 48 hours of hospital admission.

Exclusion Criteria

- Initial hospitalization in ICUs or surgical wards
- Inability to digest oral nutrition
- Already receiving nutritional support at the time of admission
- Terminal condition
- Admission to hospital due to anorexia nervosa
- Acute pancreatitis and acute liver failure
- Cystic fibrosis or stem cell transplantation
- Received gastric bypass surgery
- Relative contraindications for nutritional support
- Being previously included in trial

This study protocol was approved by the Ethic Committee of Northwest and Central Switzerland in January 2014.

INTERVENTION STUDIED

Randomization

Patients were randomly assigned (1:1) to either the intervention group or the control group.

Intervention Group

- *Participants*:
    - *Total enrolled:* 1,050 patients
    - *Final inclusion:* 114 patients (after excluding 901 patients with no serum metabolite measurements).
- *Nutrition protocol:*
    - Nutrition support initiated within 48 hours of hospital admission
    - Therapy was individualized using a nutritional treatment algorithm.
    - Patients received personalized nutritional therapy from trained and registered dietitians to achieve caloric and protein targets.
    - *Protein target:*
        - 1.2–1.5 g/kg bodyweight
        - Reduced to 0.8 g/kg bodyweight for patients with acute renal failure
    - If patients could not meet 75% of caloric and protein targets within 5 days via oral feeding, enteral or parenteral feeding was introduced.

Control Group

- *Participants:*
    - *Total enrolled:* 1,013 patients
    - *Final inclusion:* 120 patients (after excluding 893 patients with no serum metabolite measurements)
- *Nutrition protocol:*
    - Patients were provided regular hospital food without additional nutritional support or dietary counseling.
    - They were allowed to eat based on appetite alone.

Key Features of Study Design

- *Monitoring*:
    - Nutritional intake reassessed every 24–48 hours during the hospital stay
    - Intervention discontinued upon discharge
- *Blood samples*:
    - Collected upon study inclusion, processed, and stored at −80°C for later analysis
    - *Glutamate-to-glutamine ratio*: Calculated to estimate GLN consumption.
- *Blinding*: Structured telephone interviews conducted by trained, blinded nurses to assess clinical outcomes after discharge.
- *Nutritional adjustment*: Escalation to enteral or parenteral feeding was recommended if oral intake was insufficient (<75% of targets).

This structured approach ensured meticulous monitoring of nutritional intervention and control, while capturing key metabolic data for analysis **(Tables 1 and 2 and Fig. 1)**.

Outcome Evaluated

- *Primary endpoint:* All-cause short-term mortality measured at 30 days
- *Secondary endpoint* ***(Table 3)****:*
    - Mid- and long-term mortality evaluated at 180 days, 1 year, 3 years, and 5 years
    - Occurrence of adverse events within 30 days of admission
    - Transfer from medical wards to the ICU
    - Nonelective readmissions to the hospital after discharge
    - Major complications include critical health issues such as respiratory failure, cardiovascular events, acute renal failure, and gastrointestinal failure

TABLE 1: Baseline characteristics overall and stratified by high versus low glutamine.

	Overall (n = 234)	***Low glutamine (n = 159)***	***High glutamine (n = 75)***	***p-value***
Sociodemographic				
Male sex	135 (57.7%)	87 (54.7%)	48 (64.0%)	0.18
Mean age in years (SD)	73.6 (13.3)	73.5 (13.6)	73.9 (13)	0.81
Nutritional assessment				
Mean body mass index in kg/m^2 (SD)	24 (5)	24 (5)	25 (5)	0.32
Mean bodyweight in kg (SD)	69 (15)	68 (15)	71 (14)	0.11
Mean height in cm (SD)	168.1 (8.6)	167.5 (8.6)	169.3 (8.4)	0.15
NRS total score				0.75
3 points	60 (25.6%)	39 (24.5%)	21 (28.0%)	
4 points	79 (33.8%)	56 (35.2%)	23 (30.7%)	
≥5 points	95 (40.6%)	64 (40.3%)	31 (41.3%)	
CRP, day 1, mg/L	84.1 (79.8)	85.1 (78.2)	82.0 (83.4)	0.78
Admission diagnosis				
Infection	63 (26.9%)	40 (25.2%)	23 (30.7%)	0.38
Cancer	74 (31.6%)	58 (36.5%)	16 (21.3%)	*0.020*
Cardiovascular disease	24 (10.3%)	15 (9.4%)	9 (12.0%)	0.55
Frailty	13 (5.6%)	11 (6.9%)	2 (2.7%)	0.19
Lung disease	10 (4.3%)	6 (3.8%)	4 (5.3%)	0.58
Gastrointestinal disease	13 (5.6%)	9 (5.7%)	4 (5.3%)	0.92
Renal disease	15 (6.4%)	9 (5.7%)	6 (8.0%)	0.50
Comorbidity				
Charlson comorbidity index	6.4 (2.8%)	6.4 (2.9%)	6.3 (2.7%)	0.76
Hypertension	137 (58.5%)	92 (57.9%)	45 (60.0%)	0.76
Malignant disease	110 (47.0%)	77 (48.4%)	33 (44.0%)	0.53
Chronic kidney disease	81 (34.6%)	51 (32.1%)	30 (40.0%)	0.23
Coronary heart disease	54 (23.1%)	36 (22.6%)	18 (24.0%)	0.82
Diabetes mellitus	43 (18.4%)	23 (14.5%)	20 (26.7%)	*0.025*
Congestive heart failure	45 (19.2%)	33 (20.3%)	12 (16.0%)	0.39
Chronic obstructive pulmonary disease	26 (11.1%)	20 (12.6%)	6 (8.0%)	0.30
Peripheral arterial disease	26 (11.1%)	16 (10.1%)	10 (13.3%)	0.46
Cerebrovascular disease	27 (11.5%)	17 (10.7%)	10 (13.3%)	0.56
Dementia	11 (4.7%)	8 (5.0%)	3 (4.0%)	0.73

Contd...

Contd...

	Overall (n = 234)	***Low glutamine (n = 159)***	***High glutamine (n = 75)***	***p-value***
Metabolites				
Mean plasma glutamine concentration (µmol/L)	522.5 (196.2)	423.4 (130.2)	732.7 (138.3)	<0.001
Mean plasma glutamate concentration (µmol/L)	152.10 (110.35)	166.34 (124.38)	121.91 (62.87)	0.004
(CRP: C-reactive protein; NRS: nutritional risk screening; SD: standard deviation)				

TABLE 2: Association of nutritional parameters with a decrease in plasma glutamine levels.

	Unadjusted	***Adjusted****
Glutamine (decrease of 10 µmol/L)	Coef (95% CI) *p*-value	Coef (95% CI) *p*-value
Nutritional assessment		
Bodyweight (kg)	0.06 (–0.11 to 0.23) $p = 0.459$	0.06 (–0.11 to 0.24) $p = 0.474$
Body mass index (kg/m^2)	0.13 (–0.38 to 0.64) $p = 0.620$	0.12 (–0.39 to 0.63) $p = 0.640$
NRS total score		
3 points	reference	reference
4 points	–456 (–11.15 to 2.04) $p = 0.175$	–4.80 (–11.51 to 1.91) $p = 0.160$
≥5 points	–1.45 (–7.77 to 4.87) $p = 0.651$	–2.47 (–8.96 to 4.01) $p = 0.453$
CRP, day 1, mg/L	0.00 (–0.03 to 0.03) $p = 0.948$	–0.01 (–0.08 to 0.05) $p = 0.659$
NRS score components		
Loss of appetite**	–3.99 (–11.66 to 3.67) $p = 0.306$	–5.82 (–13.80 to 2.15) $p = 0.152$
Bodyweight loss (kg)		
<5% in 3 months	reference	reference
>5% in 3 months	6.00 (–1.03 to 13.03) $p = 0.094$	6.07 (–0.99 to 13.14) $p = 0.092$
>5% in 2 months	–3.83 (0.293 to –11.00) $p = 0.293$	–4.25 (–11.44 to 2.93) $p = 0.245$
>5% in 1 month	–3.94 (–10.52 to 2.64) $p = 0.239$	–3.55 (–10.18 to 3.07) $p = 0.292$
Reduced dietary intake**		
>75%	reference	reference
50–5%	–5.54 (–14.72 to 3.65) $p = 0.236$	–5.57 (–14.83 to 3.69) $p = 0.237$
25–50%	–7.27 (–16.00 to 1.47) $p = 0.102$	–6.95 (–15.83 to 1.92) $p = 0.124$
<25%	–0.14 (–9.77 to 9.49) $p = 0.977$	–0.26 (–9.98 to 9.47) $p = 0.958$

Contd...

Contd...

	Unadjusted	***Adjusted****
Severity of disease		
1	reference	reference
2	−2.89 (−8.16 to 2.38) $p = 0.281$	−3.29 (−8.82 to 2.25) $p = 0.243$
3	−7.04 (−45.16 to 31.09) $p = 0.716$	−7.69 (−46.53 to 31.14) $p = 0.697$

Note: Unadjusted and adjusted regression analyses were performed to identify associations of glutamine concentrations at admission with nutritional parameters. The regression coefficients (95% CI) indicate the change in glutamine concentration by 10 units (10 μmol/L). For binary parameters, patients with the characteristics are compared to patients without the characteristic.
*Adjusted for CCI, CRP, sex, and intervention.
**In the week preceding hospitalization compared to usual appetite and intake.
(BMI: body mass index; CI: confidence interval; Coef: coefficient; CRP: C-reactive protein; NRS 2002: nutritional risk screening 2002)

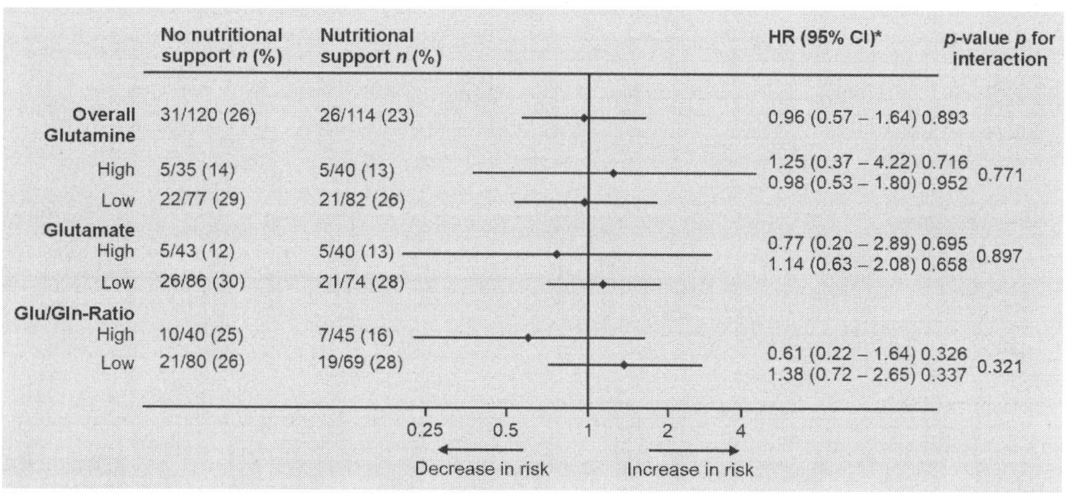

Fig. 1: Forest plot illustrating the impact of nutritional support on overall risk, as well as stratified by glutamine levels, glutamate levels, and the glutamate/glutamine ratio. Hazard ratios (HRs) with 95% confidence intervals (CIs) are presented, along with *p*-values and interaction *p*-values.
*v:Forest plot for 30-day mortality and subgroup analysis for response to nutritional support.

- Functional status decline exceeding 10% during the follow-up period
- Reduction in total length of hospital stay
- In secondary analysis, no significant differences were observed between high and low GLN group. Low glutamate level associated with adverse clinical outcome within 30 days. It was also linked to higher incidence of major complications, including respiratory failure, cardiovascular issues, and renal failure.

▪ *Association of glutamine and glutamate with nutritional parameters and inflammation:*
- *Glutamine and glutamate levels*:
  - No significant association was observed between plasma GLN or glutamate levels (or their ratio) and:
    - NRS total score

TABLE 3: Short- and long-term all-cause mortality rates stratified by glutamine and glutamate levels at 180 days, 1 year, 2 years, 3 years, and 5 years. The table includes the number of events (%), unadjusted hazard ratios (HRs) with 95% confidence intervals (CIs), and *p*-values, as well as adjusted HRs with 95% CIs and *p*-values.

			Unadjusted	***Adjusted****
Short- and long-term mortality	*Number of event (%)*	*Number of event (%)*	*HR (95% CI) p-value*	*HR (95% CI) p-value*
180-day all-cause mortality				
Glutamine	25/75 (36%)	73/159 (46%)	1.37 (0.88–2.13) $p = 0.163$	1.27 (0.81–1.99) $p = 0.289$
Glutamate	25/74 (34%)	75/160 (47%)	1.64 (1.05–2.59) $p = 0.031$	1.67 (1.06–2.63) $p = 0.028$
1-year all-cause mortality				
Glutamine	31/75 (41%)	83/159 (52%)	1.39 (0.92–2.10) $p = 0.119$	1.31 (0.86–1.99) $p = 0.203$
Glutamate	28/74 (38%)	86/160 (54%)	1.68 (1.10–2.58) $p = 0.017$	1.69 (1.10–2.59) $p = 0.017$
2-year all-cause mortality				
Glutamine	41/75 (55%)	95/159 (60%)	1.23 (0.85–1.77) $p = 0.269$	1.20 (0.83–1.74) $p = 0.331$
Glutamate	33/74 (45%)	103/160 (64%)	1.76 (1.19–2.60) $p = 0.005$	1.78 (1.20–2.64) $p = 0.004$
3-year all-cause mortality				
Glutamine	41/75 (55%)	99/159 (62%)	1.28 (0.89–184) $p = 0.191$	1.25 (0.86–1.80) $p = 0.238$
Glutamate	38/74 (51%)	102/160 (64%)	1.53 (1.05–2.22) $p = 0.025$	1.57 (1.08–2.28) $p = 0.019$
5-year all-cause mortality				
Glutamine	45/75 (60%)	108/159 (68%)	1.28 (0.90–1.81) $p = 0.167$	1.24 (0.87–1.77) $p = 0.224$
Glutamate	46/74 (62%)	107/160 (67%)	1.38 (0.98–1.96) $p = 0.067$	1.42 (1.00–2.01) $p = 0.050$

Note: Cox regression models reporting adjusted hazard ratios according to levels stratified by cut-off values of glutamine (595.5 µmol/L) and glutamate (167.5 µmol/L). Low levels are defined as less than or equal to the cut-off value, and high levels are defined as greater than the cut-off value.
(HR: hazard ratio)
*Adjusted for CCI, CRP, NRS total score, sex, and intervention.

- Individual components of the NRS score
- Baseline markers of inflammation

- *Prognostic value of low glutamine or low glutamate to predict clinical outcomes:*
  - *Low versus high glutamine plasma concentration:* No significant differences were found in short-term mortality (30 days) or long-term mortality (up to 5 years).

- *Clinical implication:* This suggests that GLN levels alone may not be a strong predictor of mortality outcomes or clinical prognosis in this cohort.

STRENGTHS AND LIMITATIONS

Strengths

- *Well-characterized cohort*:
  - The patient cohort was thoroughly defined and included participants with comprehensive clinical and demographic details.
  - Randomized study design ensured reduced bias and enhanced reliability of findings.
- *Prospectively collected data*: Short-term and long-term outcomes were systematically collected, allowing for robust analysis and consistent results.
- *Intention-to-treat analysis*: The analysis strategy enhanced the validity of the findings by including all randomized patients in their assigned groups, regardless of protocol adherence.

LIMITATIONS

- *Single-center study*: Limits the generalizability and external validity of findings to other populations and healthcare settings.
- *Limited temporal data*: Glutamine and glutamate levels were measured only at admission, which does not account for:
  - Changes in metabolite levels over time
  - The influence of nutritional interventions during hospitalization
- *Statistical power*: Smaller sample size in subgroup analyses reduced the ability to detect subtle differences or associations.

CONCLUSION

The secondary analysis of this prospective randomized trial highlighted that glutamate serves as an independent prognostic parameter among medical inpatients at nutritional risk. However, its association with the effectiveness of nutritional support was minimal. These findings emphasize the complexity of GLN metabolism and its potential role in improving risk assessment for adverse outcomes in malnourished medical patients. Further research into GLN and glutamate metabolism may provide deeper insights to optimize nutritional strategies and patient outcomes.

Effects of β-hydroxy-β-methylbutyrate (HMB) Supplementation on Lipid Profile in Adults: A GRADE-assessed Systematic Review and Meta-analysis of Randomized Controlled Trials

Sadeghi B, Bahari H, Jozi H, Hasanzadeh MA, Hashemi D, Bideshki MV. Effects of β-hydroxy-β-methylbutyrate (HMB) supplementation on lipid profile in adults: a GRADE-assessed systematic review and meta-analysis of randomized controlled trials.

Front Nutr. 2024;11:1451282.

CLINICAL QUESTION

This meta-analysis aims to explore the effect of β-hydroxy-β-methylbutyrate (HMB) on lipid profiles, which include important markers such as total cholesterol (TC), triglycerides (TGs), low-density lipoprotein cholesterol (LDL-C), and high-density lipoprotein cholesterol (HDL-C). The connection to lipid metabolism is critical since it plays a significant role in preventing cardiovascular diseases (CVDs), which are a major cause of global mortality.

WHAT IS ALREADY KNOWN?

Regulation of lipid metabolism is essential in maintaining cardiovascular health, as dyslipidemia is a major risk factor for CVDs. CVDs remain one of the leading causes of morbidity and mortality worldwide. Lipid imbalances, particularly elevated levels of TC, LDL-C, and TGs, are strongly associated with the development of atherosclerosis, which can lead to heart attacks, strokes, and other cardiovascular complications. HMB, a metabolite of the essential amino acid leucine, has gained attention for its potential role in metabolic regulation. Commonly utilized in sports and fitness, HMB is known for its anticatabolic effects, particularly during periods of stress, such as intense exercise or caloric restriction. It is widely recognized for its ability to preserve muscle mass, enhance muscle strength, and improve exercise recovery. HMB also helps in reducing muscle damage and promoting protein synthesis in the body. Given its beneficial effects on muscle maintenance, HMB supplementation is often used by athletes to support performance during rigorous training sessions. Beyond its effects on muscle tissue, HMB has been linked to improved body composition, including fat loss.

Several studies suggest that HMB supplementation may influence fat oxidation and fatty acid metabolism, which in turn could have a direct impact on lipid profiles. The regulation of fat utilization and fatty acid generation in skeletal muscle and adipocytes contributes to lower TG levels, potentially reducing the risk of CVD. The role of HMB in lipid metabolism is of particular interest. HMB is involved in the metabolic pathway of HMG-CoA (3-hydroxy-3-methyl-glutaryl-CoA), a key intermediate in the biosynthesis of cholesterol. By influencing the rate-limiting step of cholesterol synthesis, HMB has the potential to modulate lipid profiles, particularly through reductions in TC and LDL-C, which are key risk factors for CVDs. While several studies have shown promising results, such as a study by Nisan et al. (2000), which demonstrated that HMB supplementation significantly reduces TC and LDL-C, the current evidence remains limited and conflicting. Some studies show beneficial effects, while others report no significant changes in lipid profiles. Additionally, HMB's influence on other lipid parameters such as HDL-C and TGs remains unclear. This study aims to conduct a meta-analysis to better understand the effects of HMB supplementation on lipid profiles in adults. By synthesizing data from existing studies, the goal is to evaluate the impact of HMB on TC, LDL-C, HDL-C, and TGs, providing clearer insights into its potential as a tool for improving lipid metabolism and reducing the risk of CVDs.

STUDY DESIGN, STUDY SELECTION, AND INCLUDED STUDIES

- This meta-analysis was conducted in adherence to the Preferred Reporting Items for Systematic Reviews and Meta-Analyses (PRISMA) guidelines, ensuring a transparent and systematic approach.
- The study is registered with the International Prospective Register of Systematic Reviews (PROSPERO) to maintain protocol transparency.
- A comprehensive literature search was performed to identify studies evaluating the effect of HMB supplementation on lipid profiles. The search was conducted in major databases, including PubMed, Scopus, and Web of Science, with data collected up until January 2024.
- After conducting the literature search, all identified studies and abstracts were screened for eligibility based on the inclusion criteria.
- All studies were managed using EndNote software, which allowed for efficient organization, removal of duplicates, and tracking of eligible studies throughout the screening process.
- Open access database and university library subscriptions were used to locate full text of related articles.
- The GRADE (Grading of Recommendations, Assessment, Development, and Evaluation) system was employed to assess the certainty of the evidence, considering study design, risk of bias, inconsistency, imprecision, and directness of the data.
- The risk of bias in the included studies was assessed using the Cochrane Risk of Bias Protocol, which evaluates factors such as random sequence generation, allocation concealment, blinding, and incomplete outcome data.
- Search protocol yielded 559 studies. Out of these, 68 duplicates were removed.
- Based on inclusion and exclusion criteria, 462 studies were deemed irrelevant.
- Upon detailed review, 29 studies were assessed in full text. Of these, 19 studies were excluded due to insufficient data reporting on lipid profiles or other relevant outcomes.
- Ultimately, 10 studies with a total of 13 treatment arms were included in the meta-analysis. These studies met the eligibility criteria and provided adequate data for the outcome measures.

Inclusion Criteria

- Randomized controlled trials (RCTs) with either a cross-over or parallel design
- Studies involving adults aged 18 years or older
- HMB supplementation was administered for a minimum of 2 weeks.
- Studies that included both a suitable intervention group (HMB supplementation) and a control group
- Sufficient data on lipid profiles, including mean or median values for key outcomes

- Availability of 95% confidence intervals (CIs) for lipid profile outcomes in both the intervention and control groups, reported at both baseline and end of the intervention

Exclusion Criteria

- Studies where it was not possible to calculate the net benefit of HMB supplementation on lipid profiles.
- Trials where the duration of HMB supplementation was <2 weeks.
- The participants were younger than 18 years.
- Non-RCTs, including case–control studies, cross-sectional studies, cohort studies, or review papers
- Studies where baseline and follow-up lipid profile data were insufficient or absent.

Study Characteristics

- The included studies were conducted in diverse locations: Japan, China, Iran, Brazil, Spain, Australia, and the United States.
- All qualified studies were published between 2000 and 2024.
- Five studies were focused on men, one study involved women and the remaining studies included both men and women in their sample populations.
- The duration of HMB supplementation in the included studies ranged from 2 to 24 weeks
- In four studies, the supplement used was HMB, and in the remaining studies, HMB-CA (HMB-Ca, calcium salt of HMB) was used as the supplement form.
- The daily dosage of HMB supplementation varied across studies, ranging from 1,500 to 6,000 mg/day.
- The participants in these trials represented a broad range of populations, including healthy individuals, patients with liver cirrhosis and clinical malnutrition, noncystic fibrosis patients with bronchiectasis, Australian National Rugby players, amateur athletes, and older women with low muscle mass and older adults (>60 years) with sarcopenia.

Assessment of Quality and Certainty

- The risk of bias in the included studies was assessed using the Cochrane Risk of Bias 2 (ROB2) tool, which evaluates potential biases across various domains. The following bias types were specifically assessed:
  - *Selection bias:* Evaluation of random sequence generation and allocation concealment.
  - *Performance bias:* Assessment of blinding during the intervention phase.
  - *Detection bias:* Evaluation of blinding during outcome assessment.
  - *Attrition bias:* Addressing of participant dropout and handling of incomplete data.
  - *Reporting bias:* Analysis of whether selective reporting of outcomes occurred.
  - *Other potential sources of bias:* Any other factors that could affect the study's internal validity.
- The certainty of the evidence was categorized into four levels: (1) high, (2) moderate, (3) low, and (4) very low.
- Among the included studies, eight studies were categorized as having a low risk of bias, one study was rated as having a moderate risk of bias, and one study reported a high risk of bias.

- Additionally, the risk of bias for each outcome was independently evaluated using the ROB2 tool, which provided a detailed assessment of potential bias for the primary outcome measures.

OUTCOME EVALUATED

The effect of HMB supplementation on lipid profile was evaluated based on the following outcomes:

- TC (mg/dL)
- HDL-C (mg/dL)
- LDL-C (mg/dL)
- TGs (mg/dL)

For each outcome, the mean and standard deviation (SD) values at both baseline and end of intervention were extracted from the included studies. A 95% CI was used to express the effect size for each outcome.

The Cochrane Q test and I^2 statistic were used to assess study heterogeneity.

A *p*-value of <0.1 and an I^2 value of >50% indicated significant heterogeneity across studies.

Effect of HMB Supplementation on Total Cholesterol

- A total of 12 effect sizes were analyzed to assess the impact of HMB supplementation on TC levels. The results revealed no significant effect of HMB supplementation compared to the control group [weighted mean difference (WMD)]: 2.26 mg/dL (95% CI: 7.48–2.96, $p = 0.25$).
- *Heterogeneity:* No significant heterogeneity was observed ($I^2 = 0.0\%$, $p = 0.79$).

Effect of HMB Supplementation on Triglycerides

- A total of 11 effect sizes were evaluated for the impact of HMB supplementation on TG levels. HMB supplementation did not significantly reduce TG levels compared to the control group.
    - WMD: 2.83 mg/dL (95% CI: 9.73–4.07, $p = 0.58$)
- *Heterogeneity:* A high degree of heterogeneity was detected across the studies ($I^2 = 58.4\%$, $p = 0.01$).

Effect of HMB Supplementation on Low-density Lipoprotein Cholesterol

- 12 effect sizes were analyzed to assess the effect of HMB supplementation on LDL-C levels. The results indicated that HMB supplementation had no significant effect on LDL-C compared to the control group.
    - WMD: 0.13 mg/dL (95% CI: 2.18–2.44, $p = 0.94$).
- *Heterogeneity*: No significant heterogeneity was observed ($I^2 = 7.1\%$, $p = 0.37$).

Effect of HMB Supplementation on High-density Lipoprotein Cholesterol

- After analyzing 12 effect sizes, it was found that HMB supplementation did not significantly change HDL-C levels compared to the control group.
    - WMD: 0.78 mg/dL (95% CI: 2.14–0.58, $p = 0.22$).
- *Heterogeneity*: No significant heterogeneity was detected ($I^2 = 3.2\%$, $p = 0.41$).

CONCLUSION

This systematic review and meta-analysis suggest that HMB supplementation does not have a significant effect on the lipid profile, including TC, LDL-C, HDL-C, and TG levels. Despite evaluating multiple studies, no substantial changes were observed in these lipid indices following HMB supplementation.

STRENGTH OF THE SYSTEMIC REVIEW

- The review incorporates a sufficient number of studies, which enhance the robustness of the findings and support more reliable conclusions.
- Most of the studies included were assessed as high quality using the Cochrane risk of bias tool, indicating that the results are likely to be valid and trustworthy.
- The studies were conducted in various regions around the world, allowing the findings to be relevant and applicable to adult populations globally, enhancing the generalizability of the results.

LIMITATIONS OF THE STUDY

- There may be significant variability among the studies included in the systematic review and meta-analysis, which could affect the overall findings.
- The differences in study designs, populations, and intervention protocols may have influenced the results, making it challenging to draw definitive conclusions.
- Factors such as exercise and diet could have impacted the lipid profile changes associated with HMB supplementation, complicating the attribution of effects solely to HMB.
- Not all studies adequately controlled for these confounding factors, which may hinder the ability to isolate the effects of HMB.
- The inclusion of only English-language articles may have resulted in the exclusion of relevant studies published in other languages, potentially biasing the findings.
- Some studies did not provide clear information regarding their randomization or blinding processes for outcome assessment, raising concerns about the reliability of their results.
- Most of the outcomes were rated as moderate to low quality according to GRADE, indicating limitations in the strength of the evidence.

REVIEWER'S VIEWPOINT

The reviewer's viewpoint highlights that while HMB is a popular sports supplement among athletes due to its anticatabolic effects and its known benefits for muscle mass and strength, it does not significantly impact the lipid profile. The reviewer emphasizes the need for further research, specifically larger and more rigorously conducted studies with long-term intervention periods. This additional research is essential to thoroughly investigate the mechanisms of action and the potential clinical significance of HMB supplementation.

Impact of Early High-protein Intake in Critically Ill Patients: A Randomized Control Trial

Wang Y, Ye Y, Xuan L, Xu L, Wang P, Ma J, et al. Impact of early high protein intake in critically ill patients: a randomized controlled trial.

Nutr Metab (Lond). 2024;21:39.

CLINICAL QUESTION

This clinical question centers on understanding the impact of early high-protein intake on critically ill patients in intensive care settings. Specifically, it seeks to evaluate whether early aggressive protein supplementation improves outcomes and determines the effective and safe dosage of protein during the acute phase of critical illness.

Koekkoek et al. (2019) found increased mortality with high-protein intake in the first 3 days of intensive care unit (ICU) admission but a mortality reduction with higher protein intake after 3 days. Previous studies stated that early high-protein supplementation did not improve nutritional status, increased gastric intolerance, and showed no effect on 28-day mortality. During early critical illness, the body's stress response prioritizes endogenous glycogen and protein breakdown, and excessive external protein may result in complications (e.g., azotemia and hyperglycemia). The main objective of this study is to investigate the effect of early high-protein intake during phase of critical illness, determine the safe and effective protein dose during early and late phases of ICU care and assess the potential adverse effects associated with early high-protein intake.

WHAT IS ALREADY KNOWN?

Prior studies have demonstrated inconsistent outcomes, highlighting the complexity of determining the optimal protein dose in critically ill patients. Hartwell et al. conducted a retrospective study (274 critically ill adults) indicated that achieving protein targets within the first 4 days of ICU stay resulted in fewer complications. In contrast, Lin et al. demonstrated an association between early low- (0.38 g/kg/day) or high- (1.68 g/kg/day) protein intake and increased 28-day mortality in critically ill patients compared to moderate-protein intake (0.8 g/kg/day). In the EFFORT protein trial, administering >2.2 g/kg/day significantly exceeded the recommended range of 1.2–2 g/kg/day. Negative effects were observed in patients with kidney injury or organ failure, likely due to the inability to handle the metabolic load. Sepsis leads to severe protein breakdown, decreased synthesis, and multiorgan dysfunction. High-protein intake in this context places hepatic and renal systems under significant strain, compounding the risk of adverse outcomes.

STUDY DESIGN

- Prospective, single-blinded, and randomized controlled trial with two parallel treatment arms
- Patients were blinded to their assigned treatment group.
- Informed consents obtained from all the patients' legal guardians before inclusion in study

POPULATIONS STUDIED

- A total of 202 patients were screened, with 173 patients included in the study.

- Four patients in low-protein group and six patients in high-protein group self-discharged leading to loss to follow-up
- Patient recruitment occurred from January 1, 2021 to April 30, 2023
- *Inclusion criteria:*
  - Adults ≥18 years admitted to ICU or electronic intensive care unit (EICU)
  - Modified Nutrition Risk in Critically Ill (mNUTRIC) score >5.
  - Anticipated ICU/EICU stay of >7 days
- *Exclusion criteria:*
  - Burns
  - Inability to initiate enteral nutrition (EN) within 48 hours of ICU admission
  - Initiation of renal replacement therapy within 24–48 hours of ICU/EICU admission
  - Pregnancy or lactation
  - Advance malignant tumors
  - Severe complications of diabetes such as diabetic ketoacidosis and hyperosmolar coma
  - History of digestive tract surgery
  - Primary gastrointestinal injury or neuromuscular disease (affecting protein absorption)
  - Body mass index (BMI) >30 kg/m^2
  - Hyperthyroidism
  - Unwillingness to participate in study
- Demographic data such as age and gender and clinical characteristics such as APACHE II, weigh, BMI, sepsis, and the reason for ICU/EICU admission of all patients were collected before intervention treatment.

INTERVENTION STUDIED AND DEMOGRAPHIC DATA

- *Randomized groups:*
  - *Low-protein group (n = 87):*
    - Protein intake: 0.8 g/kg/day (ideal body weight)
    - Nonprotein calories: 20 kcal/kg/day for the first 3 days
  - *High-protein group (n = 86)*:
    - Protein intake: 1.5 g/kg/day
    - Nonprotein calories: 20 kcal/kg/day for the first 3 days
- *Nutrition protocol:*
  - Intervention began 1–2 days after admission
  - Both groups received EN
  - *From day 4 onward:*
    - Protein intake: 1.5 g/kg/day for both groups
    - Nonprotein calories: 25 kcal/kg/day for both groups
- *Supportive measures:*
  - *Primary disease treatment:* All subjects received standard care for the underlying illness, including organ support and antibiotics as needed.
  - *Hypoalbuminemia:*
    - 20% human albumin was administered to maintain colloid osmotic pressure and physiological homeostasis in patients with serum albumin <30 g/L.
  - *Pain and sedation:*
    - Regimen followed PADIS (Pain, Agitation, Delirium, Immobility, and Sleep Disruption) guidelines
    - Individualized pain and sedation targets were established, prioritizing pain management and light sedation strategies.
  - *Rehabilitation:* Tailored intensive rehabilitation plans were implemented based on the disease stage.
- *EN initiation*:
  - *Criteria for EN:*
    - Stable hemodynamics:
      - Mean arterial pressure (MAP) >65 mm Hg
      - Lactate <4 mmol/L

- Norepinephrine <0.2 μg/kg/min
- Absence of contraindications (e.g., gastrointestinal bleeding and intestinal obstruction)
- *Initial rate:* 10–15 mL/hour
- *EN tolerance assessed every 4 hours:*
  - *If tolerated*: Rate increased by 10–25 mL/hour every 4–8 hours.
  - *If intolerance occurred*: Rate maintained or reduced to half after symptomatic treatment.
- *Supplemental nutrition*: Patients failing to achieve 60% of target protein intake by day 7 received supplemental parenteral nutrition and were removed from the study.
- *Adverse event protocol*: Severe EN intolerance leading to clinical deterioration was documented as an adverse event, and the patient was considered lost to follow-up.

DEMOGRAPHIC DATA AND BASELINE CHARACTERISTICS

- *Key variables collected before intervention*:
  - *Patient characteristics*:
    - Age
    - Gender
    - APACHE II score: Reflecting disease severity and prognosis
    - Weight and BMI
    - Presence of sepsis
    - Reason for ICU/EICU admission
    - mNUTRIC score: Used to assess nutritional risk
  - *Laboratory measurements:*
    - Serum prealbumin (PA): Indicator of nutritional status and liver function.
    - Blood urea nitrogen (BUN)/creatinine ratio: To assess renal function and protein metabolism.
- *Muscle evaluation:*
  - *Muscle status:* The right thigh rectus femoris muscle thickness and cross-sectional area (CSA) were assessed at three time points:
    - Day 1 (ICU admission)
    - Day 5
    - ICU discharge
- *Measurement protocol:*
  - *Positioning:*
    - Patient in supine position with head elevated to 30°
    - Both lower limbs naturally relaxed and extended
  - *Probe placement:* A linear probe was placed vertically at the mid-lower third of the right thigh, between the anterior superior iliac spine and the upper edge of the patella.
  - *Thickness measurement:* Vertical distance measured within the high echogenic fascia.
  - *Cross-sectional area:* Outlined along the fascia using the ultrasound probe.
- *Quality assurance:* Each measurement was performed independently by two trained healthcare personnel to ensure accuracy and reliability.

OUTCOME EVALUATED

- *Primary outcome:* 28-day mortality (overall and by subgroup):
  - *Overall mortality:*
    - Low-protein group: 19.54%
    - High-protein group: 8.14%
    - Statistical significance: $p = 0.051$ (borderline significant)
  - *Subgroup analysis:*
    - Septic patients:
      - Low-protein group: 10%.
      - High-protein group: 1%
      - Statistical significance: $p = 0.018$ (statistically significant)

    - Nonseptic patients:
        - Low-protein group: 7%
        - High-protein group: 6%
        - Statistical significance: $p = 0.913$ (not significant)
- *Secondary outcome includes:*
    - *Duration of mechanical ventilation:*
        - Low-protein group: 10%
        - High-protein group: 9%
        - Statistical significance: $p = 0.039$ (statistically significant).
    - *ICU length of stay*:
        - Low-protein group: 10 days
        - High-protein group: 9 days
        - Statistical significance: $p = 0.025$ (statistically significant)
    - *Refeeding syndrome incidence rate:*
        - Statistical significance: $p = 0.442$ (not significant)
        - Definition: Refeeding syndrome defined as:
            - Blood phosphorus level <0.65 mmol/L, or
            - Decrease >0.16 mmol/L
    - *Enteral nutrition tolerance score:*
        - Statistical significance: $p = 0.129$ (not significant)

AUTHORS' VIEWPOINTS

The authors conclude that while high-protein intake did not directly reduce the overall 28-day mortality rate, it was associated with a significant reduction in 28-day mortality among septic patients. Additionally, the study demonstrated several benefits of early high-protein intake, including:

- *Enhanced recovery speed:*
    - Shorter duration of mechanical ventilation
    - Reduced ICU length of stay
- *Improved nutritional status:*
    - Increased serum PA levels
    - Mitigated rectus femoris muscle atrophy
- *Short-term recovery benefits:* High-protein intake positively influenced the overall recovery trajectory of critically ill patients, particularly in the early stages of their ICU stay.
- The findings suggest that early high-protein intake is a beneficial strategy to improve short-term recovery outcomes in critically ill patients, especially those with sepsis. This supports the use of personalized nutrition strategies in critical care settings, emphasizing the importance of addressing protein needs early during ICU admission.

STRENGTH OF STUDY

- Prospective randomized control trial ensures robust methodology and minimizes selection and allocation bias.
- The outcome analysis was conducted based on intension-to-treat (ITT) principle
- The demographic and baseline characteristics of participants showed no statistically significant differences between low-protein and high-protein groups.

DRAWBACKS OF STUDY

- This study was conducted at single center, which may limit the external validity and applicability of results to other populations and healthcare settings.
- The study included a relatively smaller sample size, particularly when differences between the groups are subtle. This may reduce the statistical power to detect clinically meaningful differences.
- 28-day observation period focuses only on short-term outcomes, leaving the long-term effects of early high-protein intake on recovery, morbidity and mortality unassessed.

AUTHORS' VIEWPOINTS AND IMPACT ON CURRENT PRACTICE

The reviewer acknowledges that while this study did not demonstrate a statistically significant reduction in overall 28-day mortality, it provided compelling evidence of the benefits of early high-protein intake in septic patients and on short-term recovery outcomes. Key observations include:

- *Significant findings:*
    - Reduced 28-day mortality in septic patients (statistically significant)
    - *Improved recovery metrics*:
        - Increased mechanical ventilation-free days
        - Shortened ICU stay
        - Enhanced nutritional status (e.g., increased serum PA levels and reduced muscle atrophy)
- *General implications:* Reinforces the importance of early nutritional support in critically ill patients, emphasizing the role of tailored protein intake in improving patient recovery.
- *Future direction*:
    - Larger, multicenter studies with extended follow-up periods are needed to validate these findings and explore the long-term effects of high-protein intake in diverse critically ill populations.
    - Such studies could provide a deeper understanding of optimal protein dosing strategies, especially in subgroups such as septic and nonseptic patients.

Nutrition Practices in Critically Ill Adults Receiving Noninvasive Ventilation: A Quantitative Survey of Australian and New Zealand Intensive Care Clinicians

Page K, Viner Smith E, Plummer MP, Ridley EJ, Burfield K, Chapple LS. Nutrition practices in critically ill adults receiving noninvasive ventilation: A quantitative survey of Australian and New Zealand intensive care clinicians.

Aust Crit Care. 2024;37:43-50.

CLINICAL QUESTION

Noninvasive ventilation (NIV) is widely employed in intensive care units (ICUs) for managing respiratory failure. However, nutrition management during NIV poses unique challenges, primarily due to the delivery method, which typically involves masks or helmets that obstruct nasal and oral access, complicating the administration of enteral nutrition (EN). Due to the absence of clear guidelines, nutrition strategies for patients on NIV often vary depending on individual clinician experience and institutional norms. This study aims to explore the perception of medical and nursing of staff regarding current practices in nutrition management for critically ill adults receiving NIV and to highlight the challenges and potential areas of improvement to inform future guideline development and optimize patient outcomes.

WHAT IS ALREADY KNOWN?

The use of NIV has significantly increased in ICUs for managing critically ill patients, offering respiratory support through an external interface like a mask or helmet. Despite its growing use, nutrition management during NIV remains an underresearched and challenging aspect of critical care. NIV requires a sealed interface (mask or helmet), making it challenging to deliver oral intake without removal of the device, which could compromise respiratory support. Enteral feeding tubes can create an air leak, potentially disrupting the effectiveness of respiratory support. Prolonged periods of fasting are common, as clinicians may hesitate to initiate nutrition for fear of exacerbating respiratory function. Evidence suggests that patients on NIV often experience insufficient caloric and protein intake, contributing to nutritional deficiencies and delayed recovery.

STUDY DESIGN

The main objective is to explore the views, perceptions, and current practices of medical and nursing staff regarding the nutrition management during NIV in ICU.

Methodology:

- *Target population:*
  - *Participants:* Medical officers and nursing staff with >12 months of ICU experience.
  - *Recruitment:* Conducted via purposive snowball sampling between August 29 and October 9, 2022.
  - *Platform:* Survey disseminated using the REDCap web platform.
- *Survey structure:*
  - *Three sections*:
    1. Demographics and ICU characteristics: Captured years of ICU experience, professional position, ICU bed capacity, and geographical location.
    2. NIV practices: Focused on commonly used NIV interfaces, decision makers for nutrition provision, and factors influencing those decisions.
    3. Views on nutrition during NIV: Assessed perceptions of nutritional adequacy, preferred routes of administration, barriers and facilitators to nutrition delivery, the role of dietitians, and the perceived importance of nutrition during NIV.
- *Design and pretesting:*
  - Developed by a multidisciplinary team of ICU clinicians and investigators
  - *Pilot testing*: Conducted with four ICU clinicians (including one medical officer and one nurse with >12 months of ICU experience) to ensure content validity, participant experience, and identify irrelevant questions.
  - Refined based on feedback, with an estimated completion time of 10–15 minutes
- *Sampling and recruitment*:
  - *Purposive snowball sampling*: Leveraged networks of relevant organizations and participants to disseminate the survey.
  - Targeted ICU professionals in Australia and New Zealand

POPULATIONS STUDIED

Participants Overview

- *Total surveys completed:* 182
- *Final analyzed responses:* 152 (after applying inclusion and exclusion criteria)
  - *Nurses:* 71 (48%)
  - *Medical officers:* 69 (45%)
  - *Others*: 12 (8%)

Demographics and Characteristics

- *Geographical distribution:*
  - *Australia*: 87% (n = 122/140)
  - *New Zealand*: 13% (n = 18/140)
- *ICU settings:*
  - *Metropolitan ICU*: 78% (n = 109/140)
  - *ICU bed capacity*: 35% worked in units with 21–30 beds
- *Clinical experience:*
  - *Most common response:* >20 years of ICU experience
  - *Nursing staff:* 63% (n = 45/71) were critical care trained or in training.
  - *Medical officers:* 80% (n = 45/69) were at the consultant level.

Inclusion and Exclusion Criteria

- *Included:* Participants who completed ≥50% of the survey (n = 152; 84%).
  - All included completed at least two of three survey sections.
  - 89% (n = 136) completed all three sections.
- *Excluded:* Participants completing <50% of the survey (n = 30; 16%).

Survey Focus Areas and Interventions Studied

- *NIV concepts:*
  - *Commonly used interfaces:*
    - Nose-mouth masks
    - Full-face masks
- *Importance of nutrition support:* Assessed the perceived significance of nutrition during NIV therapy.
- *Route of nutrition:* Explored preferred routes (oral, enteral, or parenteral) and the factors influencing these choices.
- *Nutrition adequacy*: Evaluated clinician perspectives on meeting nutritional needs during NIV.
- *Barriers and facilitators to nutrition delivery:* Identified practical challenges and enablers for effective nutrition support during NIV.

INTERVENTIONS STUDIED

- *NIV concepts:* Commonly used interfaces (nose-mouth masks and full-face masks)
- *Importance of nutrition support:* Assessed the perceived significance of nutrition during NIV therapy.
- *Route of nutrition:* Explored preferred routes (oral, enteral, or parenteral) and the factors influencing these choices.
- *Nutrition adequacy:* Evaluated clinician perspectives on meeting nutritional needs during NIV.
- *Barriers and facilitators to nutrition delivery:* Identified practical challenges and enablers for effective nutrition support during NIV.

RESULTS OF SURVEY

- Quantitative survey explored in Australia and New Zealand ICU medical and nursing staff members' views of nutrition practices in critically ill patients receiving the NIV.
- Nutrition during NIV is considered as important as nutrition during invasive mechanical ventilation (IMV). However, inadequate nutrition intake is frequently reported.
- Oral intake was the most commonly reported route of feeding.
- The least common practice was providing no nutrition at all (nil nutrition).
- 75% of patients receiving NIV consumed <80% of their energy and protein requirements through oral intake.
- Gastric EN demonstrated the potential to deliver greater calorie intake than oral feeding. However, EN is associated with higher rates of aspiration pneumonia compared to nonenterally fed patients.

Postpyloric EN is linked to lower incidents of aspiration, presenting a safer alternative to gastric EN in certain cases.

- There are multiple barriers to delivery of nutrition like potential aspiration due to gastrointestinal feeding and extended fasting period for procedures and intubation.
- The design of NIV interfaces poses significant logistical barriers to effective nutrition delivery, requiring innovative solutions or adaptations.
- These findings underline the critical need for developing evidence-based guidelines tailored to patients on NIV to address the challenges of inadequate nutrition and optimize outcomes in critically ill populations.

DRAWBACKS

- *Lack of consensus:* No clear agreement on the safest route of nutrition, the one most likely to achieve adequate nutrition, or the preferred route for patients on NIV.
- *Unexplored areas:*
    - The impact of energy deficit on patients receiving NIV was not investigated.
    - Clinicians showed varying opinions on feeding practices without definitive evidence to guide decisions.
- *Survey limitations:*
    - Errors in the REDCap branching logic excluded responses from clinicians with exactly 10 years of experience, leading to missing demographic data for 12 participants.
    - *Participant bias*: Respondents with an interest in nutrition may have been more inclined to complete the survey, potentially skewing results.
- *Influence of NIV administration reasons:* The survey questions were not adapted based on the specific indications for NIV, which could significantly influence clinician decision-making and practices.
- *Dietitian perspectives:* While dietitians are key stakeholders in nutrition management, their views and roles were not captured in this study, resulting in an incomplete picture of multidisciplinary practices.

AUTHORS' VIEWPOINTS AND IMPACT ON CURRENT PRACTICE

This survey aimed to explore the perceptions and practices of clinicians (medical officers and nursing staff) regarding nutrition management during NIV in critically ill patients, highlighting the absence of formal guidelines for this population.

- Barriers to nutrition delivery include aspiration risks, extended fasting periods, maintaining mask seal, and interface design limitations
- There is no consensus on the safest or most effective route of nutrition, with oral intake being inadequate in many cases.
- Improved NIV interfaces compatible with nasoenteric tubes could enhance nutrition delivery
- Developing evidence-based guidelines and multidisciplinary approaches may help standardize nutrition practices and improve outcomes.
- Gastric EN has shown potential to better meet nutritional targets compared to oral intake, though it comes with higher aspiration risks.
- Dietitians play an essential role in the assessment, planning, and monitoring of nutrition strategies for patients on NIV.

SECTION

12

Guidelines

***Section Editor:** Deven Juneja*

***Associate Editor:** Sahil Kataria*

SCCM/IDSA Guidelines for Evaluating New Fever in Adult Patients in the ICU

O'Grady NP, Alexander E, Alhazzani W, Alshamsi F, Cuellar-Rodriguez J, Jefferson BK, et al. Society of Critical Care Medicine and the Infectious Diseases Society of America (SCCM/IDSA) Guidelines for evaluating new fever in adult patients in the ICU.

Crit Care Med. 2023;51:1570-86.

CLINICAL QUESTION OR PROBLEM

The 2023 guidelines from the Society of Critical Care Medicine (SCCM) and the Infectious Diseases Society of America (IDSA) were developed to create a structured approach for assessing and managing new-onset fever in adult ICU patients who are not severely immunocompromised. Fever in this group can signify an infection or other underlying conditions, highlighting the need for a standardized diagnostic and treatment protocol to ensure timely and accurate care.

WHAT IS ALREADY KNOWN?

Prior to the 2023 update, the last revision of these guidelines happened in 2008. At that time, the guidelines provided a framework for handling new-onset fever in ICU patients, a symptom that can occur in 26–88% of these patients. Fever is often an early sign of infection, and initial assessments typically focus on identifying infectious causes, as early intervention can improve patient outcomes. However, with the advancement in diagnostic tools and new research, the 2008 guidelines became outdated, necessitating the current update.

STUDY DESIGN

The 2023 guidelines were drafted by a multidisciplinary panel of 12 experts, including professionals in critical care, infectious diseases, clinical microbiology, and organ transplantation. The panel organized their work into subgroups, each addressing different aspects of fever management, such as determining the presence of fever, treatment options, imaging, microbiological assessment, and rapid diagnostic testing. The Grading of Recommendations Assessment, Development, and Evaluation (GRADE) approach was used, which involved a thorough review of existing literature to evaluate the strength of evidence. Group leaders formulated specific Population, Intervention, Comparison, and Outcomes

(PICO) questions related to their area of focus. These questions underwent review and approval by consensus from the task force. The task force then identified relevant outcomes for each PICO, which were prioritized through electronic voting based on their importance, with only those scoring 7 or above on a 9-point scale being included. In total, 26 PICO questions were used to guide the recommendations. The panel reached a consensus on each recommendation through a voting process that required 80% agreement among at least 75% of the members. The recommendations were classified as strong or weak based on the quality of evidence and the balance between benefits and risks. Recommendations from the 2008 guidelines that were not specifically addressed in the 2023 update, remained in place. Notably, the development of these guidelines was free from industry influence or funding.

OUTCOME EVALUATED

The primary outcomes that the guidelines address include the accuracy and effectiveness of various temperature monitoring methods, the role of imaging and biomarkers in diagnosing fever, and the judicious use of antipyretics **(Table 1)**. The guidelines also emphasize the importance of avoiding unnecessary treatments, particularly the overuse of antibiotics, to prevent

TABLE 1: Key recommendations along with the type of recommendation and the quality of evidence supporting each.

Parameters	*Recommendation*	*Quality of evidence*
Central temperature monitoring	When central devices such as thermistors are available, they are preferred for temperature monitoring. Oral or rectal temperatures are recommended when these devices are not in place, as they are more reliable than axillary or tympanic membrane measurements	Weak recommendation
Routine antipyretic use	It is suggested to avoid routinely using antipyretic medications specifically to reduce fever	Weak recommendation
Antipyretics for comfort	For patients who prefer temperature reduction for comfort, antipyretics may be considered over nondrug methods	Weak recommendation
Chest radiograph for new fever	A chest radiograph is recommended for ICU patients who develop a new fever	Best-practice statement
CT for postsurgical fever	For patients with recent surgery in the thoracic, abdominal, or pelvic area, a CT scan is recommended if initial investigations do not reveal the fever's cause	Best-practice statement
PET/CT for persistent fever	For patients with persistent fever and no identified cause, 18F-FDG PET/CT may be considered if patient transport is safe	Weak recommendation
WBC scan	There is insufficient evidence to recommend using WBC scans for fever of unknown origin	No recommendation

Contd...

Contd...

Parameters	***Recommendation***	***Quality of evidence***
Abdominal ultrasound or POCUS	Routine use of abdominal ultrasound or POCUS is not recommended as an initial investigation unless specific clinical indications are present	Best-practice statement
Bedside ultrasound for abdominal symptoms	An abdominal ultrasound is recommended if there is a suspicion of an abdominal source of infection, especially after recent surgery	Best-practice statement
Thoracic bedside ultrasound	Thoracic ultrasound should be considered when an abnormal chest radiograph is present and expertise is available	Weak recommendation
Thoracic ultrasound without chest radiograph abnormalities	Insufficient evidence exists to recommend thoracic bedside ultrasound when the chest radiograph is normal	No recommendation
Blood cultures with central venous catheter	Blood cultures from both central venous catheters and peripheral sites are recommended to calculate differential time to positivity	Best-practice statement
Lumens for blood cultures	When culturing blood from central venous catheters, at least two lumens should be sampled	Best-practice statement
Rapid molecular tests with blood cultures	Rapid molecular tests should be used alongside blood cultures for patients with new fever of unclear origin	Weak recommendation
Number of blood cultures	It is recommended to collect at least two sets of blood cultures from different sites, one immediately after the other	Best-practice statement
Urine cultures for suspected UTI	For patients suspected of having a urinary tract infection, replacing the urinary catheter and obtaining urine cultures from the new catheter is recommended	Best-practice statement
Viral pathogen testing for suspected pneumonia	Testing for viral pathogens using nucleic acid amplification tests is suggested for patients with fever and suspected pneumonia or respiratory symptoms	Weak recommendation
Routine blood testing for viral pathogens in immunocompetent patients	There is insufficient evidence to recommend routine blood testing for viral pathogens in immunocompetent ICU patients	No recommendation
SARS-CoV-2 testing	Testing for SARS-CoV-2 by PCR is recommended based on the level of community transmission in patients with a new fever	Best-practice statement
Procalcitonin (PCT) measurement for low/ intermediate probability of bacterial infection	For patients with a low-to-intermediate probability of bacterial infection and new fever, measuring PCT along with clinical evaluation is suggested	Weak recommendation

Contd...

Contd...

Parameters	Recommendation	Quality of evidence
PCT measurement for a high probability of bacterial infection	It is suggested not to measure PCT for ruling out bacterial infection when the probability is high	Weak recommendation
C-reactive protein (CRP) measurement for low/ intermediate probability of bacterial infection	For patients with a low-to-intermediate probability of bacterial infection and new fever, measuring CRP in addition to clinical evaluation is suggested	Weak recommendation
CRP measurement for a high probability of bacterial infection	It is suggested not to measure CRP for ruling out bacterial infection when the probability is high	Weak recommendation
PCT or CRP measurement for low/intermediate probability of bacterial infection	For patients with a low-to-intermediate probability of bacterial infection, either PCT or CRP measurement is suggested to help rule out infection	Weak recommendation

(CT: computed tomography; 18F-FDG: flourine-18 fluorodeoxyglucose; ICU: intensive care unit; PET: positron emission tomography; POCUS: point-of-care ultrasound; SARS-CoV-2: severe acute respiratory syndrome coronavirus 2; UTI: urinary tract infection; WBC: white blood cell)

overtreatment and the development of antimicrobial resistance. The 2023 update provides actionable guidance that can help clinicians make informed decisions when managing fever in ICU patients. This structured approach is intended to benefit a wide range of healthcare providers, including intensivists, infectious disease specialists, and hospitalists, by promoting consistent and evidence-based patient care.

AUTHORS' VIEWPOINTS

The authors of the guidelines highlight the challenges associated with diagnosing and managing fever in critically ill patients, noting that while fever often serves as an early sign of infection, it is not always present in cases of infection and can also result from noninfectious causes. They emphasize the importance of using central temperature monitoring and appropriate imaging techniques and advocate for a careful approach to the use of antipyretics and antibiotics. The authors also underscore the need for continued research to fill the gaps in evidence, which currently limits the strength of many recommendations.

STRENGTH OF THE GUIDELINES

- These guidelines offer a thorough and methodical approach to evaluating new-onset fever in ICU patients.
- They integrate the latest evidence and provide well-defined recommendations on temperature monitoring, imaging, and the use of biomarkers.
- The application of the GRADE methodology ensures that the guideline development process is systematic and that the recommendations are grounded in the best available evidence.

DRAWBACKS OF THE GUIDELINES

- A key limitation of the guidelines is the reliance on weak evidence for many recommendations, reflecting the need for higher-quality research in this area.

- The use of the GRADE system, initially designed for therapeutic interventions, poses challenges when applied to diagnostic testing, which is often overutilized in ICU settings.
- The guidelines fall short in addressing fever management in severely immunocompromised patients, limiting their applicability to this critical subgroup.
- The focus on infectious causes results in less comprehensive guidance for evaluating noninfectious causes of fever, which can also be significant in the ICU context.

REVIEWERS' VIEWPOINTS

The SCCM and IDSA 2023 guidelines for evaluating new fever in adult ICU patients score well in stakeholder involvement, clarity, and editorial independence but are somewhat limited by the weak evidence base supporting many of their recommendations. The guidelines have a clear objective, focusing on evaluating and managing new-onset fever in adult ICU patients who are not severely immunocompromised. However, they do not fully address the needs of immunocompromised patients or delve deeply into noninfectious causes of fever.

The guidelines were developed by a diverse panel of experts, ensuring that multiple perspectives were considered. However, more explicit involvement of patient representatives and consideration of patient preferences could enhance the guidelines.

While the guidelines follow the GRADE methodology, which is systematic and rigorous, the recommendations are weakened by the low quality of evidence. Greater transparency in the development process and more robust evidence could improve this score. The guidelines are well-structured and clearly presented, with easily understandable recommendations and best-practice statements. However, the inclusion of more detailed algorithms or flowcharts could further aid clinical decision-making.

Practical recommendations are provided, particularly regarding temperature monitoring and imaging. However, the limited evidence base may affect the guidelines' applicability in varied clinical settings, and more detailed implementation guidance would be beneficial. The guidelines were developed with complete independence from industry influence, and conflicts of interest were well-managed, ensuring the credibility of the recommendations.

IMPACT ON CLINICAL PRACTICE AND TAKE-HOME MESSAGE

The 2023 SCCM/IDSA guidelines present a valuable framework for evaluating new-onset fever in adult ICU patients, emphasizing evidence-based practices in areas such as temperature monitoring, imaging, and biomarker use. Although the guidelines are comprehensive and reflect current advancements, their application is somewhat constrained by the weak evidence base supporting many recommendations. Clinicians should incorporate these guidelines into their practice with an awareness of their limitations, particularly in diverse patient populations and clinical scenarios. Continued research is essential to strengthen the evidence base, enhance noninvasive diagnostic methods, and expand the guidelines' applicability to broader patient groups.

Society of Critical Care Medicine Clinical Practice Guidelines for Rapid Sequence Intubation in the Critically Ill Adult Patient

Acquisto NM, Mosier JM, Bittner EA, Patanwala AE, Hirsch KG, Hargwood P, et al. Society of Critical Care Medicine Clinical Practice Guidelines for rapid sequence intubation in the critically Ill adult patient.

Crit Care Med. 2023;51:1411-30.

CLINICAL QUESTION OR PROBLEM

The guidelines were developed to address controversies and practice variations in the pharmacologic and nonpharmacologic management of the airway during rapid sequence intubation (RSI) in critically ill adult patients. RSI is a critical procedure often performed in emergency settings, where prompt and effective airway management is crucial to prevent complications. These guidelines are intended for clinicians who treat critically ill adult patients in the emergency department (ED), ICU, or other locations outside the operating room (OR) and who require emergency airway management with endotracheal intubation using RSI.

WHAT IS ALREADY KNOWN?

Rapid sequence intubation is widely recognized as the gold standard for securing the airway in critically ill patients due to its efficiency in preventing aspiration and facilitating rapid airway control. However, there is considerable variability in how RSI is performed, including the choice of induction agents, neuromuscular blockers, and premedication strategies. Existing practices are largely guided by clinician experience and institutional protocols, but there is a lack of standardized, evidence-based guidelines.

STUDY DESIGN

A multidisciplinary panel consisting of 20 SCCM members, with expertise in emergency medicine, critical care, anesthesiology, pharmacy, and respiratory therapy, supported by a GRADE methodologist and a librarian, was assembled to develop the RSI guidelines. The American College of Critical Care Medicine's Board of Regents (BOR) appointed the guideline leaders, ensuring diversity and subject matter expertise. Conflicts of interest were carefully managed, with all panelists completing required forms throughout the guideline development process. The BOR monitored the panel's work, ensuring adherence to SCCM's standard operating procedures. They created and refined PICO questions to review the best available evidence. The librarian collaborated with the panel to create search criteria, using a mix of text words and medical subject heading (MeSH) terms for the literature review. Comprehensive searches were conducted across PubMed, Web of Science, and Scopus, focusing on publications from 2000 to 2020. Additional studies were gathered based on panelists' suggestions and references from the identified articles. The guidelines were developed using the GRADE framework. The recommendations were categorized into strong, conditional, or best practice statements based on the quality of evidence and the level of consensus among the panelists.

OUTCOME EVALUATED

The guidelines aim to standardize RSI practices by providing evidence-based recommendations on various pharmacologic and nonpharmacologic aspects of the procedure. Panelists proposed 35 potential PICO questions focused on areas of interest or controversy in RSI for critically ill adults. Questions related to difficult airway management were excluded, as existing guidelines from the American Society of Anesthesiologists already cover this topic. After panelists voted, the scores were averaged and ranked for review. The panel then met virtually to discuss the results, ensuring the selected PICO questions aligned with the guideline's goals, which included both pharmacologic and nonpharmacologic aspects, and adhered to the SCCM BOR's limit of 10 PICO questions. High-ranking questions were included, with some being combined if they shared similar interventions or comparisons but different populations or outcomes, following consultation with a methodologist. The evaluated outcomes included the effectiveness and safety of different induction agents, neuromuscular blockers, and premedication strategies, as well as their impact on patient outcomes such as hypoxemia and aspiration **(Table 2)**.

AUTHORS' VIEWPOINTS

The authors highlight the importance of using evidence-based practices in RSI to reduce variability and improve patient outcomes. They acknowledge that while the guidelines provide a strong foundation for clinical decision-making, the quality of evidence for many recommendations is low, reflecting the need for individualized patient care and clinical judgment.

STRENGTH OF THE GUIDELINES

- The guidelines are comprehensive and reflect a strong consensus among a multidisciplinary panel of experts.

TABLE 2: Key recommendations along with the type of recommendation and the quality of evidence supporting each.

Recommendations	***Strength of recommendation***	***Quality of evidence***
Positioning: It is suggested to use a semi-Fowler position (head and torso inclined) during RSI	Conditional	Very low
Preoxygenation: • Preoxygenation with high-flow nasal oxygen (HFNO) is suggested when a difficult laryngoscopy is anticipated • Preoxygenation with noninvasive positive pressure ventilation (NIPPV) is suggested for patients with severe hypoxemia (PaO_2/FiO_2 <150)	Conditional	Low
Medication-assisted preoxygenation: Medication-assisted preoxygenation is suggested for patients undergoing RSI who cannot tolerate a face mask, NIPPV, or HFNO due to agitation or delirium	Conditional	Very low
Nasogastric tube decompression: Decompression of the nasogastric tube is advised when the benefit outweighs the risk in patients at high risk of regurgitating gastric contents during RSI	Best-practice statement	Not graded

Contd...

Contd...

Recommendations	*Strength of recommendation*	*Quality of evidence*
Peri-intubation vasopressors: There is insufficient evidence to recommend whether vasopressors or IV fluids are better for preventing hypotension or cardiac arrest in critically ill patients undergoing RSI	Insufficient evidence	Not applicable
Induction agent use: It is advised to use a sedative-hypnotic induction agent when a neuromuscular blocking agent (NMBA) is administered during intubation	Best-practice statement	Not graded
Induction agent selection: It is suggested that there is no significant difference in outcomes between etomidate and other induction agents for RSI, including mortality and incidence of hypotension	Conditional	Moderate
Etomidate and corticosteroid use: It is suggested not to use corticosteroids after RSI with etomidate to counteract potential adrenal suppression	Conditional	Low
NMBA use: It is recommended to administer an NMBA when using a sedative-hypnotic induction agent for intubation	Strong	Low
NMBA selection: It is suggested to use either rocuronium or succinylcholine for RSI, provided there are no contraindications to succinylcholine	Conditional	Low

(IV: intravenous; RSI: rapid sequence intubation)

- The use of the GRADE framework adds rigor to the guideline development process, ensuring that recommendations are based on the best available evidence.
- The guidelines also address key gaps in the literature and provide actionable recommendations where possible.

LIMITATIONS

- The primary limitation of the guidelines is the low quality of evidence supporting many of the recommendations, which limits the strength of some recommendations.
- The guidelines also identify significant gaps in the literature, particularly regarding the optimal choice of agents and strategies for specific patient populations.
- The recommendations may not be applicable in all clinical settings, particularly where resources or expertise may be limited.

REVIEWERS' VIEWPOINTS

Overall, these guidelines are a significant contribution to the field, providing a structured approach to RSI in critically ill patients, with the potential to enhance clinical practice and patient outcomes. The guidelines clearly define the scope, purpose, and clinical questions they intend to address. Multidisciplinary composition of the guidelines panel ensured diverse perspectives. The guidelines were developed using the GRADE framework, but the low quality of evidence for some recommendations limits the rigor. The guidelines are well-organized and provide clear recommendations. However, the recommendations may not be fully applicable in all clinical settings, particularly where resources are constrained. There is no conflict of interest management and there is transparency in the guideline development process.

IMPACT ON CLINICAL PRACTICE AND TAKE-HOME MESSAGE

The guidelines for RSI in critically ill adults offer a systematic approach to a complex and high-risk procedure frequently performed in emergency and intensive care settings. These evidence-based recommendations aim to standardize practices across different healthcare settings, reducing inconsistencies and enhancing patient outcomes. However, the reliance on low-quality evidence for many recommendations is a limitation, and the guidelines should be applied with clinical judgment and consideration of individual patient circumstances. Further research is needed to fill the identified gaps and strengthen the evidence base for RSI practices.

European Society of Intensive Care Medicine Clinical Practice Guideline on Fluid Therapy in Adult Critically Ill Patients. Part 1: The Choice of Resuscitation Fluids

Arabi YM, Belley-Cote E, Carsetti A, De Backer D, Donadello K, Juffermans NP, et al.; European Society of Intensive Care Medicine. European Society of Intensive Care Medicine clinical practice guideline on fluid therapy in adult critically ill patients. Part 1: the choice of resuscitation fluids.

Intensive Care Med. 2024;50:813-31.

CLINICAL QUESTION

Multiple factors determine the choice of resuscitation fluid in critically ill patients. These factors include: availability, cost, underlying disease condition, physiological characteristics of the fluid, and even physician preferences. This leads to wide variability in clinical practices which may affect patient outcomes. Which fluid should be preferred in a particular clinical scenario remains a matter of debate. Through this clinical practice guideline, the European Society of Intensive Care Medicine (ESICM) aims to provide physicians guidance regarding the choice of fluid to be used for resuscitation. ESICM aims to follow these guidelines with two more parts to address the issues of the amount of fluids to be used for resuscitation and fluid removal in the postresuscitation phase.

WHAT IS ALREADY KNOWN?

Intravenous fluid resuscitation is frequently required for critically ill patients. Multiple options of fluids are available for this purpose. These are broadly classified as colloids and crystalloids, with each having their own advantages and limitations. Patients with different clinical conditions may benefit from fluids with different physiological characteristics. Colloids, such as albumin, are promoted as being more effective for expanding intravascular volume because they are believed to be more effectively retained in the intravascular space and help in maintaining the intravascular oncotic pressure. However, high cost and limited availability affect their widespread use. Moreover, large-scale trials have reported ambiguous results with many trials showing them to be only equally effective as the crystalloids, offering no additional advantage.

Normal saline (NS) is arguably the most commonly prescribed intravenous fluid. However, the use of large volumes of NS has been shown to be associated with the development of hyperchloremic metabolic acidosis. Further, reports suggest an increased incidence of acute kidney injury in patients with sepsis resuscitated with large volumes of isotonic saline. Balanced fluid solutions are theoretically more physiological and have a constitution more in sync with the human plasma. This has increased their clinical application in recent years.

Various concentrations of hypertonic saline have been evaluated in animal models. However, only 3% of hypertonic saline has mainly been evaluated in human studies. Several observational studies have shown that it may provide immediate intravascular volume expansion, thereby reducing the total volume of fluid required for resuscitation. Further, a few studies have reported favorable hemodynamics and additional anti-inflammatory effects with the use of hypertonic saline. However, at present, there exist no guidelines recommending their routine use for resuscitating critically ill patients.

STUDY DESIGN

The ESICM designed a panel of experts with 2 guidelines co-chairs, 1 clinical chair, and 2 methods co-chairs along with 11 clinical experts from different specialties. After initial deliberations, the expert panel prioritized a set of 11 questions based on the PICO format. Further, the GRADE methodology was used to make the recommendations for the predecided set of questions **(Table 3)**.

TABLE 3: Summary of recommendations for the choice of resuscitation fluids.

Disease/condition	***Favored fluid***	***Level of evidence***
Crystalloids vs. colloids (albumin):		
• General critically ill • Sepsis • Acute respiratory failure • Traumatic brain injury • Perioperative period and patients at risk for bleeding • Cirrhosis	• Crystalloids • Crystalloids • Crystalloids • Crystalloids • Crystalloids • Albumin	• Moderate certainty of evidence • Moderate certainty of evidence • Very low certainty of evidence • Very low certainty of evidence • Very low certainty of evidence • Very low certainty of evidence
Which crystalloid (normal saline vs. balanced salt solutions):		
• General critically ill • Sepsis • Kidney injury • Traumatic brain injury	• Balanced crystalloids • Balanced crystalloids • Balanced crystalloids • Normal saline	• Low certainty of evidence • Low certainty of evidence • Very low certainty of evidence • Very low certainty of evidence
Isotonic vs. hypertonic crystalloids:		
General critically ill	Isotonic crystalloids	Very low certainty of evidence

POPULATION STUDIED, INCLUDING DEMOGRAPHICS

All systematic analyses, meta-analyses, and randomized control trials (RCTs) conducted in adult critically ill patients up to April 2022 were included for data analysis.

INTERVENTION

None

COMPARATOR USED

Data from trials comparing colloids (albumin) with crystalloids, NS with balanced salt solutions, and isotonic with hypertonic solutions were considered for analysis.

OUTCOMES EVALUATED

Clinically relevant outcomes including short-term mortality, need for renal replacement therapy, ventilator-free days or duration of mechanical ventilation, ICU-free days or ICU length of stay, hospital-free days or hospital length of stay, quality of life, and functional outcomes were given high priority while devising the recommendations.

AUTHOR'S VIEWPOINT

These guidelines present 11 evidence-based recommendations related to the use of albumin, balanced crystalloids, and isotonic saline as a resuscitation fluid in adult critically ill patients. In most of the clinical conditions (general critical care, sepsis, acute respiratory failure, traumatic brain injury and perioperative period and patients at risk for bleeding), crystalloids should be preferred over albumin, but albumin should be preferred in patients with cirrhosis. Compared to isotonic saline, balanced crystalloids should be preferred in all the clinical scenarios considered (general critical care, sepsis, and in patients with kidney injury and traumatic brain injury). Finally, the authors suggest using isotonic saline over small volume hypertonic saline in the resuscitation of critically ill adult patients.

STRENGTHS

- The guidelines were framed by a reputed panel of international clinical experts and methodologists. All measures were undertaken to reduce bias and internationally accepted GRADE methodology was used to formulate the recommendations.
- Outcomes considered for making recommendations were all clinically relevant.
- The recommendations are all evidence based. All relevant literature up to April 2022 was analyzed to devise the recommendations. All systematic analyses, meta-analyses, and RCTs were included for data analysis. Even data from observational studies were included for panel discussions while formulating the recommendations.
- These guidelines are in sync with other international guidelines like the surviving sepsis guidelines 2021.
- The development of these guidelines was free from industry influence or funding.

DRAWBACKS

- The role of other colloids including hydroxyethyl starch or gelatin was not discussed.
- Several other important clinical conditions requiring aggressive fluid resuscitation, such as severe burns and diabetic ketoacidosis, were also not discussed.
- Utility and efficacy of different concentrations of albumin solutions also remain unanswered.
- Another common indication of hypertonic solutions, i.e., management of

increased intracranial pressure was also not discussed.

- Indication of albumin infusions to increase serum albumin levels was also not discussed.
- All the recommendations were "conditional" recommendations with only two recommendations having moderate certainty of evidence. This may impact the level of confidence the readers may have while applying these recommendations in their routine clinical practice.

REVIEWER'S VIEWPOINTS

Resuscitation is an important component of acute care of critically ill patients and plays a vital role in determining the final outcome. These guidelines provide critical care physicians with recommendations for the choice of fluid for resuscitation for different critically ill patient subsets. It may help the physicians to provide a more individualized care, as per the patient's underlying clinical condition. Preferring crystalloids over albumin may also help in curtailing the cost of therapy. With increasing evidence and ease of availability, the use of balanced crystalloids may become more routine which may help in preventing the development of potentially serious complications of hyperchloremic metabolic acidosis secondary to large-volume isotonic saline usage.

Further, these guidelines have highlighted the gaps in the current understanding and identified research priorities for future studies. This may serve as a platform for further studies. Additionally, the subsequent guidelines, regarding the amount of resuscitation fluid and the removal of fluid in the postresuscitation phase, will provide further clarity regarding the resuscitation of adult critically ill patients.

IMPACT ON CURRENT PRACTICES AND TAKE-HOME MESSAGE

These guidelines will provide an easy reckoner for critical care physicians regarding the choice of fluids for resuscitating different subsets of patients. It may lead physicians to take informed decisions and further improve the quality of care and patient outcomes. As these guidelines are practical and easy to apply, they may find widespread acceptability and application.

2024 Focused Update: Guidelines on Use of Corticosteroids in Sepsis, Acute Respiratory Distress Syndrome, and Community-acquired Pneumonia

Chaudhuri D, Nei AM, Rochwerg B, Balk RA, Asehnoune K, Cadena R, et al. 2024 Focused Update: Guidelines on use of corticosteroids in sepsis, acute respiratory distress syndrome, and community-acquired pneumonia.

Crit Care Med. 2024;52:e219-33.

CLINICAL QUESTION OR PROBLEM

The use of corticosteroids in critically ill patients has remained a topic of discussion and clinical research for long. With these guidelines, the Society of Critical Care Medicine (SCCM) aimed to develop evidence-based recommendations for the use of corticosteroids in hospitalized patients with severe diseases such as sepsis, acute respiratory distress syndrome (ARDS), and community-acquired pneumonia (CAP) and update the 2017 corticosteroids insufficiency in critical illness (CIRCI) guidelines. As these conditions have been shown to be associated with a dysregulated inflammatory response, corticosteroids due to their anti-inflammatory actions may be potentially beneficial in these conditions.

WHAT IS ALREADY KNOWN?

Corticosteroids are double-edged swords and have always remained a topic of contention among the critical care physicians. Their use may be associated with serious and sometimes life-threatening complications, but their judicious use may help salvage patient's lives in many potentially lethal conditions.

STUDY DESIGN

The SCCM appointed a committee of experts including chairs, co-vice chairs, clinician methodologists, and methodology team members along with a panel of 22 experts to devise these guidelines. After the required deliberations, the panel of experts identified five focused PICO questions. Subsequently, the panel conducted systematic reviews of the available studies, to identify the best available evidence addressing each question and formulated recommendations using the GRADE approach. Where the evidence was strong, the panel gave a strong recommendation by using the phrase "we recommend". On the other hand, where the evidence was lacking, the panel used the "we suggest" while making the recommendations. Ultimately, all the recommendations were reviewed and approved by all the panelists by using a formal web-based voting system. Consensus was defined as consensus as 80% agreement among at least 75% of panel members. Out of the five selected PICO questions, recommendations could be made only on four, as adequate literature was not available for the fifth topic **(Table 4)**.

POPULATION STUDIED INCLUDING DEMOGRAPHICS

All the relevant studies conducted on hospitalized adults and pediatric patients with sepsis, ARDS, and CAP were included by the panelists in the systematic reviews.

INTERVENTION(S) STUDIED

Use of corticosteroids, different doses of corticosteroids, and different types of corticosteroids.

COMPARATOR USED

- Corticosteroids versus no corticosteroids, and high dose/short duration corticosteroids versus low-dose/long-duration corticosteroids in patients with sepsis.
- Corticosteroids versus no corticosteroids, and methylprednisolone versus dexamethasone or hydrocortisone in patients with ARDS.
- Corticosteroids versus no corticosteroids in patients with CAP.

OUTCOMES EVALUATED

- *Septic shock:* Hospital/long-term mortality, ICU/short-term mortality, ICU/hospital length of stay, and adverse effects of corticosteroids
- *ARDS:* Survival rates, days on invasive mechanical ventilation (IMV), days in hospital/ICU, and adverse effects of corticosteroids
- *CAP:* Hospital mortality, need for IMV, hospital and ICU length of stay, and adverse effects of corticosteroids

TABLE 4: Summary of recommendations.

Patient population	*Recommendation*	*Level of recommendation*	*Level of evidence*
Adults with septic shock	It is "suggested" to administer corticosteroids to adult patients with septic shock	Conditional recommendation	Low certainty evidence
Adults with septic shock	It is "recommended" to administer high doses/short duration corticosteroids (>400 mg/day hydrocortisone equivalent for <3 days) for adult patients with septic shock	Strong recommendation	Moderate certainty evidence
Adults with ARDS	It is "suggested" to administer corticosteroids to adults hospitalized with ARDS	Conditional recommendation	Moderate certainty evidence
Adults with CAP	It is "recommended" to administer corticosteroids to adults hospitalized with severe bacterial CAP	Strong recommendation	Moderate certainty evidence
Adults with CAP	"No recommendation" for administering corticosteroids for adults hospitalized with less severe bacterial CAP	No recommendation	NA

(ARDS: acute respiratory distress syndrome; CAP: community-acquired pneumonia; NA: not applicable)

AUTHORS' VIEWPOINTS

The selected panel made five recommendations regarding the use of corticosteroids in hospitalized patients with septic shock, ARDS, and CAP. They suggested to use corticosteroids for patients with septic shock and critically ill patients with ARDS. They recommended to administer steroids in patients hospitalized with severe bacterial CAP. Further, it is not recommended to use high dose/short duration of steroids for the management of septic shock. However, no recommendation could be made regarding the use of steroids in the management of less severe bacterial CAP or pediatric patients with septic shock, ARDS, or CAP. Additionally, no specific recommendations could be made regarding the choice of corticosteroids, dosage, or even duration of treatment due to lack of clinical evidence.

STRENGTHS

- This focused guideline has a robust methodology, including the most relevant and most recent trials for systemic analysis.
- The previous 2017 SCCM/ESICM guidelines recommended initiation of corticosteroids in septic shock not responsive to fluids requiring moderate-to-high doses of vasopressors. As the dosage criteria were vague, it may potentially lead to a delay in starting corticosteroids. The present guidelines suggest initiating corticosteroids in patients with septic shock requiring vasopressors, irrespective of the dosage,

which removes the ambiguity and may help in the early initiation of steroids.

- The authors have identified the research gaps and have suggested the agendas for future research.

DRAWBACKS

- Even though the data was analyzed for pediatric patients too, no recommendations were made, as adequate evidence was found lacking.
- Certain types of sepsis such as postsurgical sepsis and neutropenic sepsis were underrepresented in the included studies; hence, the applicability of this guideline may be doubtful in these patients.
- There are significant discrepancies from the previous guidelines regarding the dose of vasopressors at which steroids should be initiated. Even the recent surviving sepsis guidelines (2021) recommend adding steroids in patients with ongoing requirements for vasopressor therapy (dose of norepinephrine or epinephrine ≥0.25 μg/kg/min at least 4 hours after initiation). Although initiating steroids irrespective of the dose of vasopressors is simpler, these differences from previous guidelines may make it confusing for clinicians.
- No recommendation was made regarding the severity of ARDS in which corticosteroids should be initiated, compared to previous guidelines.
- No recommendations on the timing, duration, and dose of corticosteroids in patients with severe CAP, as was mentioned in the previous guidelines.
- No specific corticosteroid or dosing regimen is advocated and has been left to physician's discretion. This again may lead to confusion and disparities. Already, wide variations have been reported in the dosing regimens, especially in ARDS patients (intravenous methylprednisolone 40 mg/day to 2 mg/kg/day) with duration ranging from 7 to 30 days. Some guidance would have helped the physicians to maintain uniformity and avoid unnecessarily excessive dosing.
- The issue of adding fludrocortisone still remains unresolved.
- Criteria for defining severe CAP were different in the included studies, which may affect the applicability of these recommendations.
- The impact of a new definition for ARDS on these guidelines is difficult to determine.

REVIEWERS' VIEWPOINTS

The panel assembled by SCCM has provided updated recommendations regarding the use of corticosteroids in patients hospitalized with sepsis, ARDS, and CAP. The recommendation to initiate corticosteroids in patients with septic shock, requiring vasopressors (irrespective of their dose) to maintain the required mean arterial pressure, is a practical recommendation. The need for a "moderate-to-high dose" of vasopressors or "ongoing" vasopressor requirement for initiating corticosteroids, as advocated in the previous guidelines, may lead to ambiguity and delay in starting steroids.

However, ambiguity exists in the other recommendations made by the panel. For ARDS, the panel has simply "suggested" using corticosteroids in hospitalized patients without making any comment regarding which steroid, the timing of initiation, the severity of ARDS, or the dosage of steroids. All these decisions have been left to the clinician's discretion, defeating the purpose of making the guidelines. Even for CAP, they have made a strong recommendation for initiating corticosteroids in severe bacterial CAP, but the issues regarding dosage, type, timing, and duration are still unanswered. Overall, this guideline, although tackles a few pertinent issues, refrains from addressing many other matters regarding the use of steroids in critically ill patients.

IMPACT ON CURRENT PRACTICE AND TAKE-HOME MESSAGE

The take-home message from this guideline is mainly that steroids, if judiciously used, may be useful in many critical clinical situations. This guideline will encourage acute care physicians to initiate corticosteroids early while managing patients with vasopressor-dependent septic shock. Further, it will also enhance the confidence of physicians to administer steroids in patients with ARDS and severe bacterial CAP, but it would not have much impact on their current practices regarding the choice of steroids, their dosage, and duration. Additionally, this guideline will not aid the physicians managing ARDS, regarding patient selection for initiating corticosteroids. Finally, the huge list of "research agenda" recommended by the panel highlights the existing wide knowledge gaps and the urgent need for further large-scale trials on these relevant topics.

Society of Critical Care Medicine Guidelines on Glycemic Control for Critically Ill Children and Adults 2024

Honarmand K, Sirimaturos M, Hirshberg EL, Bircher NG, Agus MSD, Carpenter DL, et al. Society of Critical Care Medicine Guidelines on Glycemic Control for Critically Ill Children and Adults 2024.

Crit Care Med. 2024;52:e161-81.

CLINICAL QUESTION OR PROBLEM

Poor glycemic control has been shown to be associated with increased morbidity and mortality in critically ill patients. However, the questions regarding the target serum levels, frequency of monitoring, and how to monitor, still remain unanswered.

WHAT IS ALREADY KNOWN?

Maintaining glucose control in ICU patients is of paramount importance. Critically ill patients are at high risk of developing glycemic abnormalities. It is widely agreed that extremes of blood glucose levels are associated with poor outcomes. On one hand, the development of hypoglycemia may lead to immediate complications and may even be life-threatening, and on the other hand, the development of hyperglycemia is associated with long-term complications including secondary infections and high ICU mortality rates. Even wide fluctuations in sugar levels (glycemic variability) have been shown to be associated with poorer clinical outcomes. Through this update of the 2012 Society of Critical Care Medicine (SCCM) and American College of Critical Care Medicine (ACCM) guidelines, the authors aimed to review the literature and provide evidence-based guidance to critical care physicians.

STUDY DESIGN

The SCCM created a multiprofessional task force of 22 experts, including 2 chairs and

2 vice chairs, who identified the relevant questions based on PICO format. Further, a systematic review was conducted including the relevant studies (published between January 2000 and January 2023) for each PICO question. The clinical evidence was statistically summarized and the evidence-based recommendations were made as per the GRADE methodology. The recommendations were classified as "strong" or "weak" or as a "good practice statement", depending on the level of evidence available. Additionally, a fourth category of recommendations was added "In our practice", where the evidence was not sufficient but the practice was deemed appropriate by the expert panel based on their experience. Ultimately, all the expert panel members voted on each recommendation, and consensus was defined as 80% agreement among at least 75% of voting panel members.

POPULATION STUDIED INCLUDING DEMOGRAPHICS

Relevant studies conducted in critically ill children (above 42-week-old age to 18-year-old) and adults were included for the systematic analysis. Neonates were excluded. The primary population was identified as unspecified or mixed critically ill patients including patient subpopulations (e.g., medical, surgical, neurologic, trauma, etc.).

INTERVENTIONS STUDIED

Triggers for initiation of insulin therapy, route of administration, monitoring frequency, the role of an explicit decision support tool for protocol maintenance, and methodology for glucose testing.

COMPARATORS USED

- *Trigger blood glucose for insulin initiation*: Comparing lower glucose threshold 6.1–10 mmol/L (110–180 mg/dL) versus higher glucose threshold >10 mmol/L (>180 mg/dL)
- *Intensive versus conventional glucose targets*: Lower blood glucose target 4.4–7.7 mmol/L (80–139 mg/dL) versus a higher glucose target 7.8–11.1 mmol/L (140–200 mg/dL)
- Continuous intravenous (IV) infusion versus intermittent subcutaneous insulin
- *Frequency of blood glucose monitoring*: ≤1 hour, continuous or near-continuous versus longer intervals (>1 hour), during the period of glycemic instability
- Use of explicit clinical decision support tools versus standard care
- Glucose monitoring with a meter

OUTCOMES EVALUATED

Important outcomes evaluated were hospital mortality, ICU mortality, pediatric developmental outcomes, quality of life, seizures, long-term cognitive impairment, new infections, acute kidney injury, and need for renal replacement therapy.

AUTHORS' VIEWPOINTS

A total of 7 recommendations each were made for glycemic control in adult and pediatric critically ill patients. In adults, 4 recommendations were conditional, 2 were good practice statements, and 1 was a research statement **(Table 5)**. In pediatric patients, 2 statements each were "good practice" and "in our practice", while 1 statement each was a strong recommendation, conditional recommendation, and research statement, respectively **(Table 6)**.

The expert panel could achieve consensus for adults and pediatric critically ill patients regarding a preference for an insulin infusion, rather than intermittent subcutaneous insulin for the acute management of hyperglycemia with titration guided by an

TABLE 5: Recommendations for adult critically ill patients.

Recommendation	*Type of statement*	*Level of evidence*
Initiate glycemic management protocols and procedures for treating persistent hyperglycemia, ≥10 mmol/L (180 mg/dL)	Good practice statement	NA
Glycemic management protocols and procedures used should have a low risk of hypoglycemia and hypoglycemia should be treated immediately	Good practice statement	NA
To reduce the risk of hypoglycemia, it is suggested not to titrate insulin infusion to a lower BG target INT: 4.4–7.7 mmol/L (80–139 mg/dL) compared with a higher BG target range, CONV: 7.8–11.1 mmol/L (140–200 mg/dL)	Conditional recommendation	Moderate
It is recommended to conduct high-quality interventional trials of individualized glycemic targets	Research statement	NA
It is suggested to use continuous IV insulin infusion over intermittent subcutaneous insulin in the acute management of hyperglycemia	Conditional recommendation	Very low
It is suggested to monitor BG frequently (≤1 hour, continuous, or near-continuous) in patients on IV insulin, during periods of glycemic instability	Conditional recommendation	Low
It is suggested to use a protocol that includes explicit decision-support tools	Conditional recommendation	Moderate

(BG: blood glucose; CONV: conservative; INT: intensive; IV: intravenous; NA: not applicable)

explicit clinical decision support tool and frequent (≤1 hour) monitoring intervals during glycemic instability to minimize the risk of hypoglycemia and against targeting intensive glucose levels (80–139 mg/dL).

STRENGTHS

- The guidelines methodology was robust, and the recommendations are grounded in scientific evidence.
- Recommendations made were clear and specific.
- Suggestion of a more individualized approach to glycemic control is a step in the right direction.
- The authors were able to identify some knowledge gaps and have suggested future research areas.

DRAWBACKS

- Other parameters of glycemic control such as glycemic variability are largely ignored, even though there is emerging evidence which suggests that preventing glycemic variability may be as important as preventing hypo- and hyperglycemia and can affect patient outcomes.
- Newer blood glucose monitoring techniques, including continuous glucose monitors, are becoming increasingly popular. They may also aid in providing more individualized glycemic control. However, recommendations regarding their use were also lacking in these guidelines.
- Even though a more individualized glycemic control was advocated, no

TABLE 6: Recommendations for pediatric critically ill patients.

Recommendation	***Type of statement***	***Level of evidence***
Initiate glycemic management protocols and procedures to treat persistent hyperglycemia, ≥10 mmol/L (180 mg/dL)	Good practice statement	NA
Glycemic management protocols and procedures used should have a low risk of hypoglycemia and hypoglycemia should be treated immediately.	Good practice statement	NA
It is recommended not to use INT BG control, 4.4–7.7 mmol/L (80–139 mg/dL) compared with CONV BG control, 7.8–11.1 mmol/L (140–200 mg/dL)	Strong recommendation	Moderate
"No recommendation" could be made in regard to continuous IV insulin infusion over intermittent subcutaneous insulin, in the acute management of hyperglycemia. However, based on expert opinion, continuous IV infusion may be preferred	"In our practice" statement	NA
"No recommendation" could be made with regard to the frequency of BG monitoring. However, based on expert experience, frequent (interval ≤1 hour) or continuous/near-continuous monitoring systems may be preferred	"In our practice" statement	NA
It is suggested to use explicit decision support tools in patients receiving IV insulin infusions	Conditional recommendation	Very low
It is strongly recommended to conduct high-quality research on the use of explicit decision-support tools for insulin infusion titration	Research statement	NA

(BG: blood glucose; CONV: conservative; INT: intensive; IV: intravenous; NA: not applicable)

recommendations were made for specific critically ill patient subsets such as diabetics, postoperative, neurologic, etc.

- The recommendation for conventional blood glucose targets from 140 to 200 mg/dL is different from the recommendations from the American Diabetes Association (ADA) which recommends a target range of 140–180 mg/dL. Increasing the range will add to confusion among the physicians and may allow for higher glycemic variability.
- No specific comments were made regarding glycemic monitoring in resource-limited settings where continuous intravenous insulin infusion, frequent blood glucose monitoring (≤1 hour), and computerized clinical decision support tools may not be feasible due to logistical or economic constraints.
- No recommendations were made on certain other vital issues such as capillary versus arterial/venous blood glucose monitoring and point-of-care (POC) versus blood gas analyzer/central laboratory glucose monitoring.
- Further, no recommendations are made regarding the preparation of insulin infusion and transition from intravenous infusions to subcutaneous insulin, unlike the 2012 guidelines.

- Nutritional considerations for critically ill patients on intravenous insulin are also not discussed.
- Out of the 14 recommendations, only 1 was a strong recommendation, rest were conditional/good practice or "in our practice" statements.

REVIEWERS' VIEWPOINT

These guidelines were designed to be an update of the 2012 SCCM guidelines. The 2012 guidelines primarily focused on adult critically ill patients, but these guidelines addressed glycemic issues of both adult and pediatric patients. However, the 2012 guidelines were more comprehensive and dealt with several issues related to glycemic management including the nutritional aspects, glycemic variability, economics of glycemic control, and even parameters to audit. In this regard, the current guidelines seem more superficial, managing to cover only a few basic issues. Rather than adding to the previous guidelines, it has removed vital components of glycemic monitoring from the previous guidelines.

Topics such as POC testing and capillary versus arterial/venous sampling, which form integral components of glycemic monitoring, were not adequately addressed by these guidelines. The 2012 guidelines suggested that POC devices are acceptable but advised intensivists to be aware of their limitations. Likewise, they acknowledged the limitations of finger-stick capillary sampling and suggested clinical situations where arterial or venous sampling may be more accurate.

The present guidelines are moving toward a more liberal approach to glycemic control in critically ill patients. Rather than initiating insulin infusion at a threshold of >150 mg/dL (as recommended in the 2012 SCCM guidelines) and keeping the target blood glucose levels between 140 and 180 mg/dL (as recommended by ADA) or <150 mg/dL (as recommended by 2012 SCCM guidelines), the current guidelines have suggested a target range of 140–200 mg/dL.

The 2012 guidelines suggested monitoring blood glucose levels every 1–2 hours which is more practical and widely practiced. Whereas the current guidelines suggest more frequent blood glucose monitoring (≤1 hour, continuous, or near-continuous) which may not be feasible in resource-limited settings.

Questions regarding continuous glucose monitoring, which could not be addressed adequately by the 2012 guidelines due to lack of evidence, still remain unanswered. Recommendations regarding glycemic variability, which is an important glycemic target, are also lacking. These guidelines should have also explored relatively newer glycemic targets such as time-in-target-range, which have shown promise in improving glycemic control and patient outcomes in ICU.

These guidelines sought to update the 2012 guidelines and address some pertinent issues regarding glycemic control in critically ill patients but fell short of expectations. As this guideline does not address all the pertinent issues regarding glycemic control in critically ill patients, the clinicians will have to look for other avenues (including the previous SSCM and ADA guidelines) to provide comprehensive care to their patients.

IMPACT ON CURRENT PRACTICE AND TAKE-HOME MESSAGE

The present guidelines have reiterated the need to avoid hypoglycemia and have advocated a higher target range for blood glucose levels (140–200 mg/dL). They have recommended preferring intravenous continuous insulin infusion with frequent blood glucose monitoring (≤1 hour) for both adult and pediatric critically ill patients. Further, they have recommended the use of explicit decision support tools for better glycemic control and research to personalize glycemic monitoring tailored to patient's needs. Since this update has been released after 12 years, it will encourage critical care physicians to re-look into their glycemic control protocols. However, in order to make them precise and focused, several pertinent issues have been ignored by these guidelines. This makes these guidelines seem inadequate and incomplete when compared to the previous guidelines. This will make the practicing physicians fall back on the previous guidelines for managing such issues, limiting the scope of this update.

Index

Page numbers followed by *t* refer to table.

H

I

J

K

L

M

N

O

P

Q

R

S

T

U

V

W